Case Studies in Endocrinology

Case Studies in Endocrinology

Editor: Emory Hunt

AMERICAN
MEDICAL PUBLISHERS
www.americanmedicalpublishers.com

AMERICAN
MEDICAL PUBLISHERS
www.americanmedicalpublishers.com

Cataloging-in-Publication Data

Case studies in endocrinology / edited by Emory Hunt.
p. cm.
Includes bibliographical references and index.
ISBN 979-8-88740-596-4
1. Endocrinology. 2. Internal medicine. 3. Hormones. 4. Clinical medicine.
I. Hunt, Emory.
RC648 .E53 2023
616.4--dc23

American Medical Publishers,
41 Flatbush Avenue,
1st Floor, New York,
NY 11217, USA

ISBN 979-8-88740-596-4 (Hardback)

Contents

Preface

This book has been a concerted effort by a group of academicians, researchers and scientists, who have contributed their research works for the realization of the book. This book has materialized in the wake of emerging advancements and innovations in this field. Therefore, the need of the hour was to compile all the required researches and disseminate the knowledge to a broad spectrum of people comprising of students, researchers and specialists of the field.

Endocrinology is an area of medicine that focuses on the study of hormones and the endocrine system. Hormones are chemical messengers which are produced by the different glands in the body that regulate numerous physiological processes, such as growth, metabolism, reproduction and mood. The endocrine system comprises glands such as the pituitary gland, thyroid gland, adrenal glands, pancreas, ovaries (in females), and testes (in males). Endocrinology is involved in the diagnosis of patients with hormonal disorders through a combination of clinical assessment, laboratory tests and imaging studies. It also deals with the management of medical conditions which include diabetes mellitus, thyroid disorders, adrenal disorders, disorders of the reproductive system, and pituitary disorders. This book unfolds the innovative aspects of endocrinology which will be crucial for the progress of this field in the future. It will serve as a valuable source of reference for graduate and postgraduate students.

At the end of the preface, I would like to thank the authors for their brilliant chapters and the publisher for guiding us all-through the making of the book till its final stage. Also, I would like to thank my family for providing the support and encouragement throughout my academic career and research projects.

Editor

1

Acute Renal Failure Secondary to Inadvertent Propylene Glycol Overdose with Single-Day High-Dose Vitamin D (Stosstherapy)

David H. Jelley,[1] **Deborah Zayneb Mohamad Ali**,[2] **and Michelle Condren**[3]

[1]*Pediatric Department, University of Oklahoma School of Community Medicine, Tulsa, 4444 E 41st St., Tulsa, OK 74135, 918-619-4803, USA*
[2]*Pediatric Department, University of Oklahoma School of Community Medicine, Tulsa, 4502 E 41st St, Tulsa, OK 74135, 918-660-3400, USA*
[3]*University of Oklahoma College of Pharmacy, Pediatric Department, University of Oklahoma School of Community Medicine, Tulsa, 4502 E. 41st St, Tulsa, OK 74135, 918-660-3578, USA*

Correspondence should be addressed to David H. Jelley; david-jelley@ouhsc.edu

Academic Editor: Hyunsik Kang

Globally, there has been increasing attention paid to vitamin D deficiency and its treatment. Vitamin D stosstherapy with high-dose ergocalciferol in a single day is reemerging as a potential treatment option. We present an as yet unreported complication of acute renal injury due to propylene glycol toxicity in a 7-month infant treated with vitamin D stosstherapy. The product label for the vitamin D used for this patient states it is dissolved in propylene glycol (PG), but the amount is not listed on this or other US ergocalciferol liquid products that contain PG. Caution should be used when considering vitamin D stosstherapy with liquid ergocalciferol products available in the United States.

1. Introduction

Vitamin D is essential for calcium homeostasis and bone health and is obtained from sun exposure, vitamin supplements, and foods fortified with vitamin D including dairy products, infant formula, and breakfast cereals. Once foods were fortified, nutritional or vitamin D deficiency was thought to be a disease of the past, yet it remains common. While mild vitamin D deficiency is generally asymptomatic in children, more severe deficiency can result in rickets with or without hypocalcemia. Treatment includes vitamin D supplementation plus adequate nutritional intake of calcium. Stosstherapy, or single-day high dose vitamin D therapy, has been used since the 1930s and may be warranted when patients present with acute conditions secondary to low vitamin D requiring more rapid resolution of deficiency, or when there are concerns about compliance with daily therapy. Stosstherapy has been reported to be a safe and effective method of treatment [1]; however, concerns have been raised regarding the markedly elevated vitamin D levels which occur with this form of treatment. Furthermore, unintended consequences related to other molecules in the drug formulation may occur; in this case propylene glycol results in acute renal failure following vitamin D stosstherapy in an infant with nutritional rickets.

2. Case

A previously healthy 7-month-old African-American male presented to the ER in late winter after a generalized tonic-clonic seizure. There was no history of trauma or febrile illness. He was exclusively breastfed but had only received a multivitamin supplement for the first three months of life. Physical exam revealed a postictal infant with short stature, length = 64 cm (<5th percentile) and weight of 9.2 kg (75th percentile). Neurologic exam demonstrated brisk patellar reflexes, and the remainder of his physical exam was unremarkable. Initial labs showed severe hypocalcemia with total serum calcium = 5.9 mg/dl (normal range 8.5-10.9 mg/dl) and ionized calcium = .67 mmol/L (normal range 1.18-1.29 mmol/L). He was treated with IV calcium, after which serum calcium levels rose slightly but remained significantly

TABLE 1: Serial laboratory values from admission through six-week followup appointment.

	Admission Feb 11	Post Stosstherapy Feb 14	Discharge Feb 18	Outpatient followup March 28	Normal Values
Calcium	5.9	7.0	9.8	10.2	8.0-10.5 mg/dL
Ionized calcium	0.67	0.88	1.18		1.18-1.29 mmol/L
Phosphorus	5.3	5.6	6.0		3.8-6.2 mg/dL
Magnesium	2.1	2.2	1.6		1.7-2.9 mg/dL
Vitamin D	<4	112	350	86	30-100 ng/ml
Alkaline phosphatase	876	905	746	307	150-420 U/L
PTH	404.8	582.3	40	40	7.2-111.9 pg/mL
Creatinine	0.41	3.00	0.41	.45	0.20-0.73 mg/dL
CO_2	17	14	26	21	20-24 mmol/L

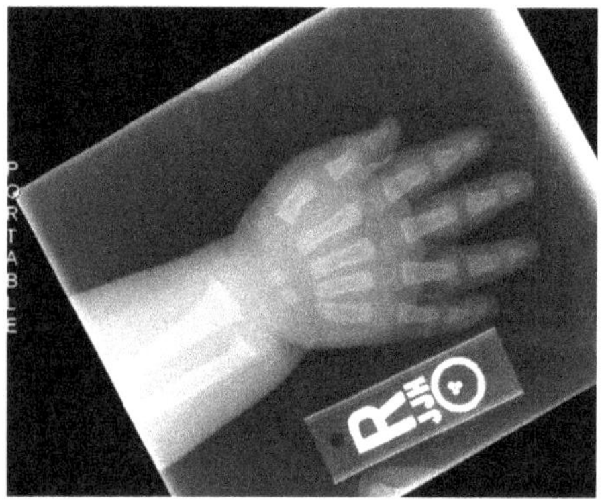

FIGURE 1: Classic rachitic changes of the wrist: fraying and widening at the radial and ulnar metaphyses.

below the normal range. Subsequent evaluation showed an undetectable 25-hydroxy vitamin D level of less than 4 ng/ml, with elevated parathyroid hormone and alkaline phosphatase levels (Table 1). Skeletal survey showed rachitic changes (Figure 1).

The patient was diagnosed with nutritional rickets and was administered vitamin D stosstherapy treatment with ergocalciferol (Virtus Pharmaceuticals, ergocalciferol oral solution, USP, 8,000 international units per mL) 100,000 international units given orally every 2 hours for a total of 600,000 international units over 12 hours. By the last dose, the patient had become lethargic and urine output was decreased from 2.1 cc/kg/hr before treatment to .7 cc/kg/hr after treatment. Labs revealed acute renal failure, metabolic acidosis, and hyperkalemia. Creatinine level rose from .41 mg/dl pretreatment to 3.0 mg/dl following stosstherapy over a 36-hour timespan. He was treated with fluid resuscitation, diuretics, sodium polystyrene sulfonate, bicarbonate, and continued IV calcium. Renal function and calcium levels normalized, and serum creatinine returned to baseline of .41 mg/dl and total calcium = 9.8 mg/dl. The patient was discharged home after 4 days on oral vitamin D and calcium supplementation.

3. Discussion

To our knowledge, this is the first reported case of renal failure due to vitamin D stosstherapy. Derived from the German word stossen, meaning "to push", stosstherapy consists of high-dose (600,000 units) ergocalciferol given over a single day. Use of this therapy for rickets was first reported over 75 years ago and is now regaining popularity [1–4]. For decades all infants in the German Democratic Republic (GDR) received 600,000 units ergocalciferol every 3 months for the first 18 months of life. While a significant percentage of these infants had elevated vitamin D levels and hypercalcemia, none were reported to have suffered renal injury or nephrocalcinosis [3, 5]. While renal failure has been associated with chronic vitamin D toxicity when dosed on a daily or weekly basis, we found no reports associated with single day stosstherapy [6].

Post hoc analysis of the ergocalciferol preparation carried by our hospital found that the side panel states it is dissolved in propylene glycol (PG), but the amount is not listed on this or other US ergocalciferol liquid products that contain PG. Further investigation revealed that the above product contains 103.6 g/100 mL of propylene glycol. The infant received 600,000 units of vitamin D2, equivalent to 75 mL of solution or 77.7 g of propylene glycol. According to the World Health Organization, this far exceeds the maximum tolerable amount of 25 mg/kg/day (or 227.5 mg for the baby in this event). In fact, the baby was exposed to 340 times the maximum amount [7]. Propylene glycol is a clear, colorless, odorless, and tasteless product used as a stabilizer, thickener, and texturizer. When given in large doses, drugs containing PG induce metabolic acidosis and reversible acute renal failure [8–11]. The primary difference between this case and previous reports using high doses of vitamin D is use of a concentrated form of ergocalciferol which did not contain propylene glycol; therefore, we suspect that acute renal failure in our patient was secondary to propylene glycol (PG) toxicity.

Caution should be used when using vitamin D stosstherapy to avoid liquid formulations of ergocalciferol solubilized with propylene glycol.

References

[1] G. O. Harnapp, "Die Stossprophylaxe der Rachitis mit Vitamin D2 und D3," *Journal of Molecular Medicine*, vol. 17, no. 11, pp. 390-391, 1938.

[2] R. W. Chesney, "Vitamin D Deficiency and Rickets," *Reviews in Endocrine and Metabolic Disorders*, vol. 2, no. 2, pp. 145–151, 2001.

[3] H. Mittal, S. Rai, D. Shah et al., "300,000 IU or 600,000 IU of oral vitamin D3 for treatment of nutritional rickets: A randomized controlled trial," *Indian Pediatrics*, vol. 51, no. 4, pp. 265–272, 2014.

[4] B. R. Shah and L. Finberg, "Single-day therapy for nutritional vitamin D-deficiency rickets: A preferred method," *Journal of Pediatrics*, vol. 125, no. 3, pp. 487–490, 1994.

[5] T. Markestad, V. Hesse, M. Siebenhuner et al., "Intermittent high-dose vitamin D prophylaxis during infancy: Effect on vitamin D metabolites, calcium, and phosphorus," *American Journal of Clinical Nutrition*, vol. 46, no. 4, pp. 652–658, 1987.

[6] B. Ozkan, M. Buyukavci, M. Energin, M. E. Dirican, H. Alp, and R. Akdag, "Nutritional rickets: Comparison of three different therapeutic approaches (300.000 U p.o., 300.000 U i.m. and 600.000 U p.o.)," *Cocuk Sagligi ve Hastaliklari Dergisi*, vol. 43, no. 1, pp. 30–35, 2000.

[7] Enterprise Directorate-General. Excipients in the label and package leaflet of medicinal products for human use. In: Secondary Enterprise Directorate-General, editor. Secondary Excipients in the label and package leaflet of medicinal products for human use. July ed 2003. http://www.ema.europa.eu/docs/en_GB/document_library/Scientific_guideline/2009/09/WC500003412.pdf.

[8] H. E. Demey, R. A. Daelemans, G. A. Verpooten et al., "Propylene glycol-induced side effects during intravenous nitroglycerin therapy," *Intensive Care Medicine*, vol. 14, no. 3, pp. 221–226, 1988.

[9] P. G. Jorens, H. E. Demey, P. J. C. Schepens et al., "Unusual D-lactic acid acidosis from propylene glycol metabolism in overdose," *Journal of Toxicology - Clinical Toxicology*, vol. 42, no. 2, pp. 163–169, 2004.

[10] P. D. Yorgin, A. A. Theodorou, A. Al-Uzri, K. Davenport, L. V. Boyer-Hassen, and M. I. Johnson, "Propylene glycol-induced proximal renal tubular cell injury," *American Journal of Kidney Diseases*, vol. 30, no. 1, pp. 134–139, 1997.

[11] H. Demey, R. Daelemans, M. De Broe, and L. Bossaert, "Propyleneglycol intoxication due to intravenous nitroglycerin," *The Lancet*, vol. 323, no. 8390, p. 1360, 1984.

2

Vitamin D-Resistant Rickets Diagnostics and Treatment Challenges at Muhimbili National Hospital, Tanzania

Evance K. Godfrey, Fatima Mussa, Parvina Kazahura, Aika Shoo, Helga Naburi, and Karim P. Manji

Department of Paediatrics and Child Health, Muhimbili University of Health and Allied Sciences (MUHAS), Dar es Salaam, Tanzania

Correspondence should be addressed to Evance K. Godfrey; gevance5@gmail.com

Academic Editor: J. Paul Frindik

Introduction. Rickets is softening of bones caused by defective mineralization of the cartilage in the epiphyseal growth plate, causing widening of the ends of long bones, growth retardation, and skeletal deformities in children. It can be classified into calciopenic and phosphopenic, each type with various subclasses. *Case Presentations.* We presented 2 cases, first of a 1 year and 4-month-old male, with a history of recurrent episodes of cough for 8 months and bowing of the legs 6 months prior to admission. Clinical and laboratory investigation was suggestive of vitamin D-dependent rickets, and he started vitamin D treatment with minimal response. The second case is of a 4 years and 7-month-old male who presented with developmental delay, poor weight gain, and recurrent chest infection and worsening of bone pain since 9 months of age. Laboratory investigation was suggestive of phosphopenic rickets, and he was started on treatment at 9 months of age with little improvement and at 4 years, he sustained multiple fractures and succumbed to severe respiratory tract infection and died at 4 years and 7 months of age. *Conclusion.* Rickets pose a diagnostic and treatment challenge in resource-limited countries, and clinical judgment and early initiation of treatment are important.

1. Introduction

Rickets is softening of bones caused by deficiency of vitamin D, calcium, or phosphate. This leads to a defective mineralization of the cartilage in the epiphyseal growth plate and subsequent widening of the ends of long bones, growth retardation, and skeletal deformities in children. Rickets is classified as calciopenic or phosphopenic according to the predominant mineral deficiency [1, 2].

Calciopenic rickets results from calcium deficiency commonly due to inadequate intake of vitamin D (essential for intestinal absorption of calcium) and rarely inadequate intake of calcium [2, 3]. Calciopenic rickets can also be caused by decreased activity of vitamin D, such as lack of conversion of 25(OH) D to the active metabolite 1, 25(OH) 2D (vitamin D-dependent rickets type 1 (VDDR-I), or resistance to the active metabolite (also known as vitamin D-dependent rickets type II (VDDR-II) due to mutations leading to dysfunction of the vitamin D receptor [2, 4–8].

Clinically, type 1 and 11 can be distinguished by presence of the following in type 11, alopecia, and elevated level of 1, 25(OH) 2D poor response to vitamin D, and hence needs treatment with infusion of calcium [1, 9, 10]. However, both types will be present with elevated ALP, low or normal calcium, low phosphorus, high-serum parathyroid hormone (PTH), and radiological changes like widening of the epiphyseal plate and cupping and fraying of the epiphyseal end of metaphysis [2].

Phosphopenic rickets is mainly due to renal phosphate wasting resulting from either the primary renal tubular defect or excess generation of phosphatonin, which inhibit phosphate reabsorption from renal tubules and also reduces vitamin D 1α-hydroxylation [10–13].

Phosphopenic rickets is usually hereditary, and X-linked dominant hypophosphatemic rickets accounts for more than

80% and remaining 20% are due to autosomal dominant hypophosphatemic rickets, autosomal recessive hypophosphatemic rickets, and hereditary hypophosphatemic rickets with hypercalciuria [11].

Rare cases of acquired phosphopenic rickets result from benign mesenchymal tumors that produce a factor that decreases the proximal renal tubular resorption of phosphate and also may be associated with renal loss of phosphate as a result of a generalized proximal tubular dysfunction such as Fanconi syndrome [11, 12].

Clinically, the patient will present with features of rickets, short stature bone pain, and dental abscess [10, 14, 15]. Laboratory findings include raised ALP, hypophosphatemia, hyperphosphaturia normal or mild decreased 1, 25 (OH) D, and normal PTH level [3, 10, 14, 15]. Treatment is palliative with a high dose of phosphorous and vitamin D [10, 14, 15].

The condition hypophosphatemic rickets was first described by Albright et al. in 1937, with a prevalence of 1 in 20,000 [14].

Calcipenic rickets can be distinguished from phosphopenic rickets by predominantly muscle weakness, involvement of all limbs, tetany, enamel hypoplasia, absence of dental abscess, low calcium, and marked elevated ALP parathyroid hormone. Treatment of calcipenic rickets is usually a high dose of vitamin D while phosphopenic rickets is by phosphorous and vitamin D [2, 11].

2. Case Presentation

We report a 1 year and 4-month-old African male, who was admitted to our hospital because of recurrent episode of cough for 8 months and bowing of the legs for 6 months prior to admission.

The recurrent episodes of dry cough were worse at night and early morning, and he also had episodes of wheezing but no bluish coloration of the mucous membrane. He attends the outpatient clinic monthly, and prior to his recent admission, he had been admitted twice in an interval of two months due cough and difficulty in breathing, which were successfully treated with nebulized salbutamol and antibiotics. There is no history of asthma or atopy on the family. During the course of his illness, he was noted to have inward bending of the lower limbs, which was more prominent when standing. He has no history of trauma, limb length discrepancy, or swelling. His anterior frontanelle closed at one year, and he had no history of hair loss or balding patches. He had his first tooth eruption at 7 months, and no report of pain or pus discharge from the teeth was noted. He attained early developmental milestones until the age of 7 months, and the delay was noted subsequently as he was unable to crawl, stand, and walk during the recent admission. He had no history of convulsions or use of anticonvulsant medications, hoarseness of voice, or history suggestive of malabsorption disorder, liver disease, or kidney disease. There is no history of consanguinity or similar disease in the family.

His mother received adequate prenatal care and had adequate sun exposure. She had no history of muscle or bone pain during pregnancy. She reports taking diet consisting of eggs and fish in here regular diet, and she had a good appetite and no reported illnesses or drug exposure apart from hematinics during the gestational period. Her pregnancy was uneventful, and she delivered by SVD at the gestational age of 38 weeks, a male baby weighing 3.1 kg and started breastfeeding on the same day. The baby was only exclusively breastfed for 2 months, formula milk was introduced at 3 months of age, and he was weaned at 6 months. Currently, he feeds on foods rich in vitamin D and had adequate intake in terms of quality and quantity and also had adequate sun exposure. Immunization is appropriate for his age, and his weight gain pattern is appropriate for his age.

On his recent admission, he was alert, had some palmar pallor, no angular stomatitis or chelitis, no craniotabes, and no dental caries. His respiratory rate was 53 cyles per minute with the lower chest in drawing, and oxygen saturation was 89% in room air. He had a dull percussion note on the left inframammary and infrascapular regions with vesicular breath sounds, and he had crackles on the left inframammary and infrascapular and axillary regions with a prolonged expiratory phase, but no obvious wheezes were heard.

Musculoskeletal findings showed no rachitic rosary or Harrison's groove, but revealed skull bossing and a widened wrist and genu varus (Figure 1).

The other systems were essentially normal.

Blood investigations which were done on the initial visit are as shown in Tables 1 and 2.

He had elevated alkaline phosphatase (ALP) and serum parathyroid hormone with normal calcium, phosphorous, and 25D OH levels, consistent with stage 2 vitamin D-dependent rickets type 1 [2, 3].

Complete blood count results showed microcytic hypochromic anemia and leukocytosis with predominant neutrophilia consistent with sepsis [16].

The C-reactive protein (CRP) level was also raised suggesting pyogenic infection. Liver and renal functions were normal.

2.1. Images Limbs and X-Ray. Radiographs of the distal radius and ulna bone (Figure 2) revealed (a) cupping/fraying in both the lower ends of the radius and ulna bone, (b) cortical thinning, epiphyseal widening, and X-ray of the proximal and distal tibia and fibula showed (c) bowing of legs and growth arrest lines. Chest X-ray showed opacification on the middle zone.

In view of the symptoms, physical examination, and investigation findings, we had a diagnosis of vitamin D-dependant rickets type 1, bronchial asthma, severe pneumonia, and moderate hypochromic microcytic anemia.

2.2. Treatment and Follow-Up. The patient was treated with salbutamol nebulization 2.5 mg 6 hrly for 48 hrs, then budenoside twice daily via a metered inhaler, then iv ceftriaxone 750 mg once daily for 3 days, and then was discharged home on syrup cefixime for 7 days. He was also started on calcitriol 0.25 μgm once daily.

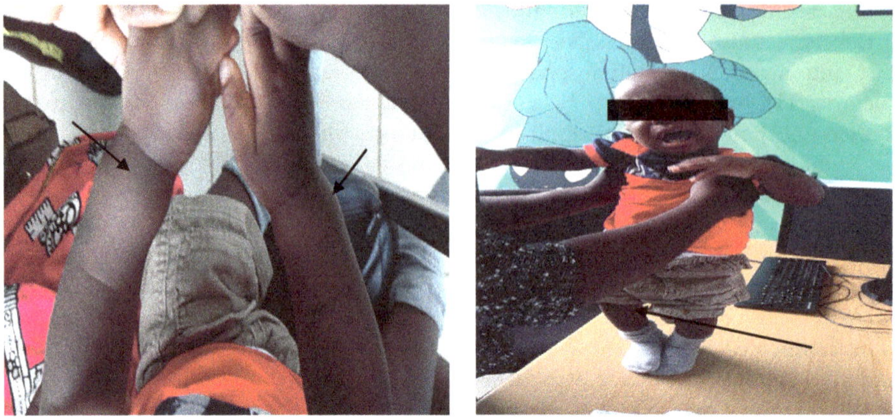

(a) (b)

FIGURE 1: Enlarged wrist (a) and genu varus (b).

TABLE 1: Results of blood investigation done on the first day of admission.

	ALP I (μ/l)	Calcium (mmol/l)	Phosphorous (mmol/l)	Magnesium (mmol/l)	Serum PTH (pg/ml)	25D OH (nmol/l)
Value	1180	2.25	0.72	0.79	182	100.75
Normal	100–644	2.1–2.6	0.7–1.3	0.7–1.2	10–55	100–250

TABLE 2: Complete blood count (CBC) results.

Hb	MCV	MCH	RDW	Plat	WBC	Neutr	Mon	LYM
9.06 gm/dl	67.4 fl	20.9 pg	24.1%	399 k/μl	19.1 k/μl	15.7 kμ/l	1.38 k/μl	1.88 k/μl

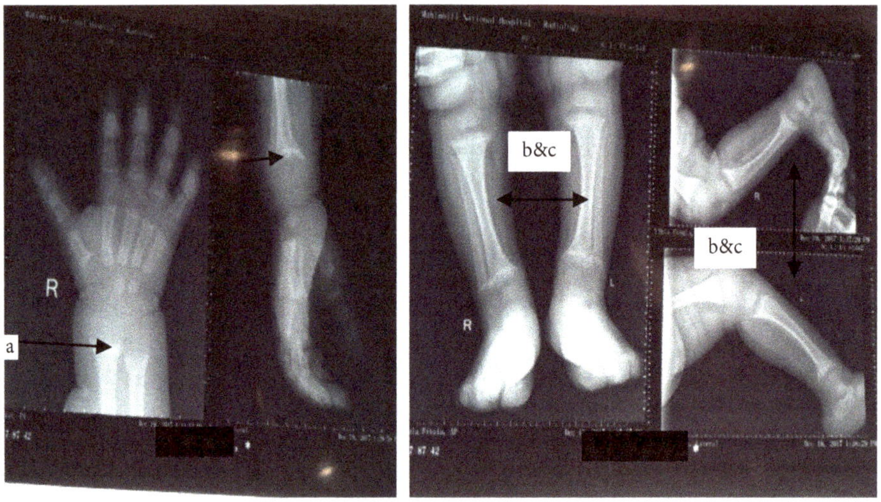

FIGURE 2: Radiological changes on the upper and lower limbs.

On subsequent outpatient follow-up clinic, his hemoglobin had returned to normal level and respiratory symptoms were improving. ALP was still high, and thus calcitriol was increased to a dose of 0.5 μgm once daily and oral calcium supplements were added. At his 6 months of follow-up visit, he had a considerable improvement in his respiratory symptoms, ALP was still remarkably high 1100 IU/L, and other tests for monitoring of serum vitamin D, calcium, phosphorous, and PTH could not be done due to financial constrains. He still had persisted genu varus and was on vitamin D and calcium.

2.3. 2nd Case. A 4-year-old male presented with developmental delay, poor weight gain, and recurrent chest infection for the past 3 years and worsening of bone pain since 9 months of age; he was delivered at the gestational age of 37 weeks, a male baby weighing 3.2 kg at birth and attained a maximum weight of 8.2 kg at 1 year. Thereafter, his weight was stagnant with a recent weight drop to 7 kg. With regard to his developmental milestone, his speech, social skills, and fine motor were appropriate for age, but he had delayed gross motor development as at age of 4 yrs he could not sit without support or stand which could be attributed to constant severe bone pain. His mother reported adequate nutrition intake and adequate sun exposure and she had optimal prenatal care with no history of bone pain. Tooth eruption was normal and no reports of abscess per oral cavity, alopecia, oliguria, or history suggesting malabsorption. He had a history of recurrent chest infection characterized by dry cough worse at night, which were being relieved by bronchodilators; he had no history of wheezes or bluish coloration of lips. His vaccination was up to date. He is the last born in a consanguineous Caucasian family of 5 children, with a history of sibling death at 1 year of age due to recurrent chest infections. Both parents were 38 years old at the time of consultation.

2.4. Physical Examination. On examination, he had normal hair distribution, his weight was 7 kg, and height was 83 cm making weight for length below -3SD and length for age below -3SD, consistent with severe wasting and stunting.

Has had widening of the wrists and genu varus on the limb, and he has no alopecia, dental abscess, or rachitic rosary.

Past investigations conducted at 9 months of age when he showed early signs revealing elevated alkaline phosphatase, low level of phosphorous calcium, and low serum vitamin D with serum parathyroid hormones within the normal range for age and sex are shown in Table 3.

These results showed elevated ALP low phosphorous, hypocalcemia, and normal PTH in keeping with phosphopenic rickets [3, 10].

2.5. Treatment and Follow-Up. He was kept on 5 μgm per day of phosphorous and calcium supplements in the previous 6 months and yet control labs revealed low calcium, low phosphorous, and elevated urinary phosphorous levels and the parathyroid hormone levels were normal.

During a year of follow-up on a high dose of vitamin D and phosphorus, though there was no clinical or biochemical improvement, he still had abnormal results as shown in Table 3.

X-ray of the limbs repeated at the age of 4 years when he presented to our hospital showed a fracture of the middle radius, with significant cortical thinning (Figure 3).

The child died at 4 years and 7 months due to severe chest infection causing septicemia and before death was kept in mechanical ventilation and antibiotics, with no improvement, and the cause of death was respiratory failure.

3. Discussion

We reported two cases with similar clinical presentation where Case 1 had classical features of vitamin D-dependent rickets both in physical examination and laboratory and radiological findings with bowing of legs, elevated ALP, hyperparathyroidism, and normal calcium. This case also had recurrent chest infection and wheezes which can be explained by the fact that vitamin D is also important in both innate and adaptive immune response [17–19]. Based on several epidemiological studies, there has been reported increased episodes of bronchospams in children with vitamin D deficiency [20, 21]. Respiratory comorbidity can be severe enough to necessitate hospital admission as was a case report from Cape-Verde of a child who stayed in hospital for 9 months due to respiratory infections [22]. Another case report from Brazil reported prolonged hospitalization for 20 months during this time which necessitated mechanical ventilation and tracheostomy [23].

Our case also presented with anemia that can be explained by the fact vitamin D has a vital role in promoting erythropoietin by downregulating proinflammatory cytokines and activating the erythropoietin hormone itself [24–26]. Other typical features of rickets like craniotabes, dental deformities, and rachitic rosary and Harisson's groove were not present in this child. Laboratory findings were in keeping with vitamin D resistance due to high ALP, normal calcium due to PTH compensation, and elevation of PTH with normal phosphorous levels. This is due to the fact that hypocalcaemia is osteopenic [3]. Clinically, we were not able to distinguish between type 1 and 2 VDD rickets because there was no distinctive feature of alopecia or dental abscess which is a common feature of type 2 vitamin D-dependent rickets from several reported cases which were reviewed [9, 27–29]. Although this is not a diagnostic criteria, there are some reported cases of type 2 VDD rickets without alopecia [1, 7]. Other markers which would help distinguish between the two forms is the level of 1, 25D OH which is highly elevated for type 2 VDD rickets and reduced in type 1 [27]; unfortunately, we were unable to access this test.

Other important tests are genetic studies to identify mutation in the CYP27B1 gene encoding for the 1-alpha hydroxylase enzyme in which the gene is mapped on chromosome 12q14 [4].

Our patient responded well to other treatments including his respiratory complaints and anemia, but had suboptimal response to vitamin D as on the next follow-up ALP was still high and Ca was low. On reviewing the literature, it was suggested to escalate the dose of vitamin D for poor response to the initial dose [3, 6]. Poor response to a high dose of vitamin D could point towards type 2.

The 2nd case we reported was of a clinical presentation of rickets with parental consanguinity and death of an older sibling with respiratory illness which suggests it could be an inherited condition. This child presented with poor weight gain and delayed motor and bone pain which are clinical characteristics of hypophosphatemic rickets; however, he has no dental manifestation as most of the published case reports reported either missing teeth or dental abscess [14, 15, 30]. Normal PTH and low phosphorous and 25 D OH and hyperphosphaturia are characteristic of phosphopenic rickets [3, 12]. Sadly, this patient had regular follow-up for 4 years with gradual deterioration of symptoms and of late had multiple fractures. There are reported cases of patients with fractures in this condition [27, 28]. These fractures pose challenge to the treatment as he already was on a high dose of vitamin D and phosphorous, but there was no clinical or biochemical response.

Table 3: Laboratory findings at 9 months and 1 year.

Serial number	Investigation	Normal level	At 9 months	1 year later
1	ALP	<281	1200 IU/L	1169
2	Calcium	2.2–2.6	2.19	2.02
3	Phosphorous	1.45–1.78	0.58	0.32
4	25D OH		66.75 nmol/l	
5	PTH	15–68.3	57.2	
6	Albumin			42 gm/dl
7	Urine phosphorous			32.21 mg/dl
8	Urine calcium	2.5–8 mmol/l		9.67 mg/dl

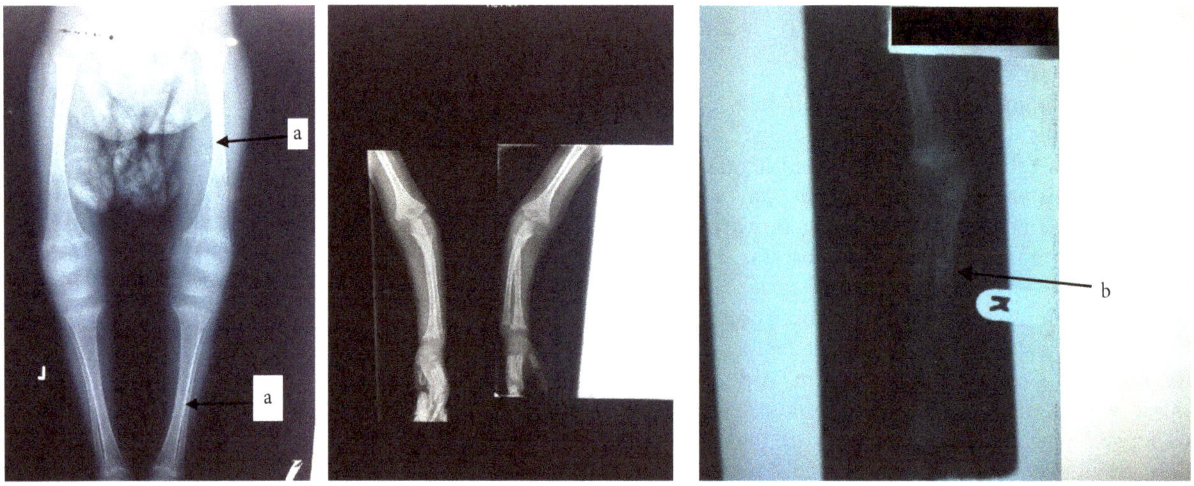

(a) (b)

Figure 3: (a) Bowing of limbs with cortical thinning; (b) X-ray findings which were done at 4 years of age showed fracture of the midradius.

4. Conclusion

Rickets pose diagnostic and treatment challenges in resource-limited countries; clinical presentation alone cannot distinguish several types of rickets, and complete laboratory and genetic studies are important.

Consent

Written informed consent was obtained from the patient's legal guardians (mother) for publication of this case report and the accompanying images.

Authors' Contributions

EG admitted the child together with FM; PK and AS participated in attending and preparation of manuscripts; KP was involved in treating the 2nd case and following up; HN was the Lecturer who provided expertise in taking care and manuscript preparation, writing and providing corrections.

References

[1] S. Ranabir, S. Choudhury, K. Jebasingh, and T. P. Singh, "Familial vitamin D resistant rickets: end-organ resistance to 1,25-dihydroxyvitamin D," *Indian Journal of Endocrinology and Metabolism*, vol. 17, no. 7, p. 224, 2013.

[2] M. Sahay and R. Sahay, "Review article Rickets—vitamin D deficiency and dependency," *Indian Journal of Endocrinology and Metabolism*, vol. 16, no. 2, 2012.

[3] C. G. D. Brook, *Handbook of Clinical Pediatric Endocrinology*, Wiley-Blackwell, Hoboken, NJ, USA, 2008.

[4] B. Özcabı, F. T. Bucak, S. Jaferova et al., "A case of vitamin d-dependent rickets type 1a with a novel mutation in the Uzbek population," *Journal of Clinical Research in Pediatric Endocrinology*, vol. 8, no. 4, pp. 484–489, 2016.

[5] M. Labuda, K. Morgan, and F. H. Glorieux, "Mapping autosomal recessive vitamin D dependency type I to chromosome 12q14 by linkage analysis," *American Journal of Human Genetics*, vol. 47, no. 1, pp. 28–36, 1990.

[6] F. H. Glorieux and J. M. Pettifor, "Vitamin D/dietary calcium deficiency rickets and pseudo-vitamin D deficiency rickets," *Bonekey Report*, vol. 3, 2014.

[7] S. Mishra, T. P. Yadav, S. Nangia, V. K. Gupta, and K. K. Sidhu, "Case reports vitamin-D dependent rickets type II," *Indian Paediatrics*, vol. 33, pp. 1995–1997, 1996.

[8] L. S. Nield, P. Mahajan, A. Joshi, and D. Kamat, "Rickets: not a disease of the past," *American Family Physician*, vol. 74, no. 4, pp. 619–626, 2006.

[9] D. Feldman and P. J Malloy, "Mutations in the vitamin D receptor and hereditary vitamin D-resistant rickets," *Bonekey Reports*, vol. 3, 2014.
[10] N. Atapattu, "Approach to a child presenting with rickets," *Sri Lanka Journal of Child Health*, vol. 42, no. 1, pp. 40–44, 2013.
[11] V. Jagtap, V. Sarathi, A. Lila, T. Bandgar, P. Menon, and N. Shah, "Hypophosphatemic rickets," *Indian Journal of Endocrinology and Metabolism*, vol. 16, no. 2, pp. 177–182, 2012.
[12] A. Angham and A. Rajaa, "Types of rickets," *Annals of Orthopedics & Rheumatology*, vol. 5, pp. 1–6, 2017.
[13] C. Xu, C. Ma, and Y. Bai, "A pediatric hypophosphatemic rickets on MRI, 99mTc-MDP bone scan and 18F-FDG PET/CT.," *Hellenic Journal of Nuclear Medicine*, vol. 20, no. 1, pp. 93–96, 2017.
[14] G. Sarat, N. Priyanka, M. P. V. Prabhat, C. Raja Lakshmi, S. M. Bhavana, and D. Ayesha Thabusum, "Hypophosphatemic rickets in siblings: a rare case report," *Case Reports in Dentistry*, vol. 2016, Article ID 4803167, 8 pages, 2016.
[15] E. C. Tumen, I. Yavuz, D. S. Tumen, and F. Atakul, "Dental and histologic findings of X-linked hypophosphataemic vitamin D-resistant rickets: a case report," *International Dental and Medical Disorders*, vol. 1, no. 1, pp. 37–42, 2008.
[16] D. S. Wheeler, "Pediatric Sepsis : markers , mechanisms , and management," *The Open Inflammation Journal*, vol. 4, pp. 1–3, 2011.
[17] O. Helve, H. Viljakainen, E. Holmlund-Suila et al., "Towards evidence-based vitamin D supplementation in infants: vitamin D intervention in infants (VIDI)—study design and methods of a randomised controlled double-blinded intervention study," *BMC Pediatrics*, vol. 17, no. 1, pp. 1–8, 2017.
[18] A. S. Najada, M. S. Habashneh, and M. Khader, "The frequency of nutritional rickets among hospitalized infants and its relation to respiratory diseases," *Journal of Tropical Pediatrics*, vol. 50, no. 6, pp. 364–368, 2004.
[19] M. Misra, D. Pacaud, A. Petryk, P. F. Collett-Solberg, and M. Kappy, "Vitamin D deficiency in children and its management: review of current knowledge and recommendations," *Pediatrics*, vol. 122, no. 2, pp. 398–417, 2008.
[20] Y. R. Alladi and J. Gopal, "Vitamin D deficiency and relation to recurrent respiratory tract infection in children less than 5 years," *Journal of Dental and Medical Sciences*, vol. 16, no. 8, pp. 88–96, 2017.
[21] J. Charan, J. Goyal, D. Saxena, and P. Yadav, "Vitamin D for prevention of respiratory tract infections: a systematic review and meta-analysis," *Journal of Pharmacology and Pharmacotherapeutics*, vol. 3, no. 4, p. 300, 2012.
[22] A. S. Fernandes, S. Lobo, A. R. Sandes, C. Simão, L. Lobo, and T. Bandeira, "Vitamin D-dependent rickets: a resurgence of the rachitic lung in the 21st century," *BMJ Case Reports*, vol. 2015, 2015.
[23] M. L. A. Maia, A. L. S. Abreu, P. C. K. Nogueira, M. L. M. Val, J. T. A. Carvalhaes, and M. C. Andrade, "Hypophosphatemic rickets: case report," *Revista paulista de pediatria*, vol. 36, no. 2, pp. 242–247, 2018.
[24] S. Uwaezuoke, "Vitamin D deficiency and anemia risk in children: a review of emerging evidence," *Pediatric Health, Medicine and Therapeutics*, vol. 8, pp. 47–55, 2017.
[25] L. Chang, X. Liu, H. Shi, W. Dai, H. Wang, and Y. Jiang, "Association of 25-hydroxyvitamin D with Hb and lead in children: a Chinese population-based study," *Public Health Nutrition*, vol. 17, no. 4, pp. 827–832, 2014.
[26] T. Liu, S. Zhong, L. Liu et al., "Vitamin D deficiency and the risk of anemia: a meta-analysis of observational studies," *Renal Failure*, vol. 37, no. 6, pp. 929–934, 2015.
[27] P. Inamdar, R. Bellad, and V. Herekar, "Vitamin D-dependent rickets type 2: alopecia responding to 1,25 hydroxy vitamin D," *Journal of the Scientific Society*, vol. 43, no. 3, pp. 155–157, 2016.
[28] M. Azemi, M. Berisha, V. IsmailiJaha et al., "Vitamin D—dependent rickets, type II case report," *Materia Socio Medica*, vol. 26, no. 1, pp. 68–70, 2014.
[29] A. A. Ghazi, A. Zadeh-Vakili, M. Z. Yeganeh et al., "Hereditary vitamin D resistant rickets: clinical, laboratory, and genetic characteristics of 2 Iranian Siblings," *International Journal of Endocrinology and Metabolism*, vol. 15, no. 3, 2017.
[30] M. Yavropoulou, K. Kotsa, A. Gotzamani Psarrakou et al., "Cinacalcet in hyperparathyroidism secondary to X-linked hypophosphatemic rickets: case report and brief literature review," *Hormones*, vol. 9, no. 3, pp. 274–278, 2010.
[31] H. Suhaimi and M. Muslim, "Teenager with severe bowing of limbs," *Journal of Clinical Case Reports*, vol. 6, no. 2, pp. 2–4, 2016.
[32] H. Juneja, M. Yadav, and I. Pahuja, "Case report X-linked linked hypophosphatemic RICKETS : a case report," *International Journal of Current Research*, vol. 8, pp. 56598–56600, 2017.

3

Myxedema Coma Associated with Macroprolactinoma: Case Report and Review of the Literature

Elizabeth Jasola Omoniyi[1,2] **and Richard J. Robbins**[1,2]

[1]*From the Division of Endocrinology, Diabetes and Metabolism, Department of Medicine, Houston Methodist Hospital, Houston, TX, USA*
[2]*Weill Cornell Medical College, New York, NY, USA*

Correspondence should be addressed to Richard J. Robbins; rjrobbins@houstonmethodist.org

Academic Editor: Toshihiro Kita

Myxedema coma is a rare life-threatening presentation of severe hypothyroidism associated with a high mortality rate. Although most cases are due to primary thyroid failure, a minority have central hypothyroidism as the underlying cause. We report the case of a 69-year-old man who presented with obtundation, hypoglycemia, and hyponatremia. The patient's initial thyroid-stimulating hormone (TSH) was within normal limits. Subsequent evaluation revealed critical anterior pituitary insufficiency due to a macroprolactinoma and a diagnosis of myxedema coma after appropriate workup The finding of a normal serum TSH should not eliminate the possibility of myxedema coma.

1. Introduction

We report a very unusual case of myxedema coma (MC). Severe hypothyroidism meeting the definition of MC is associated with a significant mortality rate (30–50%), even with standard therapy [1, 2]. The underlying causes of myxedema coma vary but usually involve a primary pathological process in the thyroid gland. Commonly, a patient with primary hypothyroidism either stops taking or stops absorbing their thyroid supplements for some time, resulting in fatigue and confusion. Mental status can gradually deteriorate; however, if precipitated by a severe infection, trauma, central nervous system depressants, or a sudden cardiovascular event, rapid onset of stupor or obtundation may ensue, termed myxedema coma. MC has also been reported rarely in patients with central hypothyroidism due to hypothalamic or pituitary diseases. We report a case of myxedema coma with central hypothyroidism associated with a macroprolactinoma.

2. Case Report

Following a rare series of three winter storms affecting Houston, TX, at the end of February 2021, there was widespread loss of power and water, and daily temperatures stayed below 0 degrees Celsius for 17 days. An estimated 250–700 Texans died from cold exposure during this period.

A 69-year-old male was brought to the emergency department in early March 2021 for evaluation of deteriorating mental status leading to disorientation and unresponsiveness. Initial laboratory tests revealed a blood glucose of 45 mg/dl and a serum sodium of 120 mEq/L. His lactic acid level was elevated at 4.2 mmol/L. He was started on intravenous 10% dextrose with no improvement of mental status, though his serum glucose rose to 102 mg/dl. A chest CT revealed a large area of infiltration in the right upper lung consistent with pneumonia. A CT scan of the head revealed calcification of the basal ganglia, thalamus, and cerebral hemispheres bilaterally. A 2 cm mass arising from the sella turcica was also noted (Figure 1). Additional laboratory studies on the day of admission (when he was hypoglycemic) revealed a serum insulin of 1.4 mU/L with normal C-peptide, IGF-2, and proinsulin levels.

He also had a significant medical history of hypertension and iron deficiency anemia that required frequent erythropoietin injections. He also had a history of daily tobacco use but had discontinued that two years prior. There was no history of illicit drug use. His only home medication was lisinopril 20 mg daily. His family reported that he had been increasingly confused and lethargic for one week prior to his emergency room presentation. His family also reported that he had not complained of headaches, nausea, vomiting, or any visual impairment.

Clinically, he was obtunded and only partially responsive to auditory stimuli. His skin was very dry and flaking off; he had generalized edema and macroglossia, but he did not have expressible galactorrhea or gynecomastia. He was variably hypothermic, with body temperature ranging from 94.8–96.1 degrees Fahrenheit. His heart rate ranged from 75 to 86 bpm. An ECG revealed a first-degree AV block. On 2 liters of nasal oxygen, his arterial pO2 was 95 mm·Hg, and his pCO2 was elevated at 48 mm·Hg. In previous medical visits, he had never been diagnosed with thyroid dysfunction, hyponatremia, or hypoglycemia. He had no prior brain imaging.

Given the newly found pituitary lesion and the patient's clinical presentation, pituitary function labs were ordered for further evaluation. His prolactin level was 1,033 ng/ml (4–15 ng/ml); free T4 was 0.2 ng/dl (0.9–1.7 ng/dl); total T3 was low at 35 ng/dl (80–200 ng/dl) with an inappropriately normal thyroid-stimulating hormone (TSH) of 2.35 uIU/ml (0.27–4.2 uIU/ml). His initial (2 PM) serum cortisol was 5 ug/dl with an ACTH of 9.6 pg/ml (7.2–63.3 pg/ml). Following intravenous cosyntropin, his cortisol rose to 10 ug/dl at 30 minutes and 11 ug/dl at 60 minutes. There was no notable change in his mental status after the cosyntropin administration. His IGF-2 was normal at 206 ng/ml (180–580 ng/ml). His initial serum parathyroid hormone level was low at 9 pg/ml.

The patient's serum follicle-stimulating hormone (FSH) was 1.0 mIU/mL (1.6–8.0 mIU/ml), and his serum luteinizing hormone (LH) was 0.3 mIU/ml (1.6–15.2 mIU/ml). An MRI of the brain confirmed a sellar and suprasellar enhancing mass, likely a pituitary adenoma, measuring 1.2 × 1.8 × 2.3 cm, with no sphenoid or cavernous sinus invasion.

The patient's total score of 85 on the widely accepted Popoveniuc et al. diagnostic scoring system [3] confirmed the diagnosis of myxedema coma. He would have received 7 points on Chiong's screening tool [4], making myxedema coma "Likely." His clinical presentation, history, and multiple laboratory and imaging findings were consistent with myxedema coma and hypopituitarism, likely secondary to a macroprolactinoma.

3. Discussion and Literature Review

We report the case of a man who had underlying central hypopituitarism, including partial TSH deficiency, as the cause of his hypothyroidism. He then developed myxedema coma, possibly due to a combination of cold exposure and pneumonia. The cause of his hypopituitarism was most likely a macroprolactinoma. As far as we can determine, this is the first documented case of myxedema coma due in part to a macroprolactinoma. We found no other case reports of this phenomenon in our literature review.

There are many potential underlying causes of MC. Two of the most common are autoimmune thyroid failure (e.g., Hashimoto thyroiditis) and post-thyroidectomy hypothyroidism. Reports of MC due to hypopituitarism with secondary hypothyroidism are quite rare and have been estimated to account for much less than 5% of all MC cases [2]. The earliest case of MC due to central hypothyroidism that we found in our literature review was reported in 1940 by Means, Hertz, and Herman, who reported MC due to Sheehan's disease hypopituitarism. An autopsy revealed atrophy of the pituitary, thyroid, adrenals, and ovaries [5]. In a 1991 literature review, Pinchera et al. estimated that hypothyroidism arising solely from hypopituitarism accounted for approximately 0.005% of all cases of hypothyroidism [6].

The most common precipitating factors in MC are hypothermia, cessation of thyroid supplements, severe infections, anesthetics, tranquilizers, respiratory failure, and stroke [1, 7]. In 2008, Dutta et al. reported on 29 cases of MC. Four (17%) likely had underlying central hypothyroidism, three of which were due to Sheehan syndrome and the last of which was due to a nonfunctioning pituitary adenoma. The precipitating cause of MC was pneumonia in three of the four patients and cold exposure in the fourth patient [8].

Several well-documented cases of MC associated with hypopituitarism have been reported in PubMed over the past 60 years [9–16]. A case with both Hashimoto thyroiditis and Sheehan syndrome leading to MC has also been reported [17], as has a case with Hashimoto thyroiditis and TSH deficiency [18]. In pediatric medicine, Thompson and Henry reported a rare case of MC due to central hypothyroidism in a 7-year-old boy with a chromosome 1q deletion [19].

Given that the vast majority (>95%) of MC cases are due to primary hypothyroidism, it can be difficult to diagnose MC when TSH is not elevated. In patients with MC due to central hypothyroidism, the TSH is typically low or normal, and these patients often have other features of hypopituitarism [8]. Additionally, given that a small but significant percentage of thyroid hormone production from the thyroid gland is TSH-independent (10–15%), these patients often also present with free T4 levels that are higher than in patients with primary hypothyroidism [8].

Although patients with MC due to central hypothyroidism typically present with altered mental status as the first symptom, their neurological impairments may be more subtle than MC due to primary hypothyroidism, in part because there is some minimal TSH-independent T4 production in central hypothyroidism. However, the mortality rate for MC appears to be similar in both central and primary hypothyroidism [8, 20].

Notably, patients with macroprolactinomas have various patterns of hypopituitarism. In a large retrospective review

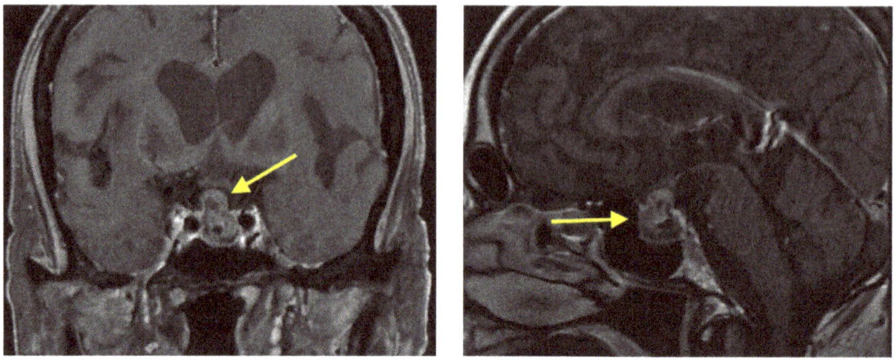

(a) (b)

Figure 1: (a) Coronal and (b) sagittal views of the 2 cm pituitary adenoma.

of men with macroprolactinomas (between 20–39 mm in size), 93% had central hypogonadism, 7% had central hypoadrenalism, and 18% had central hypothyroidism [21, 22]. Hyperprolactinemia is commonly associated with diminished or absent pulsatile LH and FSH secretion, likely due to endocrine inhibition of GnRH pulses [23]; however, there is no evidence that it suppresses TSH secretion in men. By contrast, dopamine agonists, which are often used to treat hyperprolactinemia, have been shown to suppress TSH [24].

Regardless of the etiology of the MC, management with high-dose intravenous levothyroxine as a loading dose, followed by a weight-based daily dose, remains the gold standard for therapy to help reverse the severe hypometabolic state in MC patients. Intravenous hydrocortisone should also be administered initially or concurrently, as patients with MC often have relative adrenocortical deficiency, which can worsen as the replacement thyroid hormone increases the metabolic rate [1].

4. Conclusion

Myxedema coma is an endocrine emergency that requires a high index of suspicion given its high mortality rate. Unusual underlying causes, such as tumoral hypopituitarism, can impede diagnosis due to the lack of elevated TSH levels. This can potentially delay time-sensitive management therapies. From our literature review and to the best of our knowledge, this is the first report of macroprolactinoma associated with MC and is worth noting, as it highlights the extensive range of complications that can arise from pituitary tumors. Overall, this case highlights the critical importance of careful and thorough clinical assessment in patients with seemingly incongruent clinical and laboratory findings.

References

[1] K. D. Burman and L. Wartofsky, "Myxedema coma," in *Werner and Ingbar's the Thyroid*, L. E. Braverman, D. S. Cooper, and P. Kopp, Eds., Wolters Kluwer, Alphen aan den Rijn, Netherlands, 2020.

[2] L. Wartofsky, "Myxedema coma," *Endocrinology and Metabolism Clinics of North America*, vol. 35, no. 4, pp. 687–698, 2006.

[3] G. Popoveniuc, T. Chandra, A. Sud et al., "A diagnostic scoring system for myxedema coma," *Endocrine Practice*, vol. 20, no. 8, pp. 808–817, 2014.

[4] Y. V. Chiong, E. Bammerlin, and C. N. Mariash, "Development of an objective tool for the diagnosis of myxedema coma," *Translational Research*, vol. 166, no. 3, pp. 233–243, 2015.

[5] J. H. Means, S. Hertz, and J. Lerman, "The pituitary type of myxedema or Simmond's disease masquerading as myxedema," *Transactions of the Association of American Physicians*, vol. 55, no. 32, 1940.

[6] A. Pinchera, E. Martino, and G. Faglia, "Central hypothyroidism," in *The Thyroid. A Fundamental and Clinical Text*, L. E. Braverman and R. D. Utiger, Eds., pp. 968–984, Lippincott Company, JB Lippincott Company, Philadelphia, PA, USA, 1991.

[7] V. Mathew, R. A. Misgar, S. Ghosh et al., "Myxedema coma: a new look into an old crisis," *Journal of Thyroid Research*, vol. 2011, Article ID 493462, 7 pages, 2011.

[8] P. Dutta, A. Bhansali, S. Masoodi, S. Bhadada, N. Sharma, and R. Rajput, "Predictors of outcome in myxoedema coma: A study from a tertiary care centre," *Critical Care*, vol. 12, no. 1, 2008.

[9] S. Bhogal, N. Patel, K. Mawa, V. Ramu, and T. Paul, "A rare case of myxedema coma presenting as bradycardia and hypotension secondary to pituitary apoplexy," *Cureus*, vol. 13, no. 5, Article ID e15196, 2021.

[10] M. J. Cullen, P. D. Mayne, and I. Sliney, "Myxoedema coma," *Irish Journal of Medical Science*, vol. 148, no. 1, pp. 201–206, 1979.

[11] S. Fischli, C. Stettler, and E. Christ, "Kardiogener Schock und psychotisches Zustandsbild seltener Ursache," *DMW—Deutsche Medizinische Wochenschrift*, vol. 131, no. 42, pp. 2333–2336, 2006.

[12] R. Hanslik, L. Kaspar, A. Kroiss, and J. Slany, "Myxödem als Ursache eines QT-Syndroms und rezidivierender Kammertachykardien [Myxedema as a cause of QT syndrome and recurring ventricular tachycardia]," *Zeitschrift für Kardiologie*, vol. 76, no. 1, pp. 58–61, 1987.

[13] L. Langeron, L. Croccel, G. Routier, and P. Choteau, "Myxedematous coma, thyroid involution and eosinophilic adenoma of the hypophysis," *Annales d'Endocrinologie*, vol. 20, pp. 490–493, 1959.

[14] T. Murase, A. Mukoyama, N. Ohsawa, S. Nagataki, T. Yamaji, and T. Tsushima, "A survival case of myxedema coma of pituitary origin," *Endocrinologia Japonica*, vol. 20, no. 3, pp. 331–334, 1973.

[15] M. Perlmutter and H. Cohn, "Myxedema crisis of pituitary or thyroid origin," *The American Journal of Medicine*, vol. 36, no. 6, pp. 883–892, 1964.

[16] W. Reinhardt and K. Mann, "Häufigkeit klinisches Bild und Behandlung des hypothyreoten Komas," *Medizinische Klinik*, vol. 92, no. 9, pp. 521–524, 1997.

[17] S. Benvenga, S. Squadrito, F. Saporito, A. Cimino, F. Arrigo, and F. Trimarchi, "Myxedema coma of both primary and secondary origin with non-classic presentation and extremely elevated creatine kinase," *Hormone and Metabolic Research*, vol. 32, no. 09, pp. 364–366, 2000.

[18] K. Iida, Y. Hino, T. Ohara, and K. Chihara, "A case of myxedema coma caused by isolated thyrotropin stimulating hormone deficiency and Hashimoto's thyroiditis," *Endocrine Journal*, vol. 58, no. 2, pp. 143–148, 2011.

[19] M. D. Thompson and R. K. Henry, "Myxedema coma secondary to central hypothyroidism: a rare but real cause of altered mental status in pediatrics," *Hormone Research in Paediatrics*, vol. 87, no. 5, pp. 350–353, 2017.

[20] I. Rodriguez, E. Fluiters, L. Perez-Mendez, R. Luna, C. Paramo, and R. Garcia-Mayor, "Factors associated with mortality of patients with myxoedema coma: Prospective study in 11 cases treated in a single institution," *Journal of Endocrinology*, vol. 180, no. 2, pp. 347–350, 2004.

[21] P. Iglesias and J. J. Diez, "Macroprolactinoma: A diagnostic and therapeutic update," *An International Journal of Medicine*, vol. 106, no. 6, pp. 495–504, 2013.

[22] A. Tirosh, C. Benbassat, A. Lifshitz, and I. Shimon, "Hypopituitarism patterns and prevalence among men with macroprolactinomas," *Pituitary*, vol. 18, no. 1, pp. 108–115, 2015.

[23] G. Page-Wilson, P. C. Smith, and C. K. Welt, "Prolactin suppresses GnRH but not TSH secretion," *Hormone Research in Paediatrics*, vol. 65, no. 1, pp. 31–38, 2006.

[24] B. R. Haugen, "Drugs that suppress TSH or cause central hypothyroidism," *Best Practice and Research Clinical Endocrinology and Metabolism*, vol. 23, no. 6, pp. 793–800, 2009.

4

Hypertension Accompanied by Hyperaldosteronism, Hyperkalemia and Hyperchloremic Acidosis: A Case Report and Literature Review

Yunyun Yang, Yang Ou, Yan Ren, Haoming Tian, and Tao Chen

Department of Endocrinology and Metabolism, Adrenal Center, West China Hospital of Sichuan University, Chengdu, Sichuan 610041, China

Correspondence should be addressed to Tao Chen; dr.chentao@qq.com

Academic Editor: Toshihiro Kita

This study reported on a 24-year-old woman who complained of a paroxysmal headache for six months and elevated blood pressure for four months. Laboratory examination revealed increased serum potassium and chloride levels, metabolic acidosis, suppressed renin activity, and increased plasma aldosterone concentration. Whole-exome sequencing revealed a heterozygous mutation in exon 11 of the KLHL3 gene: c.1298G > A. After treatment with low-dose hydrochlorothiazide, her clinical problems were controlled. This patient is the first case of Gordon syndrome (GS) within the Chinese population caused by a heterozygous KLHL3 mutation. A systematic review of the published literature identified 27 patients with GS caused by a KLHL3 mutation. These patients had a mean age of 28.2 ± 22.0 years; 74.1% presented with hypertension, 76.9% with hyperkalemia, and 59.1% with metabolic acidosis. The patients also had varying levels of plasma renin activity and plasma aldosterone concentrations.

1. Introduction

Gordon syndrome (GS), also known as familial hyperkalemic hypertension or pseudohypoaldosteronism type II (PHA II), is a rare type of familial hypertension. GS results from excessive activation of the thiazide-sensitive Na/Cl cotransporter (NCC) in the distal convoluted tubules, which leads to an increase in NaCl reabsorption and decreases in K^+ and H^+ excretion, eventually resulting in high blood pressure, hyperkalemia, hyperchloremic metabolic acidosis, suppressed renin levels, and variable aldosterone levels. Other clinical manifestations of GS include growth disorders, myasthenia, periodic paralysis, skeletal abnormalities, and psychomotor delay [1]. Mutations in at least four genes are responsible for GS, including the WNK1, WNK4, KLHL3, and CUL3 genes. A large cohort study of PHA II kindreds illustrated that mutations in KLHL3 and CUL3 were the leading causes (approximately 79%), and mutations in WNK1 or WNK4 only accounted for a small number of PHAII kindreds (approximately 13%).

The present case was a 24-year-old young woman with hypertension, hyperkalemia, hyperchloremia, metabolic acidosis, low renin, and elevated aldosterone. Whole-exome sequencing of the patient revealed a KLHL3 heterozygous mutation: c.1298G > A. After treatment with low-dose hydrochlorothiazide, the patient's high blood pressure, hyperkalemia, and hyperchloremic metabolic acidosis gradually normalized. In addition, the present study systematically reviewed the published literature about the Gordon syndrome with KLHL3 mutations and summarized the clinical characteristics of genetically confirmed GS cases.

2. Case Presentation

The patient was a 24-year-old young woman complaining of a paroxysmal headache for six months and elevated blood pressure for four months. Six months ago, she experienced an episodic headache after sleep insufficiency. Four months ago, she was found with hypertension (up to 150/109 mmHg) in a health examination. The patient had regular menstruation. Her father, grandfather, and grandmother had hypertension. Physical examination of this patient showed no abnormal signs except elevated blood pressure. As shown in Table 1, the patient had elevated levels of serum potassium and chloride, decreased arterial blood pH, standard bicarbonate concentration, and normal serum creatinine and glomerular filtration rate. The patient had suppressed plasma renin activity, elevated plasma aldosterone concentration, normal cortisol circadian rhythm and levels, and normal levels of 24-hour urinary free cortisol, adrenocorticotropin, and serum catecholamine. Moreover, the captopril challenge test of the patient suggested that her plasma aldosterone was suppressed by 31.6%. Her sex hormones, thyroid hormone, and parathyroid hormone were normal. Magnetic resonance imaging (MRI) examination suggested no obvious abnormality in the bilateral adrenal glands. Ultrasound of the urinary system indicated uric acid crystals in the right kidney.

The patient's father had hypertension, and her mother's blood pressure was normal; both were unavailable for laboratory examination and genetic screening. Her elder brother had normal blood pressure, normal levels of serum potassium and serum chlorine, and normal arterial blood gas analysis results.

The peripheral blood genomic DNA of the patient and her elder brother were extracted (Tiangen DNA extraction kit). Next-generation sequencing was applied to capture suspicious mutation sites in the index patient (Illumina HiSeq 2500 system). The suspected mutation was confirmed by direct sequencing of the index patient and other available individuals (Beijing Zhiyin Oriental Transformational Medicine Research Center Co., Ltd.). The patient was identified with a heterozygous mutation in exon 11 of the KLHL3 gene, c.1298G > A, which led to 433rd amino acid serine to be replaced by asparagine (S433N). Her elder brother was wild type at this site (Figure 1). According to the genetic findings, as well as typical clinical manifestations, the patient was diagnosed with the Gordon syndrome.

After treatment with low-dose hydrochlorothiazide (25 mg/day), her blood pressure fluctuated in the range of 90–100/70–80 mmHg, her blood potassium and chlorine, plasma renin activity, and aldosterone concentration returned to normal, and metabolic acidosis was corrected (Table 1). The patient continued to take the low-dose hydrochlorothiazide treatment after discharge. Her blood pressure and serum potassium were normal three months later at follow-up.

3. Review of Clinical Features and Laboratory Findings of GS Patients

To comprehensively review the clinical characteristics of GS caused by the KLHL3 gene mutation, we searched for primary studies published through December 2019 on MEDLINE (PubMed) and the Chinese Biomedical Database (CBM). The MeSH terms "Gordon syndrome," "Pseudohypoaldosteronism type II," and "familial hyperkalemic hypertension" were used for the literature search. The retrieved articles in English and Chinese languages were independently screened by two authors (YY Yang and T Chen). Full-text case studies were included only if they had available data on clinical features and laboratory findings. Clinical data, including country of origin, age at symptom onset, gender, and clinical manifestations such as blood pressure, serum potassium, arterial pH value, plasma renin activity (PRA)/concentration (PRC), and plasma aldosterone concentration (PAC), were sorted out and analyzed.

We identified 27 studies in total, then excluded 22 studies that lacked genetic tests or detailed clinical manifestations or that had mutations other than those in the KLHL3 gene, and eventually included five studies that contained 27 affected members from 8 pedigrees (Table 2). No studies in the Chinese language about the KLHL3 gene mutation were retrieved. The mean age at diagnosis was 28.2 ± 22.0 years, and 59.3% of the patients were females. The incidences of hypertension, hyperkalemia, and metabolic acidosis were 74.1%, 76.9%, and 59.1%, respectively. Among GS patients with hypertension ($n = 20$), 45% of them were diagnosed with hypertension before the age of 18 years, and the overall median age was 27.6 years (range: 0.8–62 years). Among GS patients with hyperkalemia ($n = 20$), the median age was 21.6 years. Among GS patients with metabolic acidosis ($n = 13$), the median age was 22.7 years. In addition, 73.9% of GS patients presented with suppressed PRA, 26.1% presented with normal PRA, 38.1% presented with low PAC, 52.4% presented with normal PAC, and 9.5% presented with high PAC.

4. Discussion

This study reported on a 24-year-old patient who presented with elevated blood pressure and increased serum potassium and chlorine, as well as decreased arterial blood pH, standard bicarbonate concentration, suppressed PRA, normal serum creatinine level, and normal estimated glomerular filtration rate. The above clinical clues indicated a possible diagnosis of the Gordon syndrome. Whole-exome sequencing revealed that the patient carried a heterozygous mutation in the KLHL3 gene: c.1298G > A, which led to 433rd amino acid serine to be replaced by asparagine (S433N). The patient's elder brother, who had normal blood pressure and normal serum potassium, was wild type at this site.

KLHL3 along with the WNK1, WNK4, and CUL3 genes are involved in the physiologic regulation of NCC transporter activity [1, 7–10]. Mutations in the WNK1, WNK4, KLHL3, and CUL3 genes lead to increased NCC transporter activity and membrane expression [7, 11, 12], enhance the inhibition of ROMK [7, 9, 11], and eventually lead to typical clinical features of GS. Whole-exome sequencing in this patient revealed a heterozygous mutation in exon 11 of KLHL3 (c.1298G > A). This mutation was first reported in a large cohort study of 52 European and American GS kindreds in 2012 [8]. Then, a 2017 study from South Korea reported two cases of GS carrying the same mutation, which included a 25-month-old female infant and her 30-year-old mother. The daughter had hypertension, hyperkalemia (6.9 mmol/L), and metabolic acidosis [13], and the mother

Table 1: Laboratory findings of the index patient.

Biochemical findings	Pre-HCTZ	Post-HCTZ	Reference values
Serum potassium	6.3	4.00	3.5–5.3 mmol/L
Serum sodium	142.8	138.9	137–147 mmol/L
Serum chlorine	114.7	96.4	99–110 mmol/L
Serum creatinine	60	N/A	37–110 μmol/L
eGFR	122	N/A	56–122 mL/min/1.73 m^2
Arterial blood pH value	7.286	7.400	7.35–7.45
HCO_3^-	17.6	26.2	22–27 mmol/L
PRA renin activity	0.14	1.07	0.93–6.56 ng/mL/h
PRC aldosterone	31.00	15.2	9.8–27.6 ng/dl
Serum cortisol (8 AM)	300.2	N/A	147.3–609.3 nmol/L
Serum cortisol (4 PM)	162.0	N/A	34–340 nmol/L
Serum cortisol (midnight)	57.2	N/A	<50 nmol/L
24-h UFC	43.61	N/A	20.3–127.6 μg/24 h
ACTH	21.53	N/A	5.0–78 ng/L

Note. eGFR: estimated glomerular filtration rate; ACTH: adrenocorticotropin; UFC: urinary free cortisol; HCO_3^-: serum bicarbonate; PRA: plasma renin activity; PRC: plasma aldosterone concentration; and HCTZ: hydrochlorothiazide.

- KLHL3: c. 1298 (exon11) G>A:

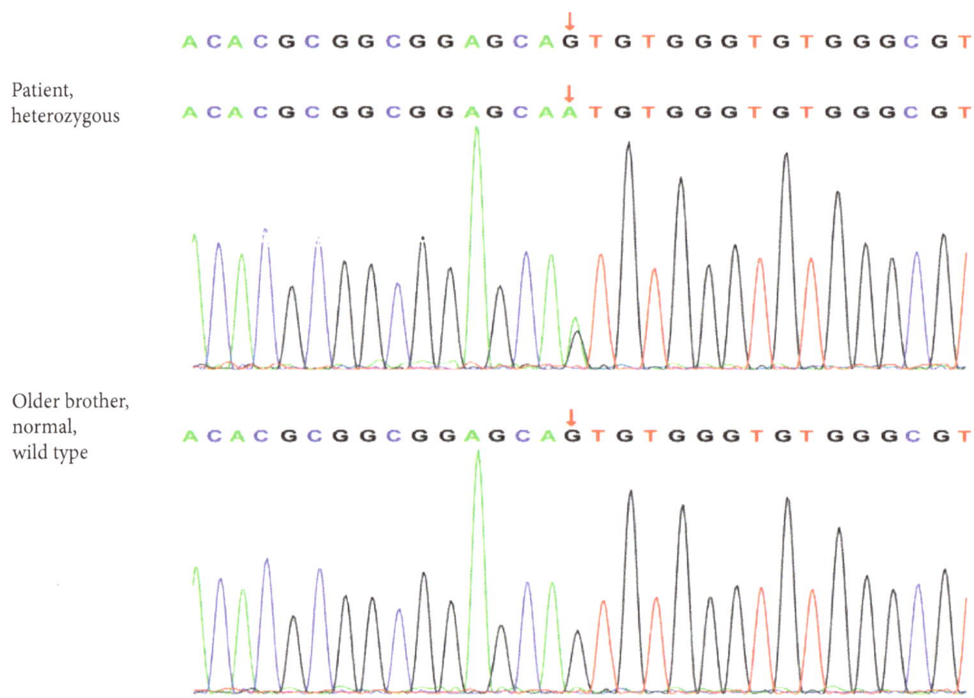

Figure 1: Whole-exome sequencing showing a novel KLHL3 mutation.

had hypertension and hyperkalemia in her twenties [4]. Previously reported GS cases from the Chinese population were mostly caused by WNK4 mutations and CUL3 mutations [14]. To date, no study has reported GS cases with KLHL3 dominant mutations among the Chinese population.

There are significant differences in the severity of clinical phenotypes among GS patients with different gene mutations. CUL3 gene mutation tends to result in much more severe clinical phenotype followed by KLHL3, WNK4, and WNK1 gene mutations. Patients with CUL3 mutations usually developed symptoms at younger ages, with more severe hyperkalemia and metabolic acidosis [7, 8], while patients with KLHL3 mutations usually developed symptoms after adulthood, with mild-to-moderate clinical manifestations.

This patient presented typical features of GS, e.g., hypertension, hyperkalemia, hyperchloremia, and metabolic acidosis, while the systematic review of published studies showed that the clinical manifestations varied among GS patients; hyperkalemia was the most common clinical symptom, which was present in 76.9% of GS patients followed by hypertension (74.1%) and metabolic acidosis (59.1%). Compared with hyperkalemia and metabolic acidosis, hypertension seemed to develop at a later stage

Table 2: Systematic review of clinical features and laboratory findings of GS patients with KLHL3 gene mutations.

ID	Mutation	Age (years)	Sex	BP	K^+	pH	HCO_3^-	PRA	PAC
Kelly et al. [2]	H498Y	18	M	150/90	7.3	7.34	18	0.2	19.1
Mitani et al. [3]	L387P	3	M	110/55	6.6	7.34	14.8	0.6	6.6
Park et al. [4]	C164F	0.8	F	115/72	6.3	7.34	19.6	<0.1	6.4
	S433N	1.7	F	110/73	6.9	7.30	12	<0.1	7.1
	S433N	23	F	Hypertension	6.4	NA	NA	NA	NA
Mayan et al. [5]	Q309R	69	F	115/78	5.4	NA	27	2.3	10.6
	Q309R	48	F	147/95	5.2	NA	25.7	0.1	4.1
	Q309R	11	M	104/61	6.4	NA	22.3	0.1	23.8
	Q309R	11	M	108/71	7.2	NA	21.5	0.1	14.0
	Q309R	10	F	103/72	5.3	NA	22.7	0.7	23.9
	R528H	38	F	154/77	5.6	NA	18	3.6	51.5
	R528H	15	F	136/77	6.0	NA	19.7	0.3	4.1
	R528H	13	F	124/77	6.2	NA	19.8	<0.3	14.8
	R528H	8	F	123/78	5.8	NA	19.1	0.7	10.7
	R528H	2	M	146/95	7.0	NA	NA	0.3	28.3
Kliuk et al. [6]	S553L	34	F	158/107	6.2	NA	NA	<0.5	15.5
	S553L	26	M	115/70	7.1	NA	NA	<0.5	6.5
	Q309R	63	M	110/80	5.6	NA	19.0	1.4	4.5
	Q309R	62	F	160/100	4.8	NA	23.6	1.7	8
	Q309R	57	M	120/90	5.1	NA	19.7	NA	16.7
	Q309R	54	M	145/105	6.4	NA	23.1	4.7	24.6
	Q309R	47	F	120/90	5.1	NA	23.8	2.5	21.8
	Q309R	47	F	145/110	5.1	NA	19.5	<1.0	NA
	Q309R	44	M	160/100	NA	NA	NA	NA	NA
	Q309R	18	M	110/70	5.2	NA	23.9	<0.5	NA
	Q309R	15	F	110/80	5.8	NA	20.2	<0.5	NA
	Q309R	12	F	114/76	5.3	NA	22	NA	NA
Present case	S433N	24	F	150/109	6.3	7.286	17.6	0.14	31.0

(median age: 27.6 versus 21.6 and 22.7 years). This evidence indicated that GS should be suspected when young patients present with hyperkalemia, even those who do not present with hypertension and metabolic acidosis.

Most of the previous studies reported that GS patients had suppressed renin activity but low or normal plasma aldosterone concentrations [2, 4, 14–17]. For instance, one of the South Korean cases of GS caused by the same mutation in the present case (S433N) had a suppressed RAAS (plasma renin activity less than 0.10 ng/mL/h and plasma aldosterone 7.1 ng/dL). Similarly, patients with other sites of KLHL3 mutations (such as Q309R, R528H, H498Y, and L387P) had low plasma renin activity and normal or decreased aldosterone levels [2–5]. The possible mechanism may be associated with increased NCC activity, which leads to increased NaCl reabsorption and volume-dependent hypertension, thus inhibiting the RAAS (decreased renin activity and aldosterone levels).

Interestingly, the present case presented with suppressed PRA and slightly increased PAC. Similarly, as shown in the results of the literature review and other published studies, there were also some cases or pedigrees with GS characterized by an elevated PAC, which was mainly caused by WNK4 or CUL3 mutations [18–20]. The possible mechanism could be related to the regulatory effects of hyperkalemia on aldosterone secretion. For example, one case with a WNK4 mutation had a potassium level of 6.4 mmol/L with a corresponding PAC of 50.7 ng/dL, while when serum potassium decreased to 5.4 mmol/L, the corresponding PAC decreased to 13.7 ng/dL [19]. This phenomenon could also be observed in our patient, whose PAC was 31.0 ng/dL when serum potassium was 6.3 mmol/L, which decreased to 15.2 ng/dL when serum potassium decreased to 4.9 mmol/L. In brief, the above evidence suggested that the RAAS among GS patients is characterized by a suppressed PRA but variable PAC that is positively associated with serum potassium level. Moreover, a suppressed PRA will lead to an increased aldosterone/renin ratio (ARR), which, in addition to elevated blood pressure, might result in inappropriate screening for primary aldosteronism.

GS patients respond to low doses of thiazide diuretics by inhibition of the activity of NCC in the distal nephrons. Previous studies have reported that thiazide diuretics could correct the clinical manifestations, including hypertension, hyperkalemia, and metabolic acidosis, in almost all GS patients [7, 8]. The present patient accepted treatment of low-dose hydrochlorothiazide (25 mg/day). Her elevated blood pressure, serum potassium, and metabolic acidosis were corrected five days later and maintained at normal levels at three months of follow-up.

5. Conclusions

This study reported on a case of the Gordon syndrome with a heterozygous mutation (c.1298G > A) in exon 11 of the KLHL3 gene. The patient had typical features of the Gordon syndrome and responded well to low-dose thiazide diuretics. GS patients with KLHL3 gene mutations present with varied clinical manifestations and might be confused with primary aldosteronism.

Abbreviations

GS: Gordon syndrome
PHA II: Pseudohypoaldosteronism type II
FHH: Familial hyperkalemic hypertension
WNK: With-no-lysine kinase
KLHL3: Kelch-like 3
CUL3: Cullin 3
OSR1: Oxidative stress-responsive gene 1
SPAK: STE20/SPS1-related proline-alanine-rich kinase
CRL: Cullin-RING E3 ubiquitin ligase
DCT: Distal convoluted tubules
NCC: Na/Cl cotransporter
ENaC: Epithelial sodium (Na+) channel
ROMK: Renal outer medullary potassium (K+) channel
RAAS: Renin-angiotensin-aldosterone system
PRA: Plasma renin activity
PAC: Plasma aldosterone concentration
AM: Acidic motif.

Consent

Informed consent was obtained from the patient and family members.

Authors' Contributions

TC conceived the study and participated in its design and coordination. YYY collected the clinical information of the participants and drafted the manuscript. YR collected the clinical information of the participants. HMT edited the manuscript. All authors read and approved the final manuscript.

Acknowledgments

This study was supported by grants from a 1.3.5 Project for Disciplines of Excellence, West China Hospital, Sichuan University (ZYGD18022 and 2018HXFH009) and a grant from the Sichuan Provincial Science and Technology Foundation (2019YJ0040).

References

[1] D. H. Ellison, "Pseudohypoaldosteronism type II," in *Gene Reviews*, R. A. Paqon, M. P. Adam, and H. H. Ardinqer, Eds., University of Washington, Seattle, WA, USA, 2017, http://www.genereviews.org.

[2] D. Kelly, M. R. Rodzlan, X. Jeunemaitre, and C. Wall, "A novel mutation in KLHL3 gene causes familial hyperkalemic hypertension," *QJM: An International Journal of Medicine*, vol. 109, no. 7, pp. 487-488, 2016.

[3] M. Mitani, M. Furuichi, S. Narumi et al., "A patient with pseudohypoaldosteronism type II complicated by congenital hypopituitarism carrying a KLHL3 mutation," *Clinical Pediatric Endocrinology*, vol. 25, no. 4, pp. 127–134, 2016.

[4] J. S. Park, E. Park, H. S. Hyun et al., "Three cases of Gordon syndrome with dominant KLHL3 mutations," *Journal of Pediatric Endocrinology and Metabolism*, vol. 30, no. 3, pp. 361–364, 2017.

[5] H. Mayan, V. Carmon, K. Oleinikov et al., "Hypercalciuria in familial hyperkalemia and hypertension with KLHL3 mutations," *Nephron*, vol. 130, no. 1, pp. 59–65, 2015.

[6] O. Kliuk-Ben Bassat, V. Carmon, A. Hanukoglu et al., "Familial hyperkalemia and hypertension (FHHt) and KLHL3: description of a family with a new recessive mutation (S553L) compared to a family with a dominant mutation, Q309R, with analysis of urinary sodium chloride cotransporter," *Nephron*, vol. 137, no. 1, pp. 77–84, 2017.

[7] K. M. O Shaughnessy, "Gordon Syndrome: a continuing story," *Pediatric Nephrology*, vol. 30, no. 11, pp. 1903–1908, 2015.

[8] L. M. Boyden, M. Choi, K. A. Choate et al., "Mutations in kelch-like 3 and cullin 3 cause hypertension and electrolyte abnormalities," *Nature*, vol. 482, no. 7383, pp. 98–102, 2012.

[9] J. K. Healy, "Pseudohypoaldosteronism type II," *Hypertension*, vol. 63, no. 4, pp. 648–654, 2014.

[10] L. Wang and J.-B. Peng, "Phosphorylation of KLHL3 at serine 433 impairs its interaction with the acidic motif of WNK4: a molecular dynamics study," *Protein Science*, vol. 26, no. 2, pp. 163–173, 2017.

[11] E. Sohara and S. Uchida, "Kelch-like 3/Cullin 3 ubiquitin ligase complex and WNK signaling in salt-sensitive hypertension and electrolyte disorder," *Nephrology Dialysis Transplantation*, vol. 31, no. 9, pp. 1417–1424, 2016.

[12] T. Moriguchi, S. Urushiyama, N. Hisamoto et al., "WNK1 regulates phosphorylation of cation-chloride-coupled cotransporters via the STE20-related kinases, SPAK and OSR1," *Journal of Biological Chemistry*, vol. 280, no. 52, pp. 42685–42693, 2005.

[13] M. Guzman-Limon and J. Samuels, "Pediatric hypertension," *Pediatric Clinics of North America*, vol. 66, no. 1, pp. 45–57, 2019.

[14] L. Shao, L. Cui, J. Lu, Y. Lang, I. Bottillo, and X. Zhao, "A novel mutation in exon 9 of Cullin 3 gene contributes to aberrant splicing in pseudohypoaldosteronism type II," *FEBS Open Bio*, vol. 8, no. 3, pp. 461–469, 2018.

[15] H. Gong, Z. Tang, Y. Yang et al., "A patient with pseudohypoaldosteronism type II caused by a novel mutation in WNK4 gene," *Endocrine*, vol. 33, no. 3, pp. 230–234, 2008.

[16] S. Tsuji, M. Yamashita, G. Unishi et al., "A young child with pseudohypoaldosteronism type II by a mutation of Cullin 3," *BMC Nephrology*, vol. 14, p. 166, 2013.

[17] A. M. Brooks, M. Owens, J. A. Sayer, M. Salzmann, S. Ellard, and B. Vaidya, "Pseudohypoaldosteronism type 2 presenting with hypertension and hyperkalaemia due to a novel mutation in the WNK4 gene," *QJM: An International Journal of Medicine*, vol. 105, no. 8, pp. 791–794, 2012.

[18] Q. Wang, B.-Y. Cao, C. Su, W.-J. Li, and C.-X. Gong, "Pseudohypoaldosteronism type II caused by CUL3 mutation

presented with visual impairment," *Chinese Medical Journal*, vol. 131, no. 15, pp. 1879–1881, 2018.

[19] T. Sakoh, A. Sekine, T. Mori et al., "A familial case of pseudohypoaldosteronism type II (PHA2) with a novel mutation (D564N) in the acidic motif in WNK4," *Molecular Genetics & Genomic Medicine*, vol. 7, no. 6, p. e705, 2019.

[20] H. Mayan, G. Munter, M. Shaharabany et al., "Hypercalciuria in familial hyperkalemia and hypertension accompanies hyperkalemia and precedes hypertension: description of a large family with the Q565E WNK4 mutation," *The Journal of Clinical Endocrinology & Metabolism*, vol. 89, no. 8, pp. 4025–4030, 2004.

5

Association of Central Precocious Puberty with a Rare Presentation of Schimmelpenning–Feuerstein–Mims Syndrome in a Peruvian Girl

Miguel Angel De los Santos-La Torre,[1] Carlos Manuel Del Águila-Villar,[1,2] Luis Rómulo Lu-de Lama,[1] Oswaldo Nuñez-Almache,[1,2] Eliana Manuela Chávez-Tejada,[1] Oscar Antonio Espinoza-Robles,[1] Paola Marianella Pinto-Ibárcena,[1] and Martha Rosario Calagua-Quispe[1]

[1]*Department of Endocrinology and Metabolism, The Child's Health National Institute (Instituto Nacional de Salud del Niño), Lima, Peru*
[2]*Faculty Member of the Medical School, Universidad Nacional Federico Villareal, Lima, Peru*

Correspondence should be addressed to Miguel Angel De los Santos-La Torre; mdlslt1983@yahoo.com

Academic Editor: Wayne V. Moore

Schimmelpenning–Feuerstein–Mims syndrome (SFM), an epidermal nevus syndrome characterized by skin lesions, has an estimated incidence of 1 per 10 000 live births. Nevus sebaceous, the most common cutaneous lesion, and verrucous nevus, the less frequent lesion, are coupled with a wide range of extracutaneous manifestations. As part of these manifestations, rarely, central precocious puberty can arise. We report the case of a 1-year-5-month-old girl who presented to the Endocrinology and Metabolism Department with breast enlargement that began at one year of age, growth of pubic and axillary hair three months later, and vaginal bleeding that occurred five months later. During clinical examination, melanocytic nevi, with a diameter ranging from 3 to 5 mm, were noted on the face. Verrucous nevi of variable size with a tendency for coalescence following the lines of Blaschko and melanocytic nevi with a diameter ranging from 3 to 6 mm were observed on the right hemibody and on the left hemibody, respectively. Right asymmetry of the lower extremities was observed. Laboratory findings showed a significant increase in the levels of follicle-stimulating hormone (FSH) and luteinizing hormone (LH) after the gonadotropin-releasing hormone (GnRH) stimulation test; additionally, imaging demonstrated advanced bone age and pubertal changes in the internal genitals. Analyses of the H-RAS, K-RAS, and N-RAS genes in the blood and in the skin were performed, and a missense mutation in exon 2 of the gene, H-RAS c37G > C (p.G13R), was detected in the latter. Treatment with triptorelin, a GnRH analog, was initiated, and it gave good clinical response. Epidermal nevus syndrome has a wide and variable systemic involvement. Thus, it is important to consider the development of precocious puberty for a prompt diagnosis and to strategize a multidisciplinary approach from the beginning.

1. Introduction

Schimmelpenning–Feuerstein–Mims (SFM) syndrome, an epidermal nevus syndrome characterized by skin lesions, has an estimated incidence of 1 per 10 000 live births [1]. Nevus sebaceous, the most common cutaneous lesion, and verrucous nevus, the less frequent lesion, occur in conjunction with several organic and systemic anomalies such as neurological, skeletal, cardiovascular, ophthalmic, and urologic disorders [2–4]. As part of these, endocrine abnormalities, such as hypophosphatemic vitamin D resistant rickets, syndrome of inappropriate antidiuretic hormone (SIADH), and more rarely central precocious puberty (CPP), are manifested; however, very few cases have been reported so far [5, 6].

The syndrome was first described by Josef Jadassohn in 1895 [5, 7]. Several years later, Gustav Wilhelm Schimmelpenning, in 1957, described the main clinical features of the syndrome in a 17-year-old adolescent and proposed it is a new phacomatosis [2]. Later, Richard C. Feuerstein and Leroy C. Mims described two cases of linear epidemic nevus with seizures and mental retardation in 1962, while Laurence Solomon, in 1968, made important contributions in expanding the characterization of the dermal component [2].

SFM syndrome is one of nine different types of epidermal nevus syndromes [7]. It has a sporadic presentation, and so far, familial cases with SFM syndrome have not been reported. Furthermore, a discordance between monochorionic twins, where one twin has the syndrome and the other is completely healthy, has been reported in both males and females [8]. The cause of the syndrome is still unknown, although Happle's hypothesis is the one that has gained the most acceptance. According to Happle, SFM syndrome would result from a genomic mosaicism where the mutated cell, as a result of a postzygotic mutation in early embryogenesis, survives only in close proximity to healthy cells. Current reports reveal that such a mutation would occur in any of the following three genes: H-RAS [9–11], K-RAS [9], and N-RAS [12]. The distribution of the skin lesions following the Blaschko lines (lines on the skin that represent the pattern of growth and development during epidermal cell migration), an important feature of the syndrome, could be explained by this hypothesis [13, 14].

The first association of SFM syndrome with CPP was described by Moss et al. in a 2-year-4 month-old boy with extensive verrucous nevi and secondary sexual characteristics [15]. Other cases with CPP have also been identified in Hong Kong [16], the United States [17, 18], Germany [19], Iran [20], and India [21]. It has been proposed that extensive verrucous nevi release factors that would lead to a premature activation of the gonadotropic axis in these patients [18, 21].

Herein, we report a case of CPP and an atypical presentation of SFM syndrome in a girl. This is the first Peruvian case and the eighth case overall, showing an association between CPP and SFM syndrome. Written informed consent was obtained for the photographs presented in this case report.

2. Case Presentation

A 1-year-5-month-old girl presented to the Endocrinology and Metabolism Department with breast enlargement that began at one year of age, pubic hair and axillary hair that appeared 3 months later, and vaginal bleeding that occurred 5 months after the onset of breast development. She was the first-born child, born at 40 weeks, weighing 3.540 kg, and a length of 51 cm. Since birth, melanocytic and verrucous nevi were noted over her face, trunk, and extremities. Her psychomotor development was normal. There was no consanguinity between the parents.

On physical examination, the child's weight and head circumference were at the 75th percentile for her age. Her length was at the 90th percentile. Skin examination revealed melanocytic nevi with a diameter ranging from 3 to 5 mm on the face (Figure 1). Verrucous nevi of variable size with a tendency for coalescence following the lines of Blaschko, stopping at the midline, were observed on the right hemibody. Furthermore, melanocytic nevi, with a diameter ranging from 3 to 6 mm, were observed on the left hemibody (Figures 2–4). According to thc Tanner stage pubertal development, the patient had breast stage IV, pubic hair stage III, and axillary hair Wolfsdorf stage II. Right asymmetry of the lower extremities was noted during the examination.

Pelvic ultrasound revealed the following: uterine size and volume, 3.75 cm × 2.4 × 1.4 cm and 6 mL, respectively; endometrium size, 5 mm; right ovarian volume, 2.8 mL; left ovarian volume, 3.3 mL; and ovarian follicles with diameter >5 mm. Bone age was 4.0 years old. Laboratory values showed a significant increase in the levels of follicle-stimulating hormone (FSH) and luteinizing hormone (LH) after the GnRH stimulation test. The results are as follows: basal LH: 3.3 IU/L and 60 min LH: 72.1 IUI/L; basal FSH: 3.9 IU/L and 60 min FSH: 18.8 IU/L. Skin biopsy, from the right hemibody lesions, showed histological features of papillomatosis, acanthosis, and hyperkeratosis, which were consistent with verrucous epidermal nevus (Figure 5). Laboratory investigation demonstrated normal levels of serum calcium, phosphorus, urinary phosphate, electrolytes, parathyroid hormone (PTH), and vitamin D. Renal and adrenal ultrasound, skeletal survey, and brain MRI showed no abnormalities.

Analyses of the H-RAS, K-RAS, and N-RAS genes in the blood and in the skin were performed, and in the latter, a missense mutation in exon 2 of the gene, H-RAS c37G > C (p.G13R), was detected. The DNA was extracted and purified using DNA binding columns (Qiagen). DNA integrity and quality were evaluated with spectrophotometry. The presence of mutations in the three genes was evaluated by the selective amplification of each gene using PCR. For sequencing, the ABI PRISM® 377 DNA fluorescent sequencer was used.

Based on these findings, a monthly treatment with long-acting GnRH analog (triptorelin) was initiated. After two months, secondary sexual characteristics reverted (Figure 2), and a decrease in the uterine and ovarian volume and suppression of the gonadotropins were observed; the bone age also stabilized.

3. Discussion

SFM syndrome associates sebaceous nevus with the involvement of other organs and systems [7]. The other form of nevus that can manifest is the keratinocytic or verrucous nevi [2]. The common anomalies in the different systems are neurological (66%), followed by ophthalmological (59%), skeletal (50%), cardiac (12%), urologic (10%), and endocrinal (<5%) [5]. This case is an atypical one because it presents with verrucous nevi instead of sebaceous nevi. Another frequent characteristic that we could appreciate in the measurement of lower limbs is a hypertrophy of bones of the right half body, ipsilateral to the verrucous nevus, as described in the scientific literature [2]. Another

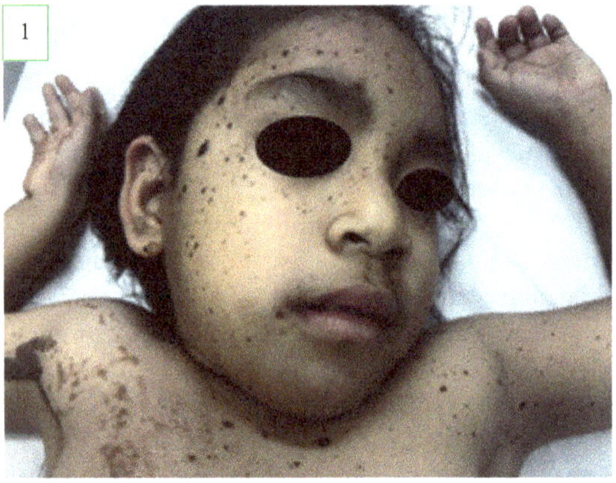

FIGURE 1: Skin patterns of the melanocytic and verrucous nevi on the face and the upper trunk

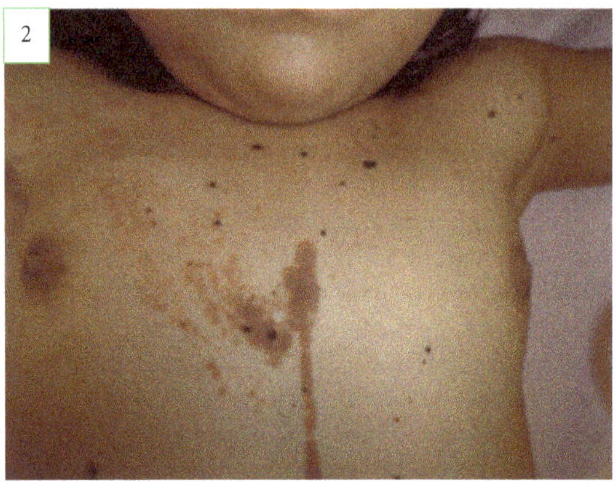

FIGURE 2: Breast development.

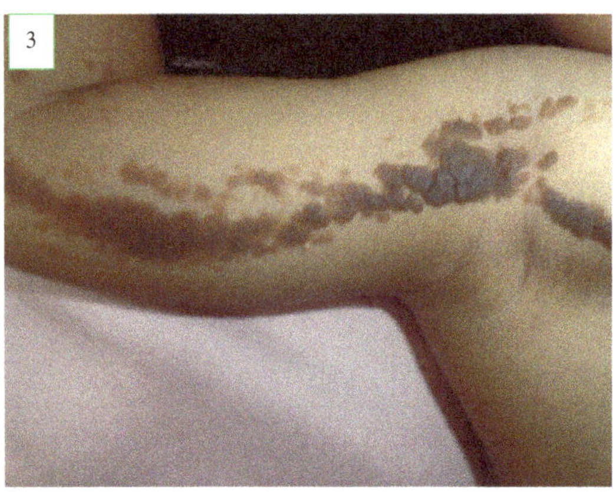

FIGURE 3: Skin patterns of the melanocytic and verrucous nevi.

accompanying extracutaneous manifestation is CPP, the suspicion of which was the reason for the endocrine consultation, without evidence of other hormonal abnormalities, such as hypophosphatemic vitamin D-resistant rickets [18, 19]; normal skeletal survey findings; normal levels of calcium, phosphorus, PTH, and vitamin D; and SIADH with normal level of electrolytes and adequate urination.

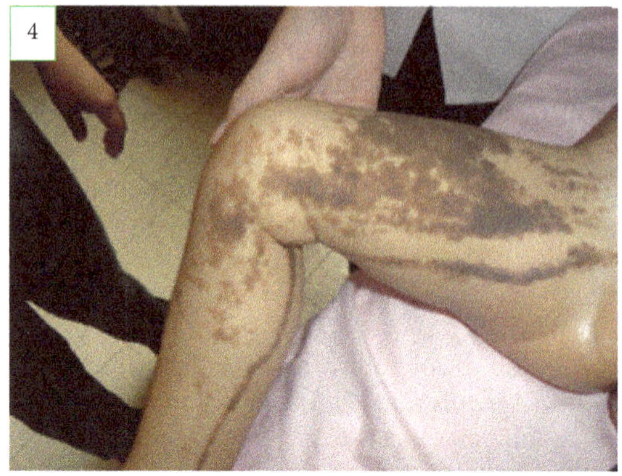

FIGURE 4: Skin patterns of the verrucous nevi on the right lower extremity

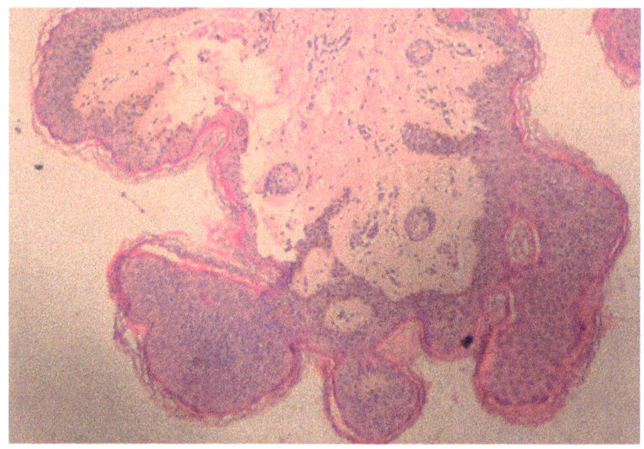

FIGURE 5: Skin biopsy: histological features of right skin lesions showed papillomatosis, acanthosis, and hyperkeratosis, which were consistent with verrucous epidermal nevus.

Mutations in the H-RAS, K-RAS, and N-RAS genes have been described previously in patients with SFM syndrome. Groesser et al. analyzed 65 sebaceous nevi and found a mutation in the H-RAS gene in 95% of the cases and the K-RAS gene in 5% of the cases; mosaicism involving H-RAS c.37G > C and K-RAS c.35G > A has also been described in two patients with SFM syndrome [9]. In our patient, genetic studies revealed a missense mutation in exon 2 of the gene, H-RAS c37G > C (p.G13R), in the skin biopsy sample; however, no mutation was detected in the blood, which confirms the occurrence of somatic mosaicism, probably as a result of a postzygotic mutation. This mutation, p.G13R, was previously described by Hafner et al. in 21 of 24 verrucous nevi with H-RAS gene involvement, reporting it as the most common mutation in a series of 72 verrucous nevi, and the H-RAS (39%) was the most affected of the three RAS genes [10]. This mutation leads to a constitutive activation of MAPK and PI3K-Akt cell signaling pathways, which translates into a higher rate of cell proliferation favoring the development of complex hamartomas in the skin and other organs [9, 11, 13].

There are few reports of SFM syndrome associated with CPP. The first association was reported by Moss et al. [15], in

1991, in a 2-year-4-month-old boy with extensive verrucous nevi and secondary sexual characteristics. The timing of diagnosis and start of treatment was similar to those of our patient; however, the management differed where the treatment in the patient described by Moss et al. involved cyproterone acetate 50–100 mg/day for 3 years; however, when an arrest in the progression of puberty was not evidenced, administration of a long-acting GnRH analog was initiated. This is probably because the GnRH analogs were not commonly used at the time of Moss's case. In our patient, triptorelin was initiated from the time of diagnosis. Similarly, Garg et al. [21] identified a 3-year-old boy with penile growth, pubic hair, increased testicular volume, and advanced bone age, with hyperpigmented verrucous plaques from 3 months of age. He was treated with monthly administration of leuprolide acetate, which is another type of GnRH analog, and a good clinical response was achieved.

Precocious puberty in our patient is due to a premature activation of the hypothalamic-pituitary-gonadal axis. This is confirmed by the hormonal profile, which revealed the levels of the LH and FSH to be in the pubertal range after the GnRH stimulation test. This was supported by advanced bone age and a uterine length and ovarian volume higher than expected for her age on the pelvic ultrasound. In this regard, Ivker et al. [18] hypothesized extensive verrucous nevi release factors that would induce puberty. It is also reasonable to assume that some time is needed for these factors to reach critical concentrations sufficient enough to stimulate the hypothalamic-pituitary axis and lead to the development of secondary sexual characteristics. It is important to perform brain MRI, particularly in cases where the H-RAS gene mutation is present, to rule out hamartomas or other CNS tumors [21]. No type of tumor was evident in our patient.

This case report highlights a fundamental characteristic of epidermal nevus syndromes that have a highly variable systemic involvement. Furthermore, it is important to remember that CPP can develop. Hence, it must be recognized promptly for optimal management, and a multidisciplinary approach must be strategized from the beginning.

Acknowledgments

The authors would like to acknowledge Marco López-Ilasaca MD and his biological molecular team for their invaluable support with the genetic studies performed for this patient.

References

[1] Linear Nevus Sebaceous Syndrome Orphanet, 2018, https://bit.ly/2SZqGlm.

[2] I. Pascual-Castroviejo and M. Ruggieri, "Schimmelpenning–Feuerstein–Mims syndrome," in *Neurocutaneous Disorders, Phakomatoses and Hamartoneoplastic Syndromes*, M. Ruggieri, I. Pascual-Castroviejo, and C. D. Rocco, Eds., Springer-Verlag/Wien, Berlin, Germany, pp. 559–573, 2008.

[3] J. Garcias-Ladaria, M. C. Rosón, and M. Pascual-López, "Nevus epidérmicos y síndromes relacionados. Parte 2: nevus derivados de estructuras anexiales," *Actas Dermo-Sifiliográficas*, vol. 109, no. 8, pp. 687–698, 2018.

[4] C. P. Lena, R. N. Kondo, and T. Nicolacópulos, "Do you know this syndrome? Schimmelpenning–Feuerstein–Mims syndrome," *Anais Brasileiros de Dermatologia*, vol. 94, no. 2, pp. 227–229, 2019.

[5] A. Asch and J. Sugarman, "Epidermal nevus syndrome," in *Handbook of Clinical Neurology-Neurocutaneous Syndromes*, M. Islam and E. Roach, Eds., pp. 293–315, Elsevier, Amsterdam, Netherland, 3rd edition, 2015.

[6] E. Alzarnougi and A. E. A. Agha, "Hypophosphatemic rickets, epidermal nevus syndrome with skeletal changes: a case report," *International Journal of Advanced Research*, vol. 5, no. 8, pp. 982–987, 2017.

[7] S.-M. Wang, Y.-J. Hsieh, K.-M. Chang, H.-L. Tsai, and C.-P. Chen, "Schimmelpenning syndrome: a case report and literature review," *Pediatrics and Neonatology*, vol. 55, no. 6, pp. 487–490, 2014.

[8] E. G. J. Rijntjes-Jacobs, E. Lopriore, S. J. Steggerda, S. G. Kant, and F. J. Walther, "Discordance for Schimmelpenning–Feuerstein–Mims syndrome in monochorionic twins supports the concept of a postzygotic mutation," *American Journal of Medical Genetics Part A*, vol. 152, no. 11, pp. 2816–2819, 2010.

[9] L. Groesser, E. Herschberger, A. Ruetten et al., "Postzygotic HRAS and KRAS mutations cause nevus sebaceous and Schimmelpenning syndrome," *Nature Genetics*, vol. 44, no. 7, pp. 783–787, 2012.

[10] C. Hafner, A. Toll, S. Gantner et al., "Keratinocytic epidermal nevi are associated with mosaic RAS mutations," *Journal of Medical Genetics*, vol. 49, no. 4, pp. 249–253, 2012.

[11] R. J. Martin, M. Arefi, M. Splitt, L. Redford, C. Moss, and N. Rajan, "Phacomatosis pigmentokeratotica and precocious puberty associated with HRAS mutation," *British Journal of Dermatology*, vol. 178, no. 1, pp. 289–291, 2018.

[12] Y. Kuroda, I. Ohashi, Y. Enomoto et al., "A postzygotic NRAS mutation in a patient with Schimmelpenning syndrome," *American Journal of Medical Genetics Part A*, vol. 167, no. 9, pp. 2223–2225, 2015.

[13] S. Asch and J. L. Sugarman, "Epidermal nevus syndromes: new insights into whorls and swirls," *Pediatric Dermatology*, vol. 35, no. 1, pp. 21–29, 2018.

[14] A. I. R. Bandera, M. F. Rodríguez, K. Vorlicka, and R. D. L. Laguna, "Líneas de Blaschko y otros mosaicismos cutáneos," *Piel*, vol. 28, no. 8, pp. 457–468, 2013.

[15] C. Moss, J. M. Parkin, and J. S. Comaish, "Precocious puberty in a boy with a widespread linear epidermal naevus," *British Journal of Dermatology*, vol. 125, no. 2, pp. 178–182, 1991.

[16] A. C. M. Yu, V. Ng, C. Dicks-Mireaux, and D. B. Grant, "Epidermal naevus syndrome associated with polyostotic fibrous dysplasia and central precocious puberty," *European Journal of Pediatrics*, vol. 154, no. 2, pp. 102–104, 1995.

[17] Y.-K. Tay, W. L. Weston, C. A. Ganong, and G. J. Klingensmith, "Epidermal nevus syndrome: association with central precocious puberty and woolly hair nevus," *Journal of the American Academy of Dermatology*, vol. 35, no. 5, pp. 839–842, 1996.

[18] R. Ivker, S. D. Resnick, and R. A. Skidmore, "Hypophosphatemic vitamin D-resistant rickets, precocious

puberty, and the epidermal nevus syndrome," *Archives of Dermatology*, vol. 133, no. 12, pp. 1557–1561, 1997.

[19] M. Zutt, F. Strutz, R. Happle et al., "Schimmelpenning–Feuerstein–Mims syndrome with hypophosphatemic rickets," *Dermatology*, vol. 207, no. 1, pp. 72–76, 2003.

[20] E. Shahgholi, M. Mollaian, Z. Haghshenas, and M. Honarmand, "Congenital rhabdomyosarcoma, central precocious puberty, hemihypertrophy and hypophosphatemic rickets associated with epidermal nevus syndrome," *Journal of Pediatric Endocrinology and Metabolism*, vol. 24, no. 11-12, pp. 1063–1066, 2011.

[21] T. Garg, R. Chander, N. Gaur, and K. Sahni, "Precocious puberty in a 3-year-old child with systematized verrucous epidermal nevus," *Indian Journal of Dermatology, Venereology, and Leprology*, vol. 81, no. 2, pp. 197-198, 2015.

6

Two Cases of Pituitary Stalk Interruption Syndrome in Syrian Children

Ibrahim Alali,[1] **Reem Saad**,[2] **and Younes Kabalan**[1]

[1]*Al-Assad University Hospital, Damascus University, Damascus, Syria*
[2]*Al-Mowassat University Hospital, Damascus University, Damascus, Syria*

Correspondence should be addressed to Ibrahim Alali; ibali2012@gmail.com

Academic Editor: J. Paul Frindik

Pituitary stalk interruption syndrome (PSIS) is an extremely rare cause of growth failure and delayed puberty. It can be diagnosed by magnetic resonance imaging (MRI) of the hypothalamus and pituitary gland, showing an ectopic or absent posterior pituitary, an absent or interrupted pituitary stalk, or small anterior pituitary, in combination with growth hormone or other pituitary hormone deficiencies. The exact etiology of PSIS is unknown. In this article, we describe two cases of PSIS in Syria which are, as far as we know, the first published cases.

1. Introduction

Growth failure is one of the most common reasons for referral to the endocrine clinic. Although the most frequent causes of short stature are constitutional and genetic, endocrine disorders, especially growth hormone (GH) deficiency, should always be considered [1]. Pituitary stalk interruption syndrome (PSIS, ORPHA 95496) is an extremely rare disorder, but its exact prevalence is still unknown [2]. This syndrome is a congenital anomaly of the pituitary gland characterized by GH deficiency (with or without other pituitary hormone deficiencies) along with radiological features of a thin or interrupted pituitary stalk, an ectopic or absent posterior pituitary, or a hypoplastic or absent anterior pituitary [3, 4].

In this article, we describe two cases of PSIS that were diagnosed in boys at different ages from Syria.

2. Case 1

A 7-year-old boy was referred to the endocrine clinic for short stature. He was born at full term without complications. His birth weight was 3 kg, and his family history was unremarkable. During childhood, he had all his vaccinations and had not been hospitalized.

On examination, he seemed well without any abnormal facial features, and he was 19 kg in weight and 101 cm in height (body mass index (BMI) 18.62 kg/m^2). Compared to his midparental predicted length (119 cm), he was 3.6 standard deviation (SD) points below expected. Heart and breath sounds were normal and so was the abdominal examination. Testicular volume was 3 ml each, measured by using a Prader orchidometer. Pubic hair distribution and penile size (3 by 1 cm) were both consistent with Tanner stage 1.

Routine blood panel and urine and stool tests were within normal range, except for mild anemia (Table 1). Plain films of the left wrist were ordered and were compatible with a bone age of a three-year-old (>2 SD below chronological age), as shown in Figure 1. A GH stimulation test conducted with 75 μcg of clonidine was consistent with GH deficiency. Other pituitary hormones were also evaluated and revealed central hypothyroidism and adrenal insufficiency (Table 2). Pituitary MRI was also performed to evaluate for anatomical abnormalities and revealed an ectopic posterior pituitary lobe along with an absent pituitary stalk (Figures 2(a) and 2(b)),

TABLE 1: Results of the complete blood count and basic metabolic panel for both patients.

Test	Normal value	First case	Second case
WBC (per mm^3)	$4.5–10.5 \times 10^3$	5.2	7.2
Hb (g/dL)	11.5–13.5	10.2	13
PLT (per mm^3)	$150–450 \times 10^3$	343	225
Creatinine (mg/dL)	0.6–1.3	0.7	0.7
Glucose (mg/dL)	60–99	71	95
ALP (U/L)	Up to 936	153	759
ALT (U/L)	Up to 41	32	—
Anti-tTG IgA (μU/mL)	<10	5.3	0.2
Total IgA (mg/dL)	61–348	—	99
Calcium (mg/dL)	8–10.5	8.3	10.4
Phosphorus (mg/dL)	2.5–5.3	4.8	5.3
Urine analysis	—	Normal	Normal
Stool analysis	—	Normal	Normal

WBC, white blood cells; Hb, hemoglobin; PLT, platelets; ALP, alkaline phosphatase; ALT, alanine aminotransferase; tTG, tissue transglutaminase; IgA, immunoglobulin type A.

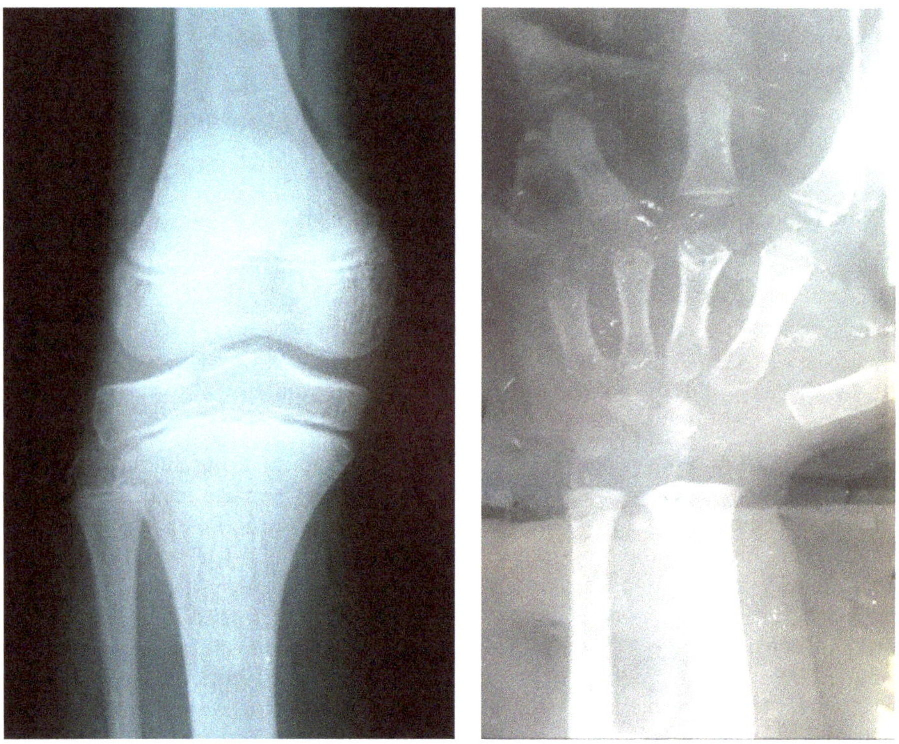

(a) (b)

FIGURE 1: (a) The left hand and wrist bones of the first patient which is consistent with a bone age of 3 years. (b) Posterior-anterior image of the left knee of the second patient reveals the open epiphysis of the growth plate.

confirming the diagnosis of pituitary stalk interruption syndrome (PSIS).

3. Case 2

A 17-year-old boy presented to the endocrine clinic for short stature as well as absence of secondary sexual characteristics.

He was born full term in a breech position without complications and had a birth weight of 2.3 kg. No hypoglycemia or other complications were reported during childhood. On examination, he had no abnormal facial features and looked well. He weighed 43 kg and was 150 cm in height (BMI 19.11 kg/m^2). Compared to his midparental predicted length (169 cm), he was 3 SD points below expected. Auscultation of the heart and lungs did not reveal any abnormalities. Abdominal exam was normal. Testicular volume was 4 ml each, measured by using a Prader orchidometer. Pubic hair was consistent with Tanner stage 1. Penile size was 2 by 1 cm, consistent with micropenis. No gynecomastia was noted.

Routine blood panel and urine and stool tests were normal (Table 1). A plain film X-ray of the left wrist was

TABLE 2: Results of hormonal evaluation for both cases along with reference range.

Hormone	Normal value	First case	Second case
TSH (μU/mL)	0.3–4.8	3.8	3.5
Free T4 (ng/dL)	0.8–1.8	0.557	0.668
IGF1 (ng/mL)	247–481	—	64.1
Basal GH (ng/mL)	—	0.506	<0.05
GH after 30 m	Any test more than 10	0.513	<0.05
GH after 60 m		0.540	<0.05
GH after 90 m		0.723	<0.05
GH after 120 m		0.719	<0.05
Testosterone (ng/mL)	2–9	—	1.98
LH (mU/L)	2–12	—	1.43
FSH (mU/L)	1.5–12.4	—	<1
8 AM cortisol (μg/dL)	5–25	3.74	3.9
ACTH (pg/mL)	7.2–63	—	24.52
Prolactin (ng/mL)	2–18	—	18.9

TSH, thyroid-stimulating hormone; LH, luteinizing hormone; FSH, follicle-stimulating hormone; ACTH, adrenocorticotrophic hormone

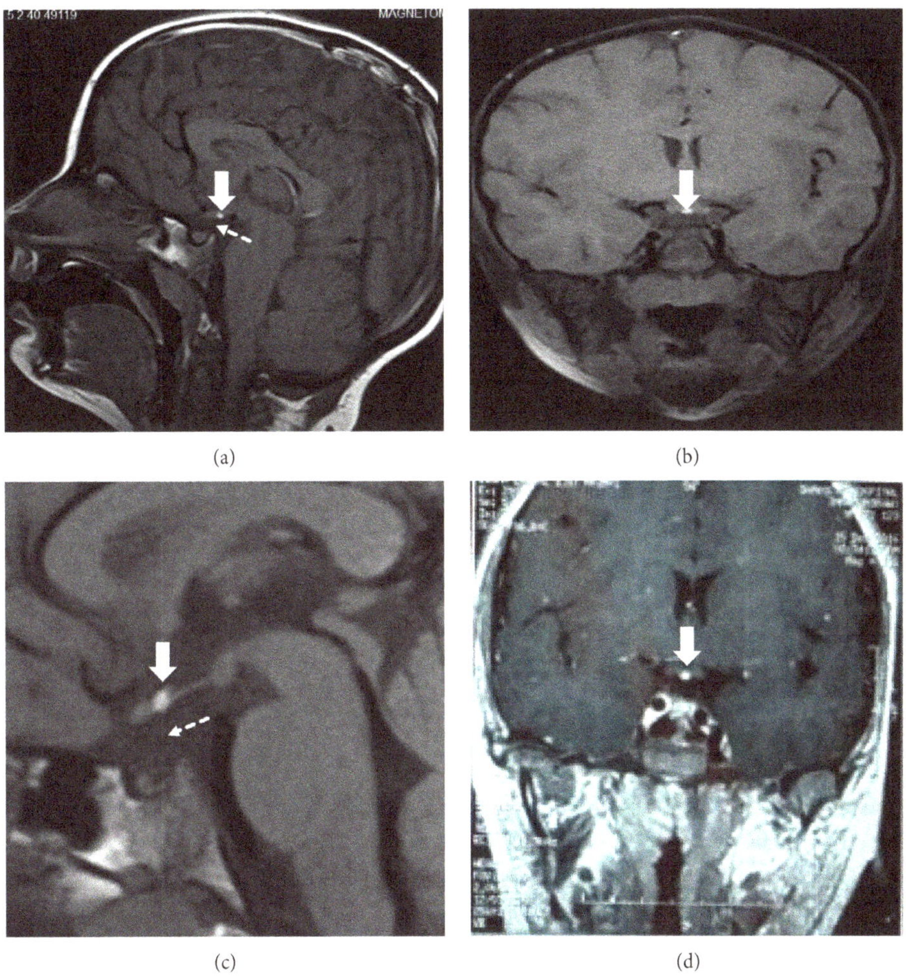

FIGURE 2: (a) The first patient's sagittal MR image without contrast for the pituitary; the solid arrowhead points to the posterior pituitary lobe (bright spot), while the dashed arrowhead points to the supposed pituitary stalk which is absent. (b) Coronal image without contrast for the first case shows the ectopic bright spot close to the optic chiasm. (c) Noncontrast sagittal view for the pituitary in the second case where the solid arrow points to the ectopic bright spot and the dashed arrowhead points to the absence of pituitary stalk. (d) Contrast coronal image for the second case.

consistent with a bone age of 13 years. Plain film X-ray of the knee showed open epiphyseal plates (Figure 1). Insulin-like growth factor 1 (IGF1) was low. Gonadal hormone assessment and GH stimulation test, conducted with 150 μcg clonidine after sex hormone priming with 100 mg IM testosterone, showed GH deficiency as well as hypogonadotropic hypogonadism (Table 2). Other pituitary hormones were also evaluated and revealed central hypothyroidism and adrenal insufficiency. Pituitary MRI was performed (Figures 2(c) and 2(d)) and again confirmed the diagnosis of pituitary stalk interruption syndrome (PSIS).

Results of echocardiography, kidney ultrasound, and ophthalmic evaluation were normal for both patients.

4. Patients Follow-Up

Our first patient was treated with hydrocortisone 15 mg daily and then levothyroxine 50 μcg daily, followed by recombinant GH 1.7 IU SC daily. Within three months, he became euthyroid and gained 3 kg weight and 3 cm height.

Our second patient was treated with hydrocortisone 15 mg daily, levothyroxine 75 mcg daily, and testosterone 100 mg monthly. He was later referred to a specialized center for recombinant GH replacement.

5. Discussion

Pituitary stalk interruption syndrome (PSIS) was initially described and defined by Fujisawa et al. in 1987 [3]. PSIS is diagnosed primarily based on the radiologic findings mentioned above along with permanent GH deficiency and one or more other pituitary hormone deficiencies [2, 3].

The exact prevalence of this syndrome remains unknown. Less than 1000 cases were reported in the literature until 2010 [2]. Its prevalence as a cause of GH deficiency is estimated to be around 4% [5]. The age at diagnosis differs according to the severity of the hormone deficiency. When PSIS presents at birth, hypoglycemia and failure to thrive are the most common symptoms. In childhood, growth retardation is usually the presenting complaint, whereas delayed puberty is usually the chief complaint when it manifests in adolescence and early adulthood [4, 6]. Although these two patients had multiple hormone deficiencies, diagnosis was established relatively later in life.

Breech delivery, cesarean section, and neonatal hypoxemia were suggested as potential causes of this syndrome [7]. However, many case series found an antenatal origin [4, 8, 9]. Genetic mutations were also detected in familial cases, such as HESX1, LHX4, SOX3, PROKR2, and OTX2 genes. Of note, genetic mutations are thought to contribute to less than 5% of PSIS cases [4, 8]. Zwaveling-Soonawala et al. found additional suggested genes for isolated PSIS (DCHS1, ROBO2, CCDC88C, and KIF14) and one for syndromic PSIS (KAT6A). Presence of many probable pathogenic genes and heritage from normal parents are implicative of polygenic etiology of sporadic cases of PSIS [10]. Similar findings were found in Guo et al.'s study in which a group of gene mutations was identified in 92% of the patients and genes NCOR2, ZIC2, and NKD2 were found to be mostly associated with Notch, Shh, and Wnt signaling pathways, respectively [11].

While our second patient had a breech delivery, our first patient underwent uncomplicated vaginal delivery and had a negative family history. The presence of multiple hormone deficiency suggests a genetic etiology. However, due to lack of availability of genetic testing assays in our country, this was not performed.

In most published series [3, 4, 8–13], PSIS exhibited a male predominance, similar to what is observed in our cases. The underlying reason behind this phenomenon is unknown, though there is a selection bias in such patients since boys, more than girls, are brought by parents for growth assessment.

TSH deficiency was the most common deficit (79.5%) alongside GH deficiency in PSIS patients, and ACTH deficiency also was common (67.5%), followed by FSH/LH deficiency in 65.1% of patients [4].

Our two cases had GH, TSH, and ACTH deficiency. LH/FSH deficiency may be detected in minipuberty or discovered later in peripuberty. Therefore, gonadal assessment should be conducted regularly in patients with PSIS [14]. While hypogonadism was detected only in the second case, gonadal axis was not assessed in the first patient given his young age.

The incidence of extrapituitary manifestations in PSIS is high [8]. Midline defects affect mainly the brain and eyes. Extracerebral abnormalities also include defects of the heart, skin, and extremities, which highlights the importance of regular examinations and cardiac, ophthalmologic, and cerebral screening [5].

The lifelong prognosis depends on the time of diagnosis and early treatment of hormonal deficiency [8].

Close monitoring of a child's growth over time helps in early detection of growth failure and early treatment of the underlying causes. Rare etiologies such as PSIS should be kept in mind especially in multiple hormonal deficiencies, as it carries good long-term prognosis if diagnosed early on and treated adequately.

Finally, these two cases are, as far as we know, the first published cases from Syria.

Consent

Informed consent was obtained from the patients' parents.

References

[1] N. Cakan and D. Kamat, "Short stature in children: a practical approach for primary care providers," *Clinical Pediatrics*, vol. 46, no. 5, pp. 379–385, 2007.

[2] Pituitary stalk interruption syndrome," *Orphanet*, 2010, https://www.orpha.net/consor/cgi-bin/OC_Exp.php?lng=en&Expert=95496.

[3] I. Fujisawa, K. Kikuchi, K. Nishimura et al., "Transection of the pituitary stalk: development of an ectopic posterior lobe assessed with MR imaging," *Radiology*, vol. 165, no. 2, pp. 487–489, 1987.

[4] R. Reynaud, F. Albarel, A. Saveanu et al., "Pituitary stalk interruption syndrome in 83 patients: novel HESX1 mutation and severe hormonal prognosis in malformative forms," *European Journal of Endocrinology*, vol. 164, no. 4, pp. 457–465, 2011.

[5] J. Vergier, F. Castinetti, A. Saveanu, N. Girard, T. Brue, and R. Reynaud, "Diagnosis of endocrine disease: pituitary stalk interruption syndrome: etiology and clinical manifestations," *European Journal of Endocrinology*, vol. 181, no. 5, pp. R199–R209, 2019.
[6] S. K. Gosi, S. Kanduri, and V. V. Garla, "Pituitary stalk interruption syndrome," *BMJ Case Reports*, vol. 12, no. 4, Article ID e230133, 2019.
[7] M. Maghnie, D. Larizza, F. Triulzi, P. Sampaolo, G. Scotti, and F. Seven, "Hypopituitarism and stalk agenesis: a congenital syndrome worsened by breech delivery?" *Hormone Research*, vol. 35, no. 3-4, pp. 104–108, 1991.
[8] C. Bar, C. Zadro, G. Diene et al., "Pituitary stalk interruption syndrome from infancy to adulthood: clinical, hormonal, and radiological assessment according to the initial presentation," *PLoS One*, vol. 10, no. 11, Article ID e0142354, 2015.
[9] M. Tauber, J. Chevrel, G. Diene et al., "Long-term evolution of endocrine disorders and effect of GH therapy in 35 patients with pituitary stalk interruption syndrome," *Hormone Research in Paediatrics*, vol. 64, no. 6, pp. 266–273, 2005.
[10] N. Zwaveling-Soonawala, M. Alders, A. Jongejan et al., "Clues for polygenic inheritance of pituitary stalk interruption syndrome from exome sequencing in 20 patients," *The Journal of Clinical Endocrinology & Metabolism*, vol. 103, no. 2, pp. 415–428, 2018.
[11] Q.-H. Guo, C.-Z. Wang, Z.-Q. Wu et al., "Multi-genic pattern found in rare type of hypopituitarism: a whole-exome sequencing study of Han Chinese with pituitary stalk interruption syndrome," *Journal of Cellular and Molecular Medicine*, vol. 21, no. 12, pp. 3626–3632, 2017.
[12] G. Pinto, I. Netchine, M. L. Sobrier, F. Brunelle, J. C. Souberbielle, and R. Brauner, "Pituitary stalk interruption syndrome: a clinical-biological-genetic assessment of its pathogenesis," *Journal of Clinical Endocrinology & Metabolism*, vol. 82, no. 10, pp. 3450–3454, 1997.
[13] M. Gutch, S. Kumar, S. Razi, S. Saran, and K. Gupta, "Pituitary stalk interruption syndrome: case report of three cases with review of literature," *Journal of Pediatric Neurosciences*, vol. 9, no. 2, pp. 188–191, 2014.
[14] D. Rottembourg, A. Linglart, C. Adamsbaum et al., "Gonadotrophic status in adolescents with pituitary stalk interruption syndrome," *Clinical Endocrinology*, vol. 69, no. 1, pp. 105–111, 2008.

7

A Case Report of Graves' Disease Induced by the Anti-Human Programmed Cell Death-1 Monoclonal Antibody Pembrolizumab in a Bladder Cancer Patient

Ken Yajima[1] **and Yushi Akise**[2]

[1]*Division of Diabetes, Endocrinology and Metabolism, Department of Internal Medicine, Federation of National Public Service Personnel Mutual Aid Associations Tachikawa Hospital, 4-2-22 Nishikicho, Tachikawa, Tokyo 190-8531, Japan*
[2]*Department of Urology, Federation of National Public Service Personnel Mutual Aid Associations Tachikawa Hospital, 4-2-22 Nishikicho, Tachikawa, Tokyo 190-8531, Japan*

Correspondence should be addressed to Ken Yajima; k.yajima@tachikawa-hosp.gr.jp

Academic Editor: Osamu Isozaki

Immune checkpoint inhibitors, such as anti-programmed cell death-1 (anti-PD-1), have been widely used in the treatment of malignancies. However, these drugs can cause immune-related adverse events resembling autoimmune diseases. There are some reports of Graves' disease (GD) induced by anti-cytotoxic T-lymphocyte-associated antigen 4 antibodies, but reports which discussed GD induced by anti-PD-1 antibodies are very rare. We report the case of a 61-year-old man with bladder cancer who presented with severe diarrhea, fatigue, palpitation, body weight loss, and hyperthyroidism after the fifth treatment with the anti-PD-1 monoclonal antibody pembrolizumab. His thyroid function prior to pembrolizumab administration had been subclinical hyperthyroidism, despite a negative thyroid-stimulating hormone receptor antibody (TRAb) level. On admission, pembrolizumab administration was discontinued. Graves' disease was diagnosed based on a positive TRAb test result and the ultrasonographic finding of increased blood flow in the superior thyroid artery. Based on colonoscopy findings, the cause of diarrhea was diagnosed as active colitis. His diarrhea was improved with prednisolone, and thyroid function was treated with potassium iodide and thiamazole. This case report of GD with positive TRAb induced by the anti-PD-1 antibody pembrolizumab may contribute to the understanding of the mechanism underlying the association between GD and autoimmune activation via PD-1.

1. Introduction

Immune checkpoint inhibitors (ICIs), including anti-programmed cell death-1 (PD-1), anti-programmed cell death-ligand 1 (PD-L1), and anti-cytotoxic T-lymphocyte-associated antigen-4 (CTLA4) monoclonal antibodies, are promising novel agents for advanced malignancies in recent years. PD-1 expressed on T cells and its ligands PD-L1 inhibit T-cell proliferation and cytokine production in activated T lymphocytes. CTLA4 is also expressed on T cells and exerts a suppressive effect on the immune response after the interaction between T-cells and antigen-presenting cells. These ICIs upregulate antitumor immune responses by blocking PD-1 and CTLA4 pathways. However, these drugs are associated with immune-related adverse events (irAEs) involving multiple endocrinology organs. Most thyroid dysfunction irAEs are destructive thyroiditis and hypothyroidism [1]. Graves' disease (GD) as an irAE is very rare; there are only a few reports of GD induced by anti-CTLA4 antibodies [2, 3]. However, to our knowledge, to date there are even fewer reports of GD caused by anti-PD-1 or anti-PD-L1 antibodies. We herein report a case of GD presenting with severe diarrhea in a patient with bladder cancer who was receiving the anti-PD-1 antibody pembrolizumab.

2. Case Presentation

A man aged 61 years was diagnosed with bladder cancer, with the primary lesion invading the prostate; he underwent total

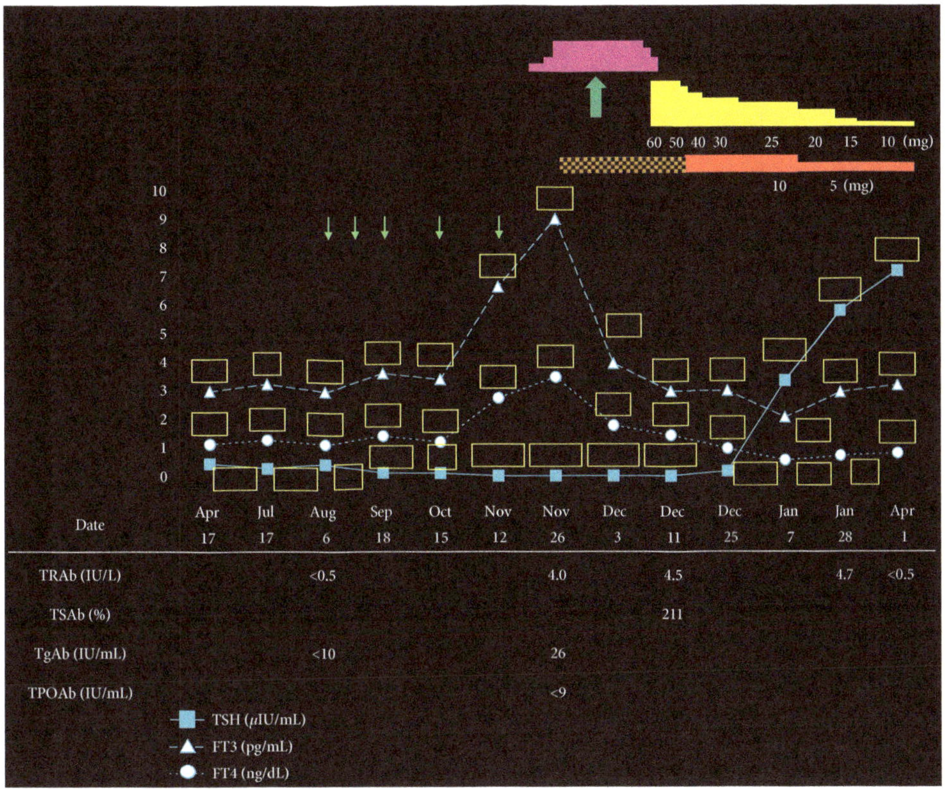

FIGURE 1: The clinical course including the patient's symptoms, medication administered, data of thyroid function tests and thyroid antibodies. The dates of pembrolizumab administration are as follows: first administration, Aug 7, 2018; second, Aug 27, 2018; third, Sep 18, 2018; fourth, Oct 15, 2018; fifth, Nov 12, 2018. Abbreviations: FT3, free triiodothyronine; FT4, free thyroxine; KI, potassium iodide; MMI, methimazole; PSL, prednisolone; TgAb, thyroglobulin antibody; TPOAb, thyroid peroxidase antibody; TRAb, thyroid stimulating hormone receptor antibody; TSAb, thyroid-stimulating antibody; TSH, thyroid stimulating hormone.

cystectomy, urethral resection, and ileal conduit two months later. After five months, computed tomography and magnetic resonance imaging showed retroperitoneal dissemination and para-aortic lymph node metastasis. Although he was treated with gemcitabine and carboplatin, he relapsed three months later. He was referred to our hospital to begin treatment with the anti-human PD-1 monoclonal antibody pembrolizumab.

Pembrolizumab (200 mg) was administered every three weeks, and it was effective. Five days after the fifth pembrolizumab administration (102 days after the first administration), he had two or three bouts of diarrhea per day. His symptoms gradually worsened; he was admitted to our hospital presenting with diarrhea 10×/day, fatigue, palpitation, and body weight loss. His blood pressure was 117/72 mmHg, body temperature was 37.0°C. Electrocardiogram showed normal sinus rhythm, and heart rate was 98/min. Laboratory data showed hyperthyroidism, that is, undetectable serum thyroid-stimulating hormone (TSH) (<0.021 μIU/mL; standard range [SR] = 0.541–4.261) associated with elevated levels of both free triiodothyronine (FT3) (8.98 pg/mL; SR = 2.39–4.06) and free thyroxine (FT4) (3.45 ng/dL; SR = 0.71–1.52), with no goiter, no cervical pain, and no thyroidal ophthalmopathy on examination (Figure 1). He was a smoker and had neither a personal nor a family history of thyroid disease. It was necessary to differentiate whether the diarrhea was caused by hyperthyroidism or by another factor. To suppress the excessive secretion of thyroid hormone, we prescribed potassium iodide (100 mg/day). Thyroid-stimulating hormone receptor antibody (TRAb) was positive (4.0 IU/L; SR = <2.0). Thyroglobulin antibody (TgAb) and thyroid peroxidase antibody (TPOAb) were both negative (26 IU/mL; SR = ≤28, <9 IU/mL; SR = ≤15.9, respectively). The thyroglobulin (Tg) level was elevated (276 ng/mL; SR = 0–33.7). Thyroid-stimulating antibody (TSAb) was positive later (211%; SR = ≤120). Thyroid ultrasonography performed the day after iodine treatment showed an increase in the superior thyroid artery flow velocity (Right 50.1 cm/s, Left 44.0 cm/s; ≥50 cm/s as a criterion for increase) and a mild increase in the intrathyroidal blood flow signal (Figure 2). Before the first pembrolizumab administration, his thyroid function was subclinical hyperthyroidism with negative TRAb (<0.5 IU/L). From these results, he was diagnosed as GD which had developed during pembrolizumab administration.

We also suggested that diarrhea had been caused by colitis, and thus we performed colonoscopy. Colonoscopy showed active colitis with granular mucosa, orange peel appearance, and loss of visible vascular pattern. Biopsy samples from terminal ileum, cecum, ascending colon, transverse colon, sigmoid colon, and rectum were active ileitis, typhlitis, and colitis with mild crypt atrophy, cryptitis, and crypt abscess. Stool culture, *Clostridium difficile* toxin, and glutamate dehydrogenase toxin were all negative. Therefore, he was diagnosed as

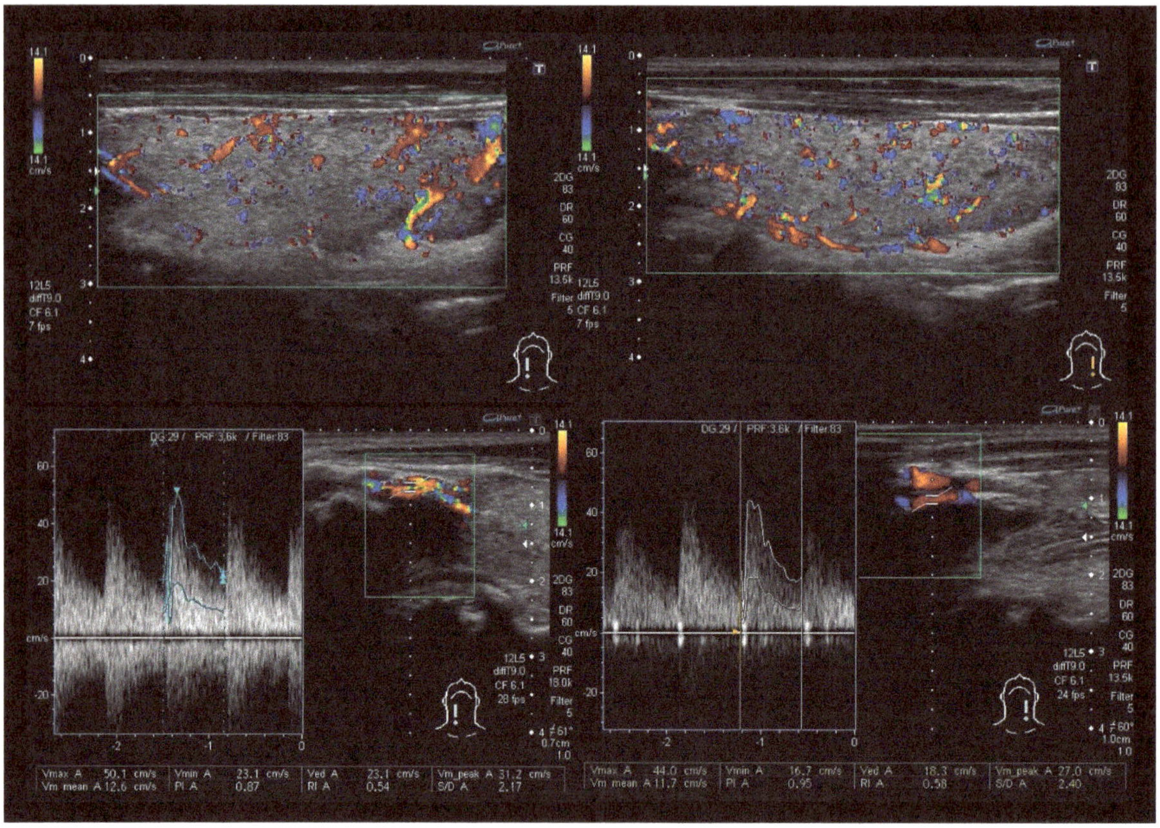

FIGURE 2: Thyroid ultrasonography performed the day after iodine treatment. Upper: Left is the intrathyroidal blood flow signal of the right lobe, Right is that of the left lobe. Lower: Left is right superior thyroid artery flow velocity, Vmax is 50.1 cm/s, Right is left superior thyroid artery flow velocity, Vmax is 44.0 cm/s.

having active colitis with diarrhea as Common Terminology Criteria for Adverse Events Grade 3. His diarrhea had not improved despite the reduction of thyroid hormone with potassium iodide treatment for 10 days. We decided that the diarrhea had been caused by immune-mediated colitis due to pembrolizumab treatment, and not by hyperthyroidism. Subsequently, his diarrhea was rapidly improved by prednisolone 60 mg (1 mg/kg/day).

On the other hand, his thyroid hormone was normalized with undetectable serum TSH for 2 weeks by iodine treatment, and thiamazole 10 mg/day was given in place of potassium iodide. TRAb was not detected after 15 weeks of thiamazole treatment. We were able to precisely document the development of GD induced by pembrolizumab, because his thyroid function was checked regularly. Although pembrolizumab administration was discontinued because of severe diarrhea, there has been no further progression of cancer to date.

3. Discussion

The incidences of thyrotoxicosis and hypothyroidism treated with the anti-PD-1 antibody pembrolizumab have been reported by de Filette et al. [4] to be 12.1% and 15.2%, respectively. According to their report, TRAb was tested in five patients and it was found to be elevated in only one patient at the time of thyrotoxicosis. In the one case of positive TRAb, thyrotoxicosis swiftly evolved into hypothyroidism without antithyroid therapy. That patient might have had GD rapidly shifting to hypothyroidism due to a switch in her antibody subpopulation.

Iadarola et al. recently reported a case of nivolumab-induced thyroid dysfunction, GD-like hyperthyroidism [5]. Their 66-year-old male patient, who was administered nivolumab, developed hyperthyroidism (FT4 was in the upper-normal range) with negative TRAb. Thyroid ultrasound showed a multinodular goiter with a normo-echoic pattern of the parenchyma and a normal pattern of vascularization. A 99 mTc scintigraphy revealed a diffuse thyroid uptake of the radionuclide suggesting GD-like hyperthyroidism, and methimazole therapy was started. TRAb test remained persistently negative. That case indicated that GD-like hyperthyroidism can also occur in nivolumab-treated patients, even in the absence of circulating TRAb. The role of thyroid autoantibodies in the pathogenesis of PD-1 inhibitor-induced thyroid dysfunction was debated, but that of TRAb was not discussed and remained unclear.

We herein reported a case in which pembrolizumab-induced hyperthyroidism (FT4 was elevated) with positively converted TRAb. We diagnosed GD considering positive TSAb and the results of thyroid ultrasonography, although thyroid scintigraphy was not evaluated because of iodine treatment. We thought this case was typical GD diagnosed based on TRAb test and thyroid ultrasound data compared to the atypical GD presented in the previous report [5]. In the present case, pembrolizumab-induced

GD was improved by potassium iodide and thiamazole and TRAb was converted to negative 15 weeks after the beginning of thiamazole treatment. Concomitantly, immune-related active colitis was also rapidly improved by prednisolone. Therefore, the use of prednisolone may further complicate the course of negatively converted TRAb.

GD is caused by failure of self-tolerance to TSH receptor. Both T cells and B cells are necessary for the development of GD. Large scale genetic analyses have identified several genes including CTLA4 conferring susceptibility of GD. There are only a few reports of GD induced by anti-CTLA4 antibodies [2, 3]. According to Azmat et al., it is plausible to hypothesize that blocking CTLA4 results in the development of activating antibodies against the TSH receptor thereby causing GD in susceptible individuals [2]. Several investigators have also suggested that this relation between CTLA4 and GD are associated with CTLA4 gene polymorphism, which is also true in Japanese [6]. However, the mechanism of GD induced by anti-CTLA4 antibodies is unclear.

In contrast, PD-1 is expressed on T cells and B cells, and PD-L1 is expressed on activated T cells, B cells, cancer cells and antigen-presenting cells. PD-1 prevents T cell proliferation, activation and cytokine release. PD-1 can inhibit B cell receptor signaling and antigen-stimulated B cell activation [7]. In addition, PD-1 is expressed on activated $CD4^{+}CD25^{+}$ regulatory T cells (Tregs) in humans [8], and the blockade of PD-1 by antagonistic anti-PD-1 antibodies inhibits the production of IL-10 from regulatory T cells [8] and thereby, enhances lymphocyte proliferation. This suggests that PD-1 may be critical in determining the activation threshold and/or suppressive activity of Tregs. In this way, the PD-1 pathway plays an important role in the down regulation of immune responses and in the prevention of autoimmune diseases. Interestingly however, PD-1 has not appeared on the stage of GD. Reports on the association between PD-1 and GD are few. We introduced two reports which investigated GD and gene polymorphisms of PD-1 [9] and PD-L1 [10]. Newby et al. documented that small effects within PD-1 may contribute towards the development of GD in the UK [9]. Hayashi et al. showed that PD-L1 gene might be one of the candidate gene polymorphisms for GD [10]. It is unclear how the polymorphism affects the development of GD in these studies.

Regarding other drug-induced GD, there was a report stating that the anti-CD52 monoclonal antibody, alemtuzumab, can induce GD in patients with multiple sclerosis [11]; 9 of 27 patients developed GD from 3–31 months after alemtuzumab treatment. The B cell and CD8 lymphocyte counts rose progressively at 15–18 months after alemtuzumab. The development of GD was associated with a quicker recovery of CD8 T cells and a low production of memory CD4 cells. The unique situation has been identified in which biochemical hyperthyroidism can be detected several months before symptoms develop, allowing access to the earliest immunological events in the pathogenesis of GD. Based on this point of view, it may be considered that anti-PD-1 antibody may induce GD by activation of the autoimmune system associated with the development of GD via PD-1/PD-L1 pathway inhibition. However, as the mechanistic profile of anti-PD-1 antibody-induced GD remains unclear, further study and the accumulation of case reports regarding ICI-induced GD is necessary.

In conclusion, this case report of GD with positive TRAb induced by the anti-PD-1 antibody pembrolizumab may contribute to the understanding of the mechanism behind the association of the development of GD and autoimmune activation via PD-1.

Acknowledgments

We would appreciate the Tama Society of Clinical Endocrinology and Metabolism for their insight and helpful advice in the management of this patient.

References

[1] S. M. Corsello, A. Barnabei, P. Marchetti, L. De Vecchis, R. Salvatori, and F. Torino, "Endocrine side effects induced by immune checkpoint inhibitors," *The Journal of Clinial Endocrinology and Metabolism*, vol. 98, no. 4, pp. 1361–1375, 2013.

[2] U. Azmat, D. Liebner, A. Joehlin-Price, A. Agrawal, and F. Nabhan, "Treatment of ipilimumab induced Graves' disease in a patient with metastatic melanoma," *Case Reports in Endocrinology*, vol. 2016, Article ID 2087525, 4 pages, 2016.

[3] E. H. Gan, A. L. Mitchell, R. Plummer, S. Pearce, and P. Perros, "Tremelimumab-h Graves hyperthyroidism," *European Thyroid Journal*, vol. 6, no. 3, pp. 167–170, 2017.

[4] J. de Filette, Y. Jansen, M. Schreuer et al., "Incidence of thyroid-related adverse events in melanoma patients treated with pembrolizumab," *The Journal of Clinical Endocrinology and Metabolism*, vol. 101, no. 11, pp. 4431–4439, 2016.

[5] C. Iadarola, L. Croce, E. Quaquarini et al., "Nivolumab induced thyroid dysfunction: unusual clinical presentation and challenging diagnosis", *Frontiers in Endocrinology*, vol. 9, 2019.

[6] T. Yanagawa, M. Taniyama, S. Enomoto et al., "CTLA4 gene polymorphism confers susceptibility to Graves' disease in Japanese," *Thyroid*, vol. 7, no. 6, pp. 843–846, 1997.

[7] T. Okazaki, A. Maeda, H. Nishimura, T. Kurosaki, and T. Honjo, "PD-1 immunoreceptor inhibits B cell receptor-mediated signaling by recruiting src homology 2-domain-containing tyrosine phosphatase 2 to phosphotyrosine," *Proceedings of the National Academy of Sciences of the United States of America*, vol. 98, no. 24, pp. 13866–13871, 2001.

[8] C. P. Gray, P. Arosio, and P. Hersey, "Heavy chain ferritin activates regulatory T cells by induction of changes in dendritic cells," *Blood*, vol. 99, no. 9, pp. 3326–3334, 2002.

[9] P. R. Newby, E. L. Roberts-Davies, O. J. Brand et al., "Tag SNP screening of the PDCD1 gene for association with Graves' disease," *Clinical Endocrinology*, vol. 67, no. 1, pp. 125–128, 2007.

[10] M. Hayashi, T. Kouki, N. Takasu, S. Sunagawa, and I. Komiya, "Association of an A/C single nucleotide polymorphism in programmed cell death-ligand 1 gene with Graves' disease in Japanese patients," *European Journal of Endocrinology*, vol. 158, no. 6, pp. 817–822, 2008.

8

Acute Heart Failure as a First Presentation of Pheochromocytoma Complicated with "Inverted" Takotsubo Syndrome

Jerrold Spapen,[1] Jeroen de Filette,[2] Stijn Lochy,[1,3] and Herbert Spapen[4]

[1] *Department of Cardiology, Universitair Ziekenhuis Brussel, Brussels, Belgium*
[2] *Department of Endocrinology, Universitair Ziekenhuis Brussel, Brussels, Belgium*
[3] *Department of Intensive Care Medicine, Universitair Ziekenhuis Brussel, Brussels, Belgium*
[4] *Development, Ageing and Pathology Research Group, Vrije Universiteit Brussel, Brussels, Belgium*

Correspondence should be addressed to Jeroen de Filette; jdefilet@vub.ac.be

Academic Editor: Wayne V. Moore

Takotsubo syndrome is a rare but emerging form of acute reversible myocardial injury characterized by transient systolic LV dysfunction, often related to emotional or physical stress. Pheochromocytoma is increasingly recognised as another possible trigger. Pheochromocytoma is a rare catecholamine-secreting tumour arising from chromaffin cells within the adrenal medulla or extra-adrenal paraganglia. The pathognomonic quartet of paroxysmal hypertension, palpitations, headache, and diaphoresis is rarely present, and diagnosis is often delayed. We describe a 43-year-old formerly healthy patient with an adrenal pheochromocytoma, presenting as an "inverted" takotsubo syndrome complicated with acute heart failure and pulmonary oedema.

1. Introduction

Takotsubo syndrome has emerged as an important cause of acute myocardial injury characterized by transient systolic left ventricular dysfunction. Multiple emotional and/or physical triggers have been identified, but the exact "stressor" remains unknown in up to 35% of patients. Pheochromocytoma is a rare neuroendocrine catecholamine-secreting tumour, originating from chromaffin cells within the adrenal medulla or extra-adrenal paraganglia. Recently, pheochromocytoma was recognised as another trigger for the syndrome. Pheochromocytoma-induced takotsubo syndrome is characterized by a more dramatic clinical presentation and higher complication rates compared to other forms. We describe a patient with an adrenal pheochromocytoma presenting as a takotsubo syndrome complicated with acute heart failure and pulmonary oedema.

2. Case Description

A 43-year-old woman without relevant medical history acutely developed nausea, severe chest pain, and dyspnoea during strenuous mountain-hiking. At a local emergency department, she was immediately intubated and initiated on intravenous nitrates because of severe arterial hypertension. At request of the family, she was transferred to our hospital. On arrival, ECG revealed an ectopic atrial rhythm, poor R-wave progression, and a prolonged corrected QT-interval. Chest X-ray showed pulmonary oedema. The troponin level was 2.42 μg/L (normally <0.005), and NT-proBNP was 39,061 ng/L (normally <125). Echocardiography documented severely impaired left ventricular (LV) function (ejection fraction (EF) 35%) with basal and midsegmental akinesis and preserved contractility of the apex. Coronary angiography ruled out significant coronary disease. Ventriculography confirmed "inverted" takotsubo cardiomyopathy (Figure 1). Because of refractory high blood pressure, a diagnostic work-up was performed. Contrast-enhanced total body CT scan identified a left adrenal heterogeneous mass measuring 59×56 mm (Figure 2). 24-hour fractionated urinary metanephrine and normetanephrine levels were 7483 and 8895 μg, respectively (normally <240 and <600). Adequate alpha-adrenergic and beta-blockade was ensured, and

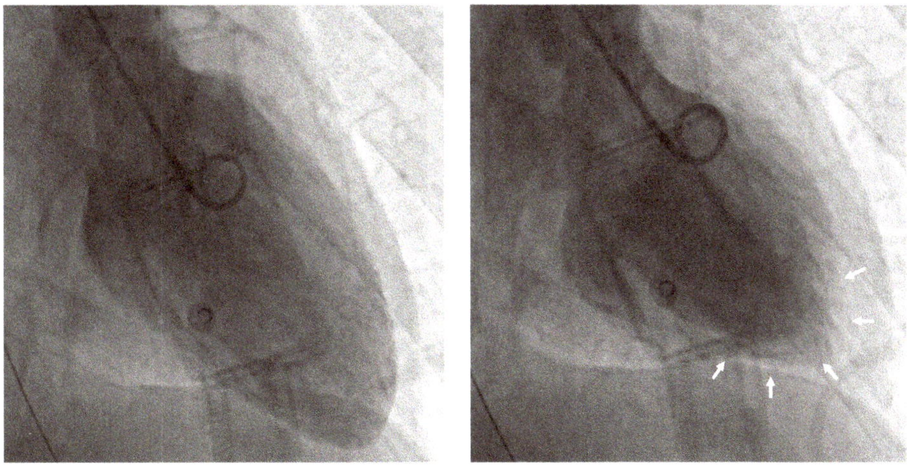

(a) (b)

FIGURE 1: Ventriculography showing akinesia of the basal and midmyocardial segments and preserved contractility of the apex (arrows). The aspect is compatible with an inverted takotsubo pattern. (a) Diastole and (b) systole.

laparoscopic adrenalectomy was performed. Pathological examination revealed nests of polygonal cells with eosinophilic cytoplasm. Immunohistochemical staining was strongly positive for chromogranin A and S100 (Figure 3), confirming the diagnosis of pheochromocytoma. After surgery, the patient's hemodynamic condition rapidly stabilized. The LV systolic function, evaluated by repeated bedside "quick look" cardiac ultrasound, gradually improved during the following weeks. She made a further uneventful recovery and was discharged from the hospital 50 days after admission. Follow-up echocardiography at the cardiology clinic 10 weeks later showed complete normalization of LV function.

3. Discussion

Takotsubo syndrome (TS) is a rare but emerging form of acute reversible myocardial injury characterized by transient systolic LV dysfunction, often related to emotional or physical stress. The prevalence is estimated at 1 to 2% of patients with suspected acute coronary syndrome. TS most typically presents as pronounced regional wall motion abnormalities with akinesis of the apex and hyperkinesis of the basal segments but may appear in other variants. Recently, pheochromocytoma was recognised as another trigger for the syndrome [1, 2]. The pathognomonic quartet of paroxysmal hypertension, palpitations, headache, and diaphoresis is rarely present, and its diagnosis is often delayed. Brain haemorrhage, aortic dissection, severe LV hypertrophy, coronary vasospasm, myocardial infarction, arrhythmias, and acute heart failure with pulmonary oedema are all life-threatening complications related to high levels of circulating catecholamines, in particular norepinephrine, released by the tumour [3]. The pathogenesis of pheochromocytoma-induced TS remains elusive. A cardiocerebral relationship in TS is well established, but the exact mechanism of "neurogenic myocardial stunning" is unknown. The spillover of norepinephrine from myocardial presynaptic terminations following intense stress may induce direct cellular damage and/or epicardial and microvascular dysfunction [1, 4, 5].

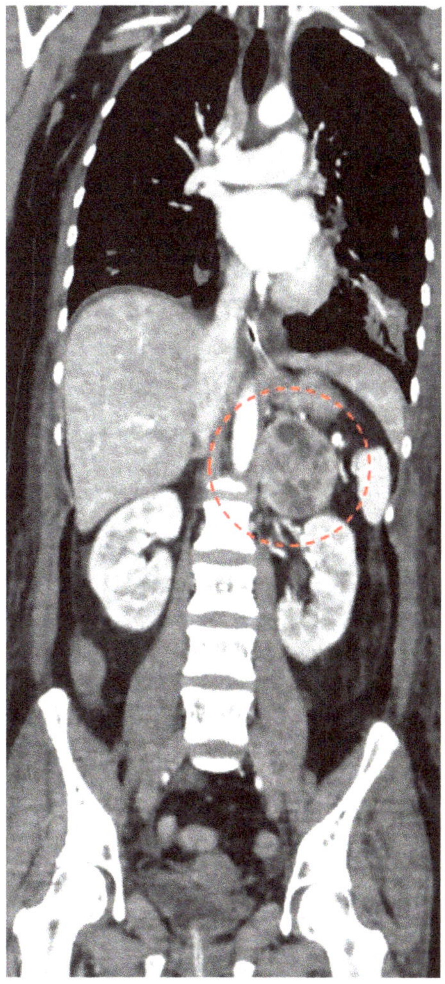

FIGURE 2: Contrast-enhanced total body CT scan revealing a left adrenal heterogeneous mass of 59 × 56 mm (red dots).

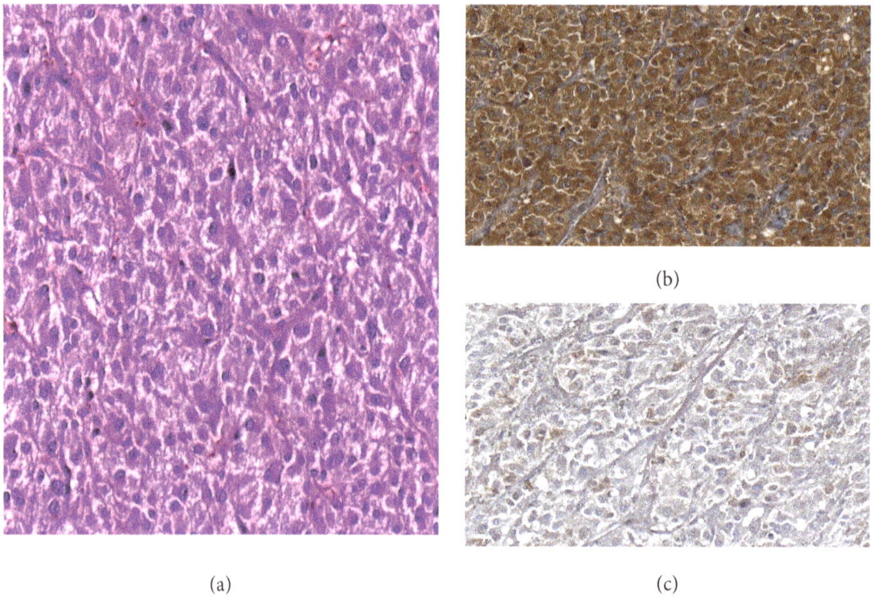

FIGURE 3: Pathological examination showing nests of polygonal cells with eosinophilic cytoplasm (a). Immunohistochemical staining is strongly positive for chromogranin A (b) and S100 (c) confirming the diagnosis of pheochromocytoma.

Recently, persisting subclinical myocardial abnormalities (systolic/diastolic dysfunction and evidence of myocardial inflammation and fibrosis) were detected despite curative tumour resection and without biochemical disease activity. These alterations do not correlate with arterial hypertension (and subsequent pressure overload) but rather suggest direct catecholamine cardiotoxicity [6]. Pheochromocytoma-induced TS follows a remarkably more dramatic clinical course with higher complication and recurrence rates than "classic" TS. Patients are approximately 20 years younger, predominantly male (30% vs. 10.2%), and almost one-third develops a basal or "inverted" TS pattern compared to 2.2% of all TS subjects. Global forms, which are rarely seen in TS, are also more frequently reported in pheochromocytoma patients [5, 7]. By definition, TS is a self-limiting disease. Treatment is focused on supportive care and elimination of the triggering factor(s). In pheochromocytoma patients, inotropic agents are contraindicated, and beta-blockers must be combined with alpha-blocking agents to avoid a hypertensive crisis [2, 5]. Extracorporeal life support may be necessary to sustain LV systolic function while awaiting hemodynamic recovery [8]. Surgical removal of the tumour is essential. This case report highlights the importance of early suspicion and diagnostic work-up for pheochromocytoma in patients with acute heart failure of unknown origin, even in the absence of clinical evidence of catecholamine excess, especially in young patients, complicated disease course, recurrent cases, and atypical (inverted/basal or global) takotsubo subtypes.

Disclosure

This manuscript has been presented as a conference abstract at the 24th Annual Congress of the Belgian Society of Internal Medicine.

Authors' Contributions

JS and JdF planned the concept of this case report and drafted the manuscript. JS and SL provided the figures. All authors critically reviewed, revised, and contributed to the final article.

References

[1] J.-R. Ghadri, I. S. Wittstein, A. Prasad et al., "International expert consensus document on takotsubo syndrome (part I): clinical characteristics, diagnostic criteria, and pathophysiology," *European Heart Journal*, vol. 39, no. 22, pp. 2032–2046, 2018.

[2] J.-R. Ghadri, I. S. Wittstein, A. Prasad et al., "International expert consensus document on takotsubo syndrome (part II): diagnostic workup, outcome, and management," *European Heart Journal*, vol. 39, no. 22, pp. 2047–2062, 2018.

[3] A. Riester, D. Weismann, M. Quinkler et al., "Life-threatening events in patients with pheochromocytoma," *European Journal of Endocrinology*, vol. 173, no. 6, pp. 757–764, 2015.

[4] H. Medina de Chazal, M. G. Del Buono, L. Keyser-Marcus et al., "Stress cardiomyopathy diagnosis and treatment," *Journal of the American College of Cardiology*, vol. 72, no. 16, pp. 1955–1971, 2018.

[5] S. Y-Hassan and H. Falhammar, "Pheochromocytoma- and paraganglioma-triggered takotsubo syndrome," *Endocrine*, vol. 65, no. 3, pp. 483–493, 2019.

[6] V. M. Ferreira, M. Marcelino, S. K. Piechnik et al., "Pheochromocytoma is characterized by catecholamine-mediated myocarditis, focal and diffuse myocardial fibrosis, and myocardial dysfunction," *Journal of the American College of Cardiology*, vol. 67, no. 20, pp. 2364–2374, 2016.

[7] S. Y-Hassan, "Clinical features and outcome of pheochromocytoma-induced takotsubo syndrome: analysis of 80 pub-

lished cases," *The American Journal of Cardiology*, vol. 117, no. 11, pp. 1836–1844, 2016.
[8] B. Flam, M. Broomé, B. Frenckner, R. Bränström, and M. Bell, "Pheochromocytoma-Induced inverted takotsubo-like cardiomyopathy leading to cardiogenic shock successfully treated with extracorporeal membrane oxygenation," *Journal of Intensive Care Medicine*, vol. 30, no. 6, pp. 365–372, 2015.

9

Adrenal Mass in a 70-Year-Old Woman

Kiana Karimi,[1,2] **Mohsen Nikzad**,[3] **Sohrab Kulivand**,[4] **and Shiva Borzouei**[5]

[1] *Student Research Committee, Hamadan University of Medical Sciences, Hamadan, Iran*
[2] *Universal Scientific Education and Research Network (USERN), Tehran, Iran*
[3] *Department of Internal Medicine, School of Medicine, Hamadan University of Medical Sciences, Hamadan, Iran*
[4] *Department of Radiology, School of Medicine, Hamadan University of Medical Sciences, Hamadan, Iran*
[5] *Department of Endocrinology, School of Medicine, Hamadan University of Medical Sciences, Hamadan, Iran*

Correspondence should be addressed to Shiva Borzouei; borzooeishiva@yahoo.com

Academic Editor: Osamu Isozaki

Introduction. Adrenocortical carcinoma is a rare endocrine malignancy with a bimodal age distribution pattern that affects women more than men. More than half of the patients present with hormone excess manifestations such as Cushing's syndrome and virilization. Non-functional tumors usually are diagnosed incidentally following imaging studies due to a mass effect or metastatic disease. Surgical resection is considered the best curative treatment for these tumors. *Case Presentation.* A 70-year-old woman presented with a 3-month history of diffuse intermittent abdominal discomfort, weight loss, and additional hair growth. Imaging investigations revealed a large 187 × 85 × 140 mm mass between the liver and upper pole of the right kidney which has displaced the adjacent structures. Hormonal evaluations detected high levels of cortisol and adrenal androgens. She underwent open adrenalectomy and right nephrectomy due to severe adhesion of the mass. Histopathological evaluations revealed adrenocortical carcinoma and the patient received adjuvant radiotherapy. *Conclusion.* Precise physical examination, hormonal evaluation, and imaging studies play a key role in differentiating malignant adrenal masses in all patients, especially in those with vague symptoms. Radical excision of the mass and appropriate adjuvant chemotherapy or radiotherapy improve the outcome for patients.

1. Introduction

Adrenocortical carcinoma (ACC) is a rare endocrine malignancy with an approximate prevalence of 1 to 2 per million. Although this malignancy can develop at any age, it has a bimodal age distribution pattern which commonly affects patients under the age of 5 or in the 4th to 5th decades of life [1]. In addition to genetic predisposition, there is no definite and known risk factor for ACC. However, some studies have shown smoking in men and the use of contraceptives in women as probable risk factors for ACC [2].

Most patients present with signs and symptoms of hormone excess, especially hypercortisolism (50–80%). About one-third of patients have clinical manifestations of local tumor growth, and 20–30% of them are diagnosed incidentally following imaging studies for other reasons [3]. The initial diagnosis of ACC is based on a careful history and physical examination, along with biochemical and endocrinological evaluations. Computed tomography (CT) scanning and magnetic resonance imaging (MRI) are choice imaging modalities for distinguishing ACCs from adrenocortical adenomas, determining local invasion, and distant metastases [4].

In the pathological evaluation of adrenal tumors, size is an important and determining factor in the diagnosis of ACCs [3]. These tumors are typically large, more than 6 cm and diameters of 4–25 cm [5, 6]. Clinical, histological, and immunohistochemical parameters are also conductive in confirming the diagnosis. The Weiss system is the most acceptable histopathological system for assessing malignancy in adrenocortical tumors [7].

Despite the limitation of knowledge about the treatment and prognosis of these patients due to its rarity, some progress has been made in this regard. Surgical resection of the tumor and suspicious lymph nodes is considered a potentially curative treatment. Adjuvant mitotane therapy is recommended for all patients who are at risk for recurrence or have high-grade or incompletely resected tumors. The addition of postoperative radiation therapy (RT) is also suggested for this group of patients [8].

Herein, we present the case of a 70-year-old woman with abdominal discomfort, weight loss, and terminal hair overgrowth that was diagnosed with adrenocortical carcinoma.

2. Case Presentation

A 70-year-old woman, a retired teacher, presented with a 3-month history of abdominal pain. The abdominal discomfort has been intermittent and diffuse without any specific pattern. She has lost her appetite and her body weight decreased about 10 kg over this period. She has complained of malaise and occasional headaches. She denied nausea or vomiting, diaphoresis, palpitation, sleep disturbance, and abnormal uterine bleeding. She has also noted some additional hair growth on her chin, between the breasts, and on the lower abdomen. In her previous medical history, she had controlled hypertension and was on losartan, and she had no history of diabetes. She has also been hospitalized due to COVID-19 one month previously.

On physical examination, she looked cachectic. Her blood pressure was 160/80 mmHg, and other vital signs were normal. On abdominal examination, she had no striae or central obesity. There was mild tenderness over the right upper quadrant and a non-pulsatile 15 cm mass was palpated under the liver. She had excessive terminal hair with a modified Ferriman–Gallwey score of 16. Lower extremities examination showed proximal myopathy in the pelvic girdle. Examination of the cardiovascular and respiratory systems was normal.

The initial laboratory tests revealed an elevation in white blood cell count, fasting glucose concentration, and lactate dehydrogenase level. Other findings were all within the normal limits (Table 1). Contrast-enhanced CT of abdomen indicated a solid retroperitoneal 187 × 85 × 140 mm mass with regular borders and heterogenous enhancement located between the upper pole of the right kidney and VI and VII segments of the liver which has pushed the right kidney down (Figure 1). According to these findings, more hormonal evaluations were performed with the abnormal results shown in Table 2. There was no evidence of bone involvement in the bone scan. Findings suggested adrenal carcinoma, and the patient underwent an exploratory laparotomy after controlling hypertension.

Laparotomy was performed, and the right adrenal mass and kidney were excised due to severe adhesion of the mass to the right renal vein. The inferior vena cava has also been repaired. Macroscopically, the adrenal removed specimen measured 23 × 15 × 9 cm and weighted 1667 g. The tumor was solid, yellowish-gray, and well-defined with an intact capsule. Cross section of the tumor revealed a non-homogenous nodular area with extensive necrosis. There was no evidence of neoplastic invasion to the capsule or external surface of the mass. Microscopic examination revealed polyhedral neoplastic cells in trabecular structures which were arranged in dense cellular sheets. Tumoral cells had giant and pleomorphic nuclei, vesicular chromatin, marked eosinophilic nucleoli, and large amounts of eosinophilic granular to clear cytoplasm. The mitotic activity was more than 6 in 50/high-power fields (HPF), and multifocal coagulation tumoral necrosis was observed. The capsular invasion was identified, but it was not extended beyond it. There was no evidence of tumoral involvement in the right kidney (Figure 2).

Table 1: Initial laboratory workup [9].

Test	Result	Normal range
WBC (white blood cells)	15740/μl	4000–11000
RBC (red blood cells)	5.9 million/μl	4.2–5.4
Hb (hemoglobin)	15.2 g/dl	12.5–16
Platelets	194000/μl	140000–450000
FPG (fasting plasma glucose)	127 mg/dl	60–110
LDH (lactate dehydrogenase)	340 IU/l	140–280
ESR 1h (erythrocyte sedimentation rate)	5 mm/h	0–30
CRP (C-reactive protein)	Negative	
Bun	14 mg/dl	5–23
Cr	1.1 mg/dl	0.6–1.4
Ca	8.6 mg/dl	8.6–11
P	3.4 mg/dl	2.9–5.1
Na	142 mEq/l	135–145
K	3.9 mEq/l	3.9–5.3

The patient was observed in the intensive care unit for a few days after surgery. She was referred to the oncology ward with no surgical complications 9 days after surgery. Since the mass was completely resected and there was no evidence of distant spread of the tumor, she underwent adjuvant radiation therapy without chemotherapy. Follow-up thoracic, abdominal, and pelvic CT 3 months after surgery revealed no recurrence or metastasis, and all hormonal and biochemistry evaluations were within normal limits. 5 months after surgery, she is alive and back to normal in good condition.

3. Discussion

Adrenocortical carcinoma is a rare malignancy in the endocrine system, usually with a poor prognosis [10]. The incidence of these tumors is about 0.7–2.0 cases per million each year, and they are more found in women in the fifth decade of life [11, 12]. They can also affect children, mostly as functional tumors [13]. Most ACC cases appear to be sporadic as in the present case. However, some cases were considered to be associated with several hereditary tumor disorders such as Li–Fraumeni syndrome, multiple endocrine neoplasia type 1, and Beckwith–Wiedemann syndrome [14].

Studies have indicated that more than 60% of ACCs are hormone-producing tumors and they can develop clinical syndromes of hormone excess. These tumors usually induce Cushing's syndrome (45%) in adults and are associated with glucocorticoid excess symptoms, such as weakness, and weight gain, which commonly develop over three to six months. About 25% of patients present with a mixed

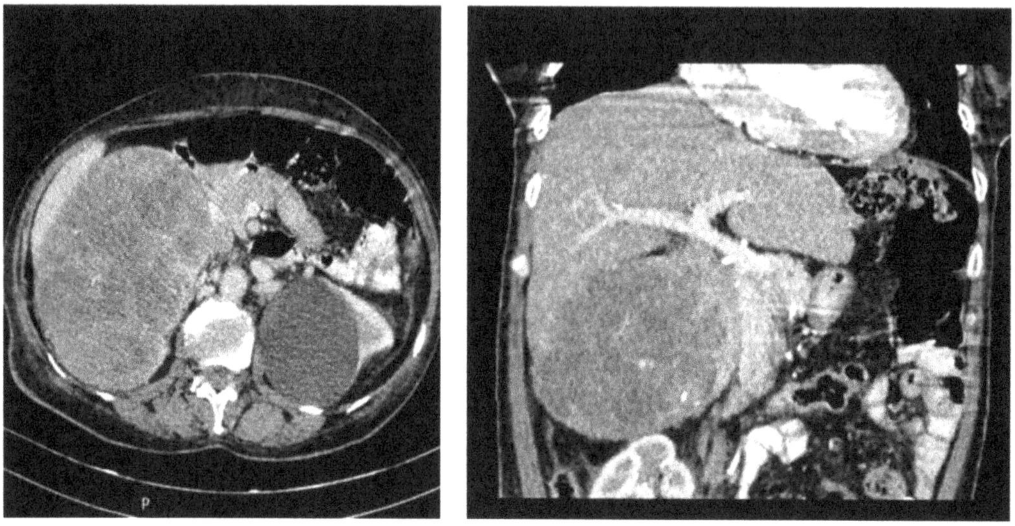

(a) (b)

Figure 1: Abdominal CT scan with IV contrast. (a) Axial view of the heterogenous well-defined mass above the right kidney. (b) Coronal view of the adrenal mass effect on the IVC and pancreatic tail.

Table 2: Hormonal and tumor marker evaluation [9].

Test	Result	Normal range
Dehydroepiandrosterone sulfate	>1000 μg/dL	Female: 30–400
Testosterone	8.810 ng/ml	>50y: 0.029–0.408
17-OH-progesterone	25.37 ng/ml	Menopause: 0.2–0.9
Estradiol	76 pg/ml	<60
Androstenedione	4.3 ng/ml	0.9–3.2
Cortisol (8 AM)	46.81 micg/dL	6.4–21
24-hour urinary free cortisol	255.1 μg/24 hrs	1.5–63
24-hour urinary metanephrine	30 μg/24 hrs	<350
24-hour urinary normetanephrine	386.9 μg/24 hrs	<600
AFP (alpha-fetoprotein)	3.74 IU/ml	Up to 5.8
CEA (carcinoembryonic antigen)	1.1 ng/ml	Non-smokers: <5.0
CA 125 (carbohydrate antigen 125)	23.48 U/ml	Up to 35

Cushing's and virilization syndrome, due to excessive secretion of both androgens and glucocorticoids and only fewer than 10% of them induce virilization symptoms, implying ACC rather than adenoma [6, 15]. Our patient's main complaint was abdominal discomfort besides recent weight loss which is related to local mass effect. She had no clinical manifestations of Cushing's or virilization syndrome which may be due to the short period from the onset of the tumor growth.

Hormonal estimation including adrenal androgens and glucocorticoids levels may help to determine the adrenal source of the patient's signs and symptoms, providing tumor markers which are useful during patient's follow-up to assess possible tumor recurrence or residual tumor after surgery [8]. In the present case, high adrenal androgens and estradiol levels were detected and made the diagnosis of adrenal carcinomas more probable than adrenal adenomas [16]. Urinary excretion of metanephrines and normetanephrines was measured, and they were within normal range which excluded the possibility of pheochromocytoma.

CT scan and MRI are preferred imaging methods for evaluating the tumor size, local invasion, or distant tumor invasion. These tumors usually have the following features on CT scan: tumor size larger than 4 cm, inhomogeneous but well-defined suprarenal mass, displacing adjacent structure, heterogenous enhancement after IV contrast administration, and less frequent calcification and IVC tumor thrombus, especially in right-sided tumors [4]. As described above, our patient had most of these features in imaging studies.

Fine-needle aspiration biopsy is not usually recommended for distinguishing adrenal carcinoma from a benign adrenal mass. However, it could be performed when there is a high suspicion of distant metastasis in adrenal glands [17]. The Weiss histopathologic system is commonly used for evaluating the probability of malignancy in adrenocortical tumors. The modified Weiss system has the following criteria: abnormal mitoses, >6 mitoses/50 HPF, ≤25% clear tumor cells in the cytoplasm, necrosis, and capsular invasion [7]. The present case had all the features, which led to establishing the diagnosis of malignancy.

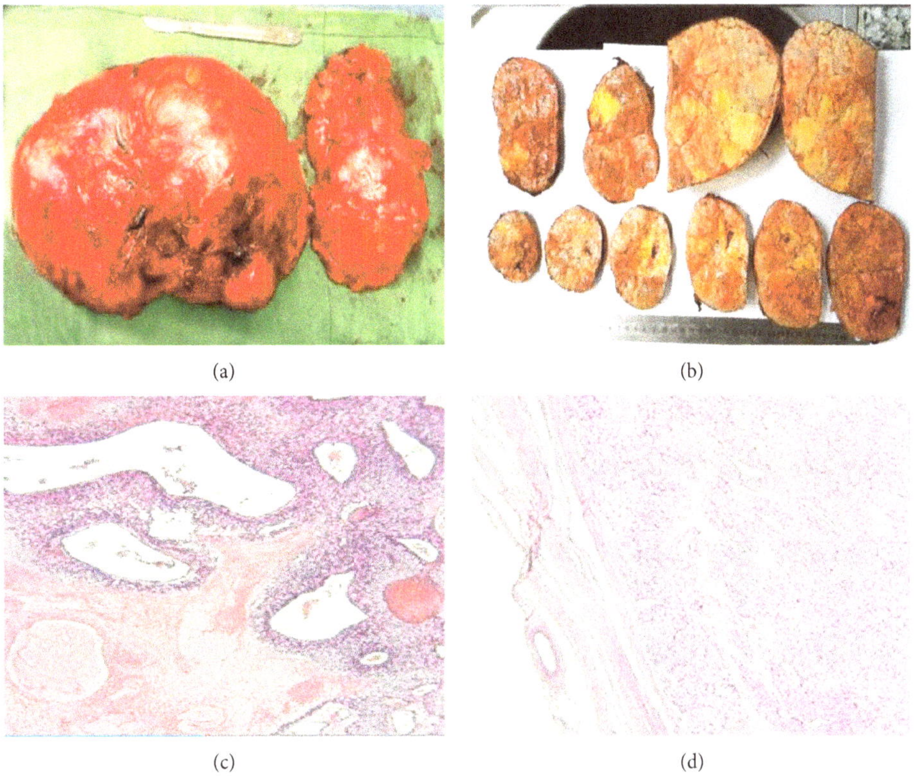

Figure 2: (a) Macroscopical view of the adrenal mass and right kidney. (b) The adrenal mass with a nodular and extensive necrotic area at sectioning. (c) High mitotic activity with multifocal necrosis. (d) Extension of the neoplastic cells to the capsule.

Table 3: Classification system for staging ACC [9, 20].

ENSAT stage	TNM stage	TNM definition
I	T1, N0, M0	T1, tumor ≤5 cm N0, no positive lymph node M0, no distant metastases
II	T2, N0, M0	T2, tumor >5 cm N0, no positive lymph node M0, no distant metastases
III	T1-T2, N1, M0 T3-T4, N0-N1, M0	N1, positive lymph node(s) M0, no distant metastases T3, tumor infiltration into surrounding tissue T4, tumor invasion into adjacent organs or venous tumor thrombus in vena cava or renal vein
IV	T1-T4, N0-N1, M1	M1, presence of distant metastases

ENSAT, European Network for the Study of Adrenal Tumors; TNM, tumor, node, metastasis.

Complete surgical resection is the only potentially curative treatment for stage I to III ACCs (Table 3). However, due to the presence of occult micrometastases, it may not be curative for many patients [15]. Adjuvant mitotane therapy is recommended for all the patients at high risk of disease recurrence after surgery, including all cases with high-grade disease, intraoperative tumor spillage or fracture, incompletely resected tumor, and vascular or capsular invasion [8, 18]. Previously, ACC was considered to be a relatively radioresistant tumor. However, some studies indicated a benefit in those who are at risk of local recurrence [19]. In the present case, the tumor was in stage III and we decided to perform open surgery rather than laparoscopic resection due to the tumor size, uncertainty about the tumor local invasion, and reducing the risk of spillage or fracture. The mass was successfully resected; after histopathologic evaluation, no invasion beyond the capsule was detected, so we preferred radiotherapy to chemotherapy as adjuvant therapy after surgery.

In conclusion, ACC as a rare neoplasm is a great challenge for diagnosis and treatment. Although most adult patients have functional tumors, precise physical examination, hormonal evaluation, and imaging studies should be conducted for all suspicious patients to diagnose both functional and non-functional tumors and differentiate them from adrenal adenomas. Despite the lack of information about a certain treatment, surgical resection is recommended as a potentially curative treatment. Adjuvant chemotherapy or radiotherapy should be considered based on staging and histopathologic evaluation after surgery.

References

[1] R. Libé, "Adrenocortical carcinoma (ACC): diagnosis, prognosis, and treatment," *Frontiers in Cell and Developmental Biology*, vol. 3, p. 45, 2015.

[2] A. W. Hsing, J. M. Nam, H. T. Co Chien, J. K. McLaughlin, and J. F. Fraumeni Jr., "Risk factors for adrenal cancer: an exploratory study," *International Journal of Cancer*, vol. 65, no. 4, pp. 432–436, 1996.

[3] T. Else, A. C. Kim, A. Sabolch et al., "Adrenocortical carcinoma," *Endocrine Reviews*, vol. 35, no. 2, pp. 282–326, 2014.

[4] N. Bharwani, A. G. Rockall, A. Sahdev et al., "Adrenocortical carcinoma: the range of appearances on CT and MRI," *American Journal of Roentgenology*, vol. 196, no. 6, pp. W706–W714, 2011.

[5] P. M. Copeland, "The incidentally discovered adrenal mass," *The Endocrinologist*, vol. 9, no. 6, pp. 415–423, 1999.

[6] L. Ng and J. M. Libertino, "Adrenocortical carcinoma: diagnosis, evaluation and treatment," *The Journal of Urology*, vol. 169, no. 1, pp. 5–11, 2003.

[7] S. Aubert, A. Wacrenier, X. Leroy et al., "Weiss system revisited: a clinicopathologic and immunohistochemical study of 49 adrenocortical tumors," *The American Journal of Surgical Pathology*, vol. 26, no. 12, pp. 1612–1619, 2002.

[8] M. Fassnacht, O. M. Dekkers, T. Else et al., "European society of Endocrinology clinical practice guidelines on the management of adrenocortical carcinoma in adults, in collaboration with the European network for the study of adrenal tumors," *European Journal of Endocrinology*, vol. 179, no. 4, pp. G1–G46, 2018.

[9] V. Chortis, *Developing New Diagnostic and Therapeutic Approaches in Adrenocortical Carcinoma*, University of Birmingham, Edgbaston, UK, 2017.

[10] S. Jasim and M. A. Habra, "Management of adrenocortical carcinoma," *Current Oncology Reports*, vol. 21, no. 3, p. 20, 2019.

[11] J. F. H. Pittaway and L. Guasti, "Pathobiology and genetics of adrenocortical carcinoma," *Journal of Molecular Endocrinology*, vol. 62, no. 2, pp. R105–R119, 2019.

[12] J. P. Luton, S. Cerdas, L. Billaud et al., "Clinical features of adrenocortical carcinoma, prognostic factors, and the effect of mitotane therapy," *New England Journal of Medicine*, vol. 322, no. 17, pp. 1195–1201, 1990.

[13] M. D. Wooten and D. K. King, "Adrenal cortical carcinoma. Epidemiology and treatment with mitotane and a review of the literature," *Cancer*, vol. 72, no. 11, pp. 3145–3155, 1993.

[14] C. A. Koch, K. Pacak, and G. P. Chrousos, "The molecular pathogenesis of hereditary and sporadic adrenocortical and adrenomedullary tumors," *Journal of Clinical Endocrinology and Metabolism*, vol. 87, no. 12, pp. 5367–5384, 2002.

[15] B. Allolio and M. Fassnacht, "Adrenocortical carcinoma: clinical update," *Journal of Clinical Endocrinology and Metabolism*, vol. 91, no. 6, pp. 2027–2037, 2006.

[16] W. Arlt, M. Biehl, A. E. Taylor et al., "Urine steroid metabolomics as a biomarker tool for detecting malignancy in adrenal tumors," *Journal of Clinical Endocrinology and Metabolism*, vol. 96, no. 12, pp. 3775–3784, 2011.

[17] N. C. Jhala, D. Jhala, M. A. Eloubeidi et al., "Endoscopic ultrasound-guided fine-needle aspiration biopsy of the adrenal glands: analysis of 24 patients," *Cancer*, vol. 102, no. 5, pp. 308–314, 2004.

[18] S. Puglisi, A. Calabrese, V. Basile et al., "New perspectives for mitotane treatment of adrenocortical carcinoma," *Best Practice & Research Clinical Endocrinology & Metabolism*, vol. 34, no. 3, Article ID 101415, 2020.

[19] B. Polat, M. Fassnacht, L. Pfreundner et al., "Radiotherapy in adrenocortical carcinoma," *Cancer*, vol. 115, no. 13, pp. 2816–2823, 2009.

[20] D. Kasper, A. Fauci, S. Hauser, D. Longo, J. Jameson, and J. Loscalzo, *Harrison's Principles of Internal Medicine*, McGraw-Hill, New York, NY, USA, 2018.

10

Primary Aldosteronism Associated with Multiple Adrenocortical Micronodules in a Patient with Renal Cell Carcinoma

Kazuhito Oba,[1] Yuko Chiba,[1] Yoko Matsuda,[2] Takeshi Kumakawa,[1] Rie Aoyama,[3] Miho Akahoshi,[1] Seiji Hashimoto,[1] Aya Tachibana,[1] Koichi Toyoshima,[1] Remi Kodera,[1] Kenji Toyoshima,[1] Yoshiaki Tamura,[1] Takashi Nagata,[4] Yuto Yamazaki,[5] Hironobu Sasano,[5] and Atsushi Araki[1]

[1]*Departments of Diabetes, Metabolism, and Endocrinology, Tokyo Metropolitan Geriatric Hospital Tokyo, Tokyo, Japan*
[2]*Department of Pathology, Tokyo Metropolitan Geriatric Hospital, Tokyo, Japan*
[3]*Department of Cardiology, Tokyo Metropolitan Geriatric Hospital and Institute of Gerontology, Tokyo, Japan*
[4]*Department of Urology, Tokyo Metropolitan Geriatric Hospital, Tokyo, Japan*
[5]*Department of Pathology, Tohoku University Graduate School of Medicine, Sendai, Japan*

Correspondence should be addressed to Atsushi Araki; aaraki@tmghig.jp

Academic Editor: Toshihiro Kita

A 47-year-old woman with a history of diabetes mellitus (DM) and obesity was admitted to our hospital for glucose control. She was detected to have hypertension (HT) and diagnosed with primary aldosteronism (PA) based on the high level of aldosterone to renin ratio and the results of the upright furosemide-loading test according to the criteria of the Japanese Society of Hypertension (JSH) guidelines. Computed tomography revealed left renal tumor and adrenocortical adenoma. She underwent left nephrectomy and adrenalectomy. The pathological findings were clear-cell renal cell carcinoma (RCC) and nonfunctional adrenocortical adenoma. Her nonneoplastic adrenal tissue histologically revealed CYP11B2-positive multiple adrenocortical micronodules (MNs) and concomitant paradoxical hyperplasia of the zona glomerulosa. Therefore, MNs were thought to be responsible for PA in this patient. After surgery, HT was improved, and the result of upright furosemide-loading test after 12 months of surgery did not fulfill the criteria of PA according to the JSH guidelines. However, the adrenocorticotrophic hormone stimulation test was positive; considering the possibility of slight aldosterone overproduction from the right adrenal gland, the administration of spironolactone was started. Herein, we report a rare case of RCC in conjunction with PA histologically associated with MNs.

1. Introduction

Primary aldosteronism (PA) is a disorder characterized by the excessive production of aldosterone from the adrenal adenoma or hyperplasia, leading to sodium retention, potassium loss, and high blood pressure, thereby causing secondary hypertension, diabetes mellitus (DM), and cardiovascular disease [1]. Previous studies have shown that PA could also be complicated with various malignancies, in particular, renal cell carcinoma (RCC), the incidence of which is associated with aldosterone levels [2]. The aldosterone-mediated upregulation of K-RAS is considered to result in the activation of the Akt and Raf pathways, which leads to tumor proliferation [3], or oxidative stress and DNA damage caused by aldosterone [4] might promote the development of RCC; however, the mechanistic details have remained largely unknown.

In contrast, some previous studies revealed that RCC was associated with adrenal tumors, including unilateral or bilateral adrenal adenoma, adrenal hyperplasia, or metastasis [5–9]. Two cases of unilateral adrenal hyperplasia with contralateral RCC have been reported [10].

PA due to multiple adrenocortical micronodules (MNs) was first reported in 2002 [11]. Subsequently, monoclonal antibodies against cytochrome P450 11B2 (CYP11B2), which recognized the enzymes involved in aldosterone synthesis, were developed [12]. CYP11B2 immunohistochemistry is useful for definitive histopathological diagnosis to detect precisely the lesions responsible for PA, such as aldosterone-producing adenoma (APA), diffuse hyperplasia (DH), and MNs [13]. MNs are defined as the presence of CYP11B2-positive cortical micronodules in the CYP11B2-negative zona glomerulosa (ZG), which has been considered to develop from the aldosterone-producing cell cluster (APCC) [14].

Herein, we report a rare case of RCC in conjunction with PA exhibiting pathological findings of MNs.

2. Case Presentation

A 47-year-old woman with a history of DM and obesity (BMI, 41.7 kg/m^2) was admitted to our hospital for the treatment of DM. Although she did not have a history of hypertension, her systolic and diastolic blood pressures were 144–169 and 82–98 mmHg, respectively, and she had a high aldosterone to renin ratio (ARR), as revealed by 0.9 ng/mL/h of plasma renin activity (PRA) and 201 pg/mL of plasma aldosterone concentration (PAC). Serum potassium and creatinine level were 3.9 mEq/L and 0.60 mg/dl, respectively. She underwent an upright furosemide-loading test; her PRA level after loading was 0.8 ng/mL/h and fulfilled the diagnostic criteria for PA according to the Japanese Society of Hypertension (JSH) guidelines [15]. Furthermore, her adrenocorticotropic hormone (ACTH) stimulation test (intravenous injection of 250 μg of tetracosactide acetate) result was positive because of high PAC max/cortisol ratio (17.6; PAC and cortisol levels were 403 pg/mL and 22.9 μg/dL, respectively) [16]. The ACTH-cortisol system was intact because the plasma ACTH level was 15.3 pg/mL; fasting and late-night serum cortisol levels were 10.7 μg/dL and 3.7 μg/dL, respectively; and the urinary cortisol level was 41.2 μg/day. Serum dehydroepiandrosterone sulfate level was 140 ng/mL, which was within the normal range. Hence, she was diagnosed with hypertension due to PA.

Abdominal computed tomography (CT) revealed a low-density tumor of 45 mm in diameter in the left kidney. In the contrast-enhanced CT, most part of the left renal tumor was enhanced in the arterial phase (Figure 1(a)) and washed out in the venous phase; furthermore, the tumor included a necrotic part, which was not enhanced by the contrast agent. This strongly suggested that the tumor was a RCC. Furthermore, a low-density left adrenocortical tumor of 10 mm in diameter was detected (Figure 1(b)). Adrenal scintigraphy showed no uptake in both the adrenal glands. The ACTH-stimulated adrenal venous sampling was unsuccessful and incomplete. The localization of PA was not known. After detailed explanation was provided, she decided to undergo surgery for the removal of both the left renal tumor and left adrenal gland.

She underwent left radical nephrectomy and left adrenalectomy. The resected left kidney included a well-circumscribed, solid, and yellow-to-red tumor measuring 43 × 39 × 29 mm. The renal tumor was well circumscribed with the fibrous membrane and was entirely composed of clear cells with relatively small round nuclei (Fuhrmann grade: Grade 2). The tumor cells were arranged in a trabecular or solid alveolar pattern with abundant vessels in their stroma (Figure 2). The renal tumor was histopathologically diagnosed as stage I, grade 2 clear-cell RCC (T1bN0M0). Macroscopically, the left adrenal tumor had xanthochromic appearance and measured 11 mm in its greatest dimension. Light microscopic examination revealed that the tumor was predominantly composed of clear cells (Figure 3(a)). Immunoreactivity of steroidogenic factor-1 was detected at the nuclear side of the tumor cells, suggesting that this tumor had originated from the adrenal cortex (data not shown) [17]. Based on the criteria of Weiss [18, 19], we histologically diagnosed the tumor as adrenocortical adenoma. This adenoma was negative for CYP11B2 immunoreactivity (Figure 3(b)), indicating that it did not have the ability to produce aldosterone. Therefore, we concluded that this adenoma was not responsible for PA.

In contrast, CYP11B2-positive MNs measuring less than 2 mm in their greatest dimension were detected predominantly at the subcapsular area of the adrenal cortex (Figure 4(a) and 4(b). The CYP11B2 immunoreactivity was predominantly noted at the subcapsular part of the micronodules and diminished inward. Based on the CYP11B2 immunoreactivity pattern in the micronodules, we considered that their zonation was preserved (Figure 4(c)); therefore, we diagnosed them as nonneoplastic adrenocortical lesions. The nonnodular part of the ZG morphologically revealed hyperplasia, but was negative for CYP11B2 immunoreactivity (Figure 4(a) and 4(b)), consistent with the paradoxical hyperplasia of the ZG, which is frequently detected in the adjacent adrenal cortex of APA [20]. Therefore, MNs were considered to be responsible for PA in this case.

Her postoperative course was uneventful, and she was discharged at 12 days after the surgery. During the follow-up of 6 months, her systolic and diastolic blood pressures and glucose control (HbA1c) were improved to 122–141 mmHg, 70–72 mmHg, and 6.0–6.5%, respectively. Her body weight had also reduced from 106.8 kg to 95.0 kg. However, after the operation, PRA level was still low (mean 0.7 ng/ml/h, range: 0.5–0.9 ng/mL/h), and PAC was relatively high (mean: 267 pg/mL, range: 182–351 pg/mL), so that ARR had a high level (mean: 452 pg/mL/ng/mL/h, range: 202–702 pg/mL/ng/mL/h) in the 2nd month after surgery. Then, spironolactone was administered and continued for 8 months.

She underwent an upright furosemide-loading test and an ACTH stimulation test 12 months after left adrenalectomy and 2 months after discontinuation of spironolactone. Her PRA level after loading was elevated to 3.1 ng/mL/h from 0.3 ng/mL/h (before loading) and did not fulfill the diagnostic criteria for PA as per the JSH guidelines [15]. However, the ACTH stimulation test was positive because of high PAC max/cortisol ratio (10.7; PAC and cortisol levels were 256 pg/mL and 24.0 μg/dL, respectively). Considering the possibility of slight aldosterone overproduction from the right adrenal gland, the administration of spironolactone was started again.

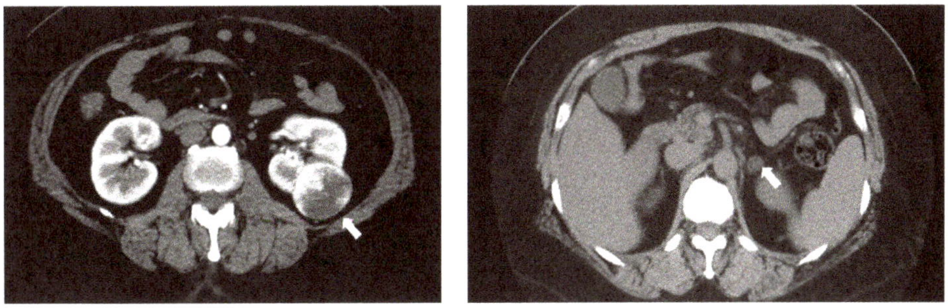

(a) (b)

FIGURE 1: The computed tomographic (CT) findings of the left adrenal tumor. (a) Renal tumor in the arterial phase. Most of the left renal tumor was enhanced using contrast medium, except the necrotic area. (b) Adrenal tumor. The left adrenal tumor was a low-density mass having a diameter of 10 mm and was suspected as adrenocortical adenoma.

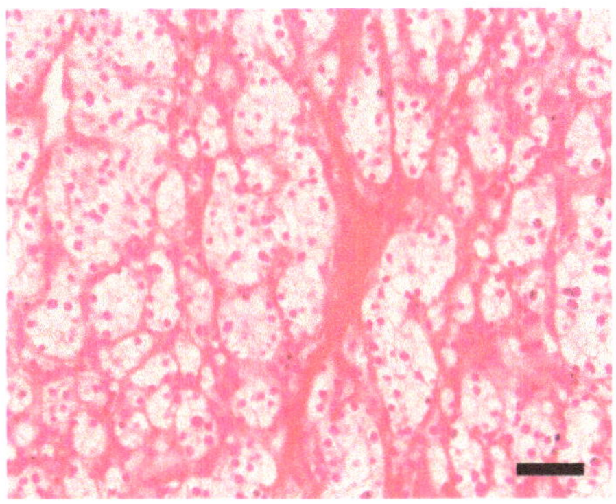

FIGURE 2: Histopathological findings of the renal cell carcinoma. Hematoxylin and eosin staining. The tumor cells had small round nuclei and clear cytoplasm with cell atypia. The tumor cells showed trabecular pattern with abundant vessels in the tumor stroma. These findings were consistent with grade 2 clear-cell renal cell carcinoma. Bar, 50 μm.

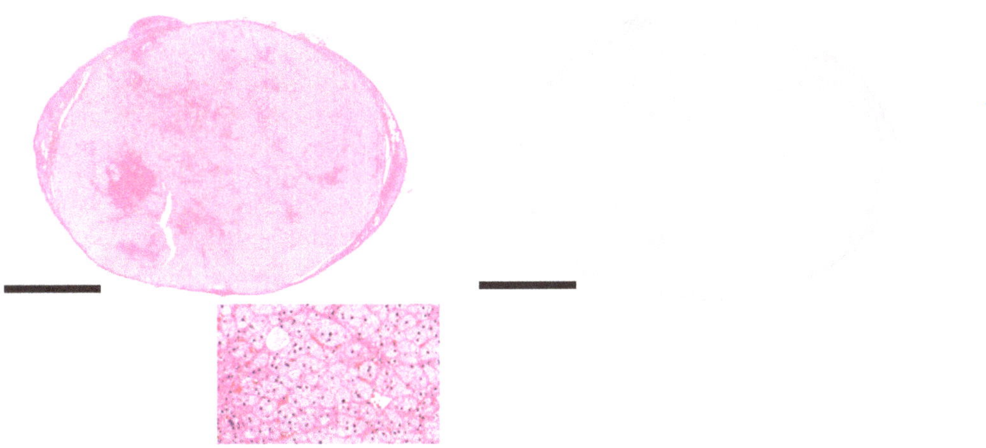

(a) (b)

FIGURE 3: Histopathological findings of the adrenocortical adenoma. (a) Hematoxylin and eosin staining. The adrenocortical tumor was predominantly composed of clear cells. These characteristics are consistent with those of adrenocortical adenoma. Bar, 3 mm. (b) Cytochrome P450 11B2 (CYP11B2) immunostaining. The tumor cells were negative for CYP11B2. Bar, 3 mm.

3. Discussion

We experienced a rare case of RCC in conjunction with PA exhibiting pathological findings of MNs. PA patients are at an increased risk of developing RCC [2]. Lang et al. showed that 5 of 335 patients with PA had RCC (13% of all malignancies), whereas no RCC was detected in the hypertensive controls [2]. Patients with PA were reported to have

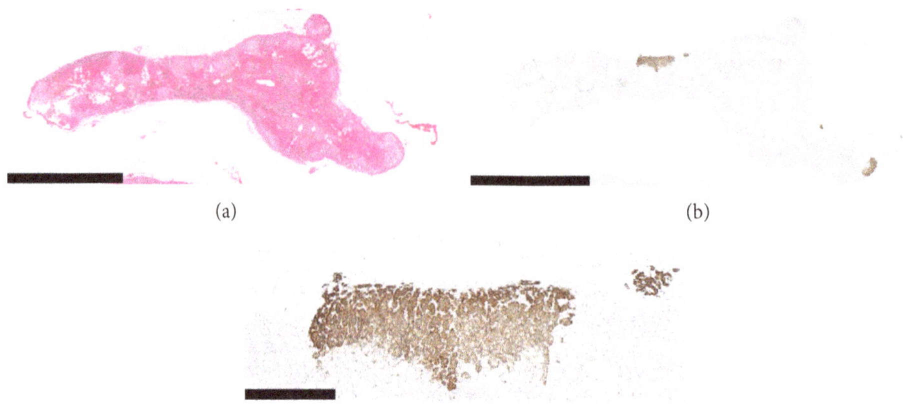

(a) (b) (c)

Figure 4: Histopathological findings of multiple micronodules and hyperplastic lesions in the left adrenal gland. (a) Hematoxylin and eosin staining. Multiple hyperplastic lesions in the left adrenal gland. Bar, 5 mm. (b) CYP11B2 immunostaining. Multiple CYP11B2-positive micronodules were detected predominantly at the subcapsular area of the adrenal cortex and showed preserved zonation. Many CYP11B2-negative hyperplastic cells were detected in the zona glomerulosa; paradoxical hyperplasia of the zona glomerulosa was noted. Bar, 5 mm. (c) CYP11B2 immunostaining. The magnified image of the CYP11B2-positive micronodules shown in (b). The CYP11B2 immunoreactivity waned from the subcapsular area to inward in the micronodules, in which zonation was preserved. Bar, 600 μm.

higher oxidative stress, which could be reduced by treating PA [4]. Previous in vitro and animal model studies suggest that high aldosterone levels can cause oxidative stress, leading to DNA damage [21–23]. In our case, high aldosterone levels could have been involved in the development of RCC. Alternatively, unknown growth factors produced by RCC might promote the growth of adrenal tumors because RCC often produces hormones, growth factors, and inflammatory cytokines such as IL-6 [24].

Because PA is associated with cardio- and cerebrovascular complications and mortality [1], making accurate diagnosis and localizing PA are important because surgically correctable lesions are characterized as unilateral. Primary lesions in PA have been classified as APA, idiopathic hyperaldosteronism (IHA), unilateral adrenal hyperplasia (UAH), primary adrenal hyperplasia (PAH), adrenal cancer, and glucocorticoid-remediable aldosteronism [25]. In addition to these, Omura et al. reported 4 cases of PA due to unilateral MNs in 2002. They concluded that the clinical and pathologic characteristics of unilateral MNs are distinct from those of APA, IHA, UAH, and PAH. Furthermore, PA induced by MNs might be frequently overlooked because MNs cannot always be detected using the standard adrenal CT or scintigraphy [11]. In our case, we could not localize the lesion responsible for PA by using CT and scintigraphy. Because specific monoclonal antibodies, which can accurately distinguish the isoforms of CYP11B1 and CYP11B2 from each other, have been developed, aldosterone-producing cells can be identified using CYP11B2 immunohistochemistry [12], which is considered to be indispensable for the histopathological diagnosis of PA subtypes classified into APA, DH, or MNs [13].

APCC was first revealed as a CYP11B2-positive cell cluster within the ZG area in the nonpathological adrenal gland [26, 27]. However, APCC has been shown to induce PA by using CYP11B2 immunostaining [13]. The APCC from PA was found to be different from that in the nonpathological adrenal gland. The prevalence of somatic mutations in the aldosterone-driver gene in multiple APCCs that caused PA was considerably higher than that in the APCC in the nonpathological adrenal gland. Multiple APCCs might cause PA when 1% of the adrenal cortex becomes positive for CYP11B2 [14]. PA with unilateral or bilateral MNs has been extensively reported [14, 28–30]. Some MN cases have common genetic mutations in *CACNA1D*, *ATP1A1*, *ATP2B3*, and *KCNJ5* to those found in APA cases [14, 26]. MNs might be involved in the genesis of APA through these mutations. Since we did not conduct gene mutation analysis in our case, further research is necessary to clarify this point.

In this study, we did not conduct pathological investigation of the right adrenal gland. After the resection of the left adrenal gland, high blood pressure, hyperglycemia, and body weight control were improved. However, ARR and PAC levels remained high in contrast to low PRA levels after left adrenalectomy. Furthermore, the result of the ACTH stimulation test showed that the PA was not completely cured by left adrenalectomy although the result of upright furosemide-loading test was negative. The ACTH stimulation test has been reported to be useful for the diagnosis of PA with the sensitivity of 98% and the specificity of 91% [16]. These results suggest that the possibility of some overproduction of aldosterone from MNs, micro-APA, or DH from the right adrenal gland cannot be neglected.

Therefore, we started medical treatment with spironolactone after surgery to prevent cardiovascular events and renal function deterioration in the long term. Several studies indicated that both surgical and medical treatment of PA could prevent organ damage and decrease the risk of cardiovascular events and renal disease progression [31]. Careful follow-up is necessary to check for the recurrence of adrenal tumors as well as RCC.

In conclusion, we report a rare case of RCC in conjunction with PA exhibiting pathological findings of MNs. This case was considered to be valuable from the viewpoint of the pathogenesis and treatment of PA due to MNs.

Acknowledgments

The authors thank all staff involved in the examination of the patient. In particular, they thank Mototsune Kakizaki and Keisuke Nonaka who contributed to histopathological diagnosis, Kanae Yoshida who operated on the patient, and Kazuhiro Takeda who performed ACTH-stimulated adrenal venous sampling.

References

[1] J. W. Funder, R. M. Carey, F. Mantero et al., "The management of primary aldosteronism: case detection, diagnosis, and treatment: an endocrine society clinical practice guideline," *The Journal of Clinical Endocrinology & Metabolism*, vol. 101, no. 5, pp. 1889–1916, 2016.

[2] K. Lang, K. Weber, M. Quinkler et al., "Prevalence of malignancies in patients with primary aldosteronism," *The Journal of Clinical Endocrinology & Metabolism*, vol. 101, no. 4, pp. 1656–1663, 2016.

[3] S. King, S. Bray, S. Galbraith, L. Christie, and S. Fleming, "Evidence for aldosterone-dependent growth of renal cell carcinoma," *International Journal of Experimental Pathology*, vol. 95, no. 4, pp. 244–250, 2014.

[4] L. Petramala, P. Pignatelli, R. Carnevale et al., "Oxidative stress in patients affected by primary aldosteronism," *Journal of Hypertension*, vol. 32, no. 10, pp. 2022–2029, 2014.

[5] M. Ambos, M. Bosniak, R. Lefleur, and H. Mitty, "Adrenal adenoma associated with renal cell carcinoma," *American Journal of Roentgenology*, vol. 136, no. 1, pp. 81–84, 1981.

[6] G. Aliaev Iu, N. D. Akhvlediani, and P. S. Blokhin, "Ipsilateral adrenalectomy is not obligatory in nephrectomy for renal cell carcinoma," *Urologiia*, vol. 2, no. 2, pp. 16–22, 2008.

[7] A. Hirose, Y. Okada, A. Fukushima, and Y. Tanaka, "A rare case of primary aldosteronism caused by bilateral functioning adrenocortical adenomas with renal cell carcinoma," *Journal of UOEH*, vol. 27, no. 4, pp. 315–323, 2005.

[8] R. Swiatkowska-Stodulska, E. Swierblewska, J. Zielonko, and K. Sworczak, "[Clear cell carcinoma of the kidney and Conn's syndrome in a patient with arterial hypertension--a case report]," *Wiadomości Lekarskie*, vol. 64, no. 2, pp. 104–108, 2011.

[9] E. Rossi, M. Foroni, G. Regolisti et al., "Combined Conn's syndrome and subclinical hypercortisolism from an adrenal adenoma associated with homolateral renal carcinoma," *American Journal of Hypertension*, vol. 21, no. 11, pp. 1269–1272, 2008.

[10] S. Kudoh, T. Kawaguchi, and T. Suzuki, "Two case reports of unilateral adrenal hyperplasia with contralateral renal cell carcinoma," *The Japanese Journal of Urology*, vol. 91, no. 6, pp. 565–569, 2000.

[11] M. Omura, H. Sasano, T. Fujiwara, K. Yamaguchi, and T. Nishikawa, "Unique cases of unilateral hyperaldosteronemia due to multiple adrenocortical micronodules, which can only be detected by selective adrenal venous sampling," *Metabolism*, vol. 51, no. 3, pp. 350–355, 2002.

[12] C. E. Gomez-Sanchez, X. Qi, C. Velarde-Miranda et al., "Development of monoclonal antibodies against human CYP11B1 and CYP11B2," *Molecular and Cellular Endocrinology*, vol. 383, no. 1-2, pp. 111–117, 2014.

[13] K. Nanba, M. Tsuiki, K. Sawai et al., "Histopathological diagnosis of primary aldosteronism using CYP11B2 immunohistochemistry," *The Journal of Clinical Endocrinology & Metabolism*, vol. 98, no. 4, pp. 1567–1574, 2013.

[14] Y. Yamazaki, Y. Nakamura, K. Omata et al., "Histopathological classification of cross-sectional image-negative hyperaldosteronism," *The Journal of Clinical Endocrinology and Metabolism*, vol. 102, no. 4, pp. 1182–1192, 2016.

[15] K. Shimamoto, K. Ando, T. Fujita et al., "The Japanese society of hypertension guidelines for the management of hypertension (JSH 2014)," *Hypertension Research*, vol. 37, no. 4, pp. 253–390, 2014.

[16] M. Omura and T. Nishikawa, "Screening tests and diagnostic examinations of hypertensives for primary aldosteronism," *Rinsho Byori The Japanese Journal of Clinical Pathology*, vol. 54, no. 11, pp. 1157–1163, 2006, (in jpn).

[17] R. El-Khairi and J. Achermann, "Steroidogenic factor-1 and human disease," *Seminars in Reproductive Medicine*, vol. 30, no. 5, pp. 374–381, 2012.

[18] L. M. Weiss, L. J. Medeiros, and A. L. Vickery Jr., "Pathologic features of prognostic significance in adrenocortical carcinoma," *The American Journal of Surgical Pathology*, vol. 13, no. 3, pp. 202–206, 1989.

[19] S. Aubert, A. Wacrenier, X. Leroy et al., "Weiss system revisited," *The American Journal of Surgical Pathology*, vol. 26, no. 12, pp. 1612–1619, 2002.

[20] H. Sasano, M. Okamoto, and N. Sasano, "Immunohistochemical study of cytochrome P-$450_{11}\beta$-hydroxylase in human adrenal cortex with mineralo-and glucocorticoid excess," *Virchows Archiv A Pathological Anatomy and Histopathology*, vol. 413, no. 4, pp. 313–318, 1988.

[21] N. Queisser, P. I. Oteiza, H. Stopper, R. G. Oli, and N. Schupp, "Aldosterone induces oxidative stress, oxidative DNA damage and NF-κB-activation in kidney tubule cells," *Molecular Carcinogenesis*, vol. 50, no. 2, pp. 123–135, 2011.

[22] N. Queisser, N. Schupp, H. Stopper, R. Schinzel, and P. I. Oteiza, "Aldosterone increases kidney tubule cell oxidants through calcium-mediated activation of NADPH oxidase and nitric oxide synthase," *Free Radical Biology and Medicine*, vol. 51, no. 11, pp. 1996–2006, 2011.

[23] N. Queisser, K. Amann, V. Hey, S. L. Habib, and N. Schupp, "Blood pressure has only minor influence on aldosterone-induced oxidative stress and DNA damage in vivo," *Free Radical Biology and Medicine*, vol. 54, pp. 17–25, 2013.

[24] K. Kamińska, A. M. Czarnecka, B. Escudier, F. Lian, and C. Szczylik, "Interleukin-6 as an emerging regulator of renal cell cancer," *Urologic Oncology: Seminars and Original Investigations*, vol. 33, no. 11, pp. 476–485, November 2015.

[25] A. Ganguly, "Primary aldosteronism," *New England Journal of Medicine*, vol. 339, no. 25, pp. 1828–1834, 1998.

[26] K. Nishimoto, K. Nakagawa, D. Li et al., "Adrenocortical zonation in humans under normal and pathological conditions," *The Journal of Clinical Endocrinology & Metabolism*, vol. 95, no. 5, pp. 2296–2305, 2010.

[27] K. Nishimoto, S. A. Tomlins, R. Kuick et al., "Aldosterone-stimulating somatic gene mutations are common in normal adrenal glands," *Proceedings of the National Academy of Sciences*, vol. 112, no. 33, pp. E4591–E4599, 2015.

[28] Y. Hirono, M. Doi, T. Yoshimoto et al., "A case with primary aldosteronism due to unilateral multiple adrenocortical micronodules," *Endocrine Journal*, vol. 52, no. 4, pp. 435–439, 2005.
[29] A. Ito, Y. Yamazaki, H. Sasano et al., "A case of primary aldosteronism caused by unilateral multiple adrenocortical micronodules presenting as muscle cramps at rest: the importance of functional histopathology for identifying a culprit lesion," *Pathology International*, vol. 67, no. 4, pp. 214–221, 2017.
[30] K. Nishimoto, T. Seki, I. Kurihara et al., "Case report: nodule development from subcapsular aldosterone-producing cell clusters causes hyperaldosteronism," *The Journal of Clinical Endocrinology & Metabolism*, vol. 101, no. 1, pp. 6–9, 2016.
[31] L. A. Sechi, G. Colussi, A. Di Fabio, and C. Catena, "Cardiovascular and renal damage in primary aldosteronism: outcomes after treatment," *American Journal of Hypertension*, vol. 23, no. 12, pp. 1253–1260, 2010.

11

Clinical Characteristics and Treatment Outcomes in Endogenous Cushing's Syndrome: A 15-Year Experience from Thailand

Wasita Warachit Parksook,[1,2] **Nitchakarn Laichuthai**,[2] **and Sarat Sunthornyothin**[2]

[1]*Division of General Internal Medicine, Department of Medicine, Faculty of Medicine, Chulalongkorn University, and King Chulalongkorn Memorial Hospital, Thai Red Cross Society, Patumwan, Bangkok 10330, Thailand*
[2]*Division of Endocrinology and Metabolism, Department of Medicine, and Hormonal and Metabolic Research Unit, Excellence Center in Diabetes, Hormone and Metabolism, Faculty of Medicine, Chulalongkorn University, and King Chulalongkorn Memorial Hospital, Thai Red Cross Society, Patumwan, Bangkok 10330, Thailand*

Correspondence should be addressed to Sarat Sunthornyothin; saratmd@gmail.com

Academic Editor: Eli Hershkovitz

The most common subtype of endogenous Cushing's syndrome (CS) is Cushing's disease (CD), with higher proportions of adrenal CS reported from Asia, compared to other continents. However, little was known about CS in this territory. This study was to investigate the distribution, clinical characteristics, and treatment outcomes of CS in a single tertiary hospital in Thailand. We performed a retrospective evaluation of 82 patients with endogenous CS during 2001–2015. The most common subtype was CD, followed by adrenal CS and ectopic ACTH syndrome (EAS), respectively. Weight gain was the most common presentation. Normal body mass index (BMI), Asian cutoff, was observed in 33% of patients. Specific features of CS (plethora, muscle weakness, bruising, and/or wide purplish striae) were documented in less than half of patients. The median age, adrenocorticotropic hormone (ACTH), and urinary free cortisol (UFC) concentrations were significantly different among 3 subtypes of CS and were highest among patients with EAS. An initial remission rate after transsphenoidal surgeries in CD was 62%, with higher rates in pituitary microadenomas compared to macroadenomas. All patients with unilateral adrenal disease achieved CS remission after adrenal surgeries. Patients with EAS achieved CS remission mostly from bilateral adrenalectomy. The highest mortality rate was observed in the EAS group. These findings were consistent with previous studies in Asia, with more proportions ACTH-independent CS.

1. Introduction

Cushing's syndrome (CS) is a state of excessive endogenous cortisol secretion. It is rare, with an estimated prevalence of 40 cases per million and an incidence of 0.7–2.4 cases per million per year [1–3]. It is more common in women and can occur at any age, even though it tends to occur during the fourth to sixth decades of life [1–3]. Worldwide, the most common cause of CS is Cushing's disease (CD), followed by adrenal CS and ectopic ACTH syndrome (EAS) [1–4]. CS is associated with deleterious effects to health [5]. A 5-year mortality rate in active CS was around 50% due to infection and cardiovascular complications in 1952 [6]. In 1979, mortality rates markedly decreased due to combination treatment [7]. Restoring eucortisolism leads to clinical and biochemical improvement regarding metabolic disturbances, bone health, immune dysfunction, hypercoagulable state, and quality of life.

Studies in Asia showed higher distribution of adrenal CS, ranging from 20–75% of CS etiology [8–12]. Outcomes of CS treatment varied among subtypes and studies. There was only one small case series from the region of Southeast Asia [10]. To date, little is known regarding CS in this region. Therefore, our primary objective is to investigate the distribution of CS in a single tertiary hospital in Thailand. Secondary objectives are to investigate clinical presentations, management, and treatment outcomes of CS in our center.

2. Materials and Methods

We performed a retrospective study in a tertiary referral hospital, King Chulalongkorn Memorial Hospital (KCMH), Bangkok, Thailand. All patients aged 18 years and over with the diagnosis of CS between the year 2001 and 2015 were included, using the ICD-10 codes for CS (E24). Description synonyms were adrenal CS, CD, CS myopathy, hypercortisolism, pituitary-dependent hypercortisolism, and pituitary-dependent CD. Diagnostic criteria that suggest CS were urinary free cortisol (UFC) concentration greater than the normal range for the assay, serum cortisol greater than 50 nmol/L after an overnight/low-dose dexamethasone suppression test (DST), and/or elevated late-night salivary cortisol (LNSC) [13]. Patients with a history of exogenous steroid use were excluded. This study protocol was approved by the local ethics committee.

2.1. Definitions. Patients with blood pressure from 140/90 mmHg, self-reported history of hypertension or taking antihypertensive agents were classified as hypertensive. Diabetes mellitus (DM) was diagnosed according to the guideline [14]. Patients with fasting plasma glucose (FPG) ≥7.0 mmol/L or HbA1C ≥6.5% or 2-hour glucose ≥11.1 mmol/L during oral glucose tolerance test (OGTT) or having treatment with antidiabetic medications were classified as diabetes. Impair fasting glucose (IFG) was defined if fasting glucose ranged from 5.6–6.9 mmol/L. Impaired glucose tolerance (IGT) was defined if a 2-hour glucose during OGTT was 7.8–11.0 mmol/L. Dyslipidemia was defined if triglyceride (TG) ≥1.7 mmol/L or low density lipoprotein (LDL) ≥3.4 mmol/L or high density lipoprotein (HDL) <1.0 mmol/L in men or <1.3 mmol/L in women or total cholesterol (TC) ≥5.2 mmol/L or having treatment with lipid-lowering agents. Venous thromboembolism (VTE) was defined as having an evidence of clot or thrombosis at any sites proven by relevant imaging. Normal body weight was classified as body mass index (BMI) of less than 23 kg/m^2 according to the World Health Organization (WHO) classification for Asians. Remission from CS was considered in only patients with both clinical and biochemical remission. Clinical remission of CS was defined by the disappearance of Cushing's stigmata (wide purplish striae, proximal muscle weakness, plethora, or bruising). Biochemical remission was defined as the need for glucocorticoid replacement or achieving normalization of dexamethasone suppression serum cortisol (<50 nmol/L) and/or UFC excretion (<414 nmol/day). Recurrence was defined if patient developed clinical signs and symptoms of overt CS after any previous remission, as well as UFC greater than the normal range for the assay, serum cortisol greater than 50 nmol/L after an overnight/low-dose DST, and/or elevated LNSC. Persistent CS was failure to demonstrate remission after treatment.

2.2. Biochemical Measurements. ACTH and serum cortisol samples were collected between 7 and 9 AM and were measured with chemiluminescent immunometric assay (Immulite/Siemens). UFC was measured with radioimmunoassay (Immulite/Siemens). All other biochemical variables were assayed in the central laboratory of KCMH, using standardized analytical methods.

2.3. Preoperative Imaging Analysis and/or Procedures. Magnetic resonance imaging (MRI) of pituitary gland was done in all patients with CD. A microadenoma was defined as an adenoma sized less than 1 cm. A macroadenoma was defined as an adenoma sized from or greater than 1 cm. Adrenal imaging using either computed tomography (CT) or MRI was done in all patients with adrenal CS.

Patients with EAS underwent CT scans of the neck, chest, abdomen, and pelvis or octreotide scans. Inferior petrosal sinus sampling (IPSS) and/or high-dose dexamethasone suppression test (HDDST) were done in patients with ACTH-dependent CS with inconclusive pituitary imaging.

2.4. Treatment. All procedures were performed by physicians in KCMH. Patients with CD underwent transsphenoidal surgery (TSS) with selective adenomectomy by neurosurgeons. Biochemical remission was defined as postoperative cortisol <138 nmol/L within 7 days after the surgery. Delayed remission was defined as hypocortisolemia (morning cortisol <138 nmol/L) or achieving normalization of dexamethasone suppression serum cortisol (<50 nmol/L) and/or UFC excretion (<414 nmol/day) within 30 days after the surgery. Patients with either persistent or recurrent Cushing's after initial TSS received second-line therapeutic options (surgery, medications, and/or radiotherapy). Patients with adrenal CS underwent unilateral adrenalectomy by urologists, followed by glucocorticoid replacement in unilateral cortisol-secreting adrenal adenomas. Subsequent adrenalectomy was done in patients with bilateral diseases and had persistent hypercortisolism. Patients with EAS underwent surgical removal if tumor localizations were successful. Patients with occult or metastatic EAS were treated with either medications or bilateral adrenalectomy as initial managements.

2.5. Statistical Analysis. Since the data were nonnormally distributed, continuous variables were presented as medians with interquartile range (IQR). Group comparisons were examined with Kruskal–Wallis test for nonparametric testing or Chi-squared tests. A p value of less than 0.05 was considered to be statistically significant. Statistical analysis was performed with SPSS statistics version 22.0.

3. Results

3.1. Subtypes of CS. There were 82 patients diagnosed with CS. There were 58 patients with unsuppressed DST, while the rest had UFC excretion greater than the normal range. None of our patients were diagnosed using LNSC because the test was unavailable at our institution at that time. None of our patients were taking medications that could affect the hypothalamic-pituitary-adrenal (HPA) axis at the time of testing. These medications included strong CYP3A4 inducers or inhibitors, oral contraceptive pills, and medical therapies used in clinical practice for the treatment of CS. The most common subtype was CD (45%), followed by adrenal CS (32%) and EAS (13%). All patients with CD had benign ACTH-producing pituitary adenomas. For adrenal CS, the most common etiology was unilateral cortisol-producing adrenal adenoma (62%). Malignant adrenal tumors accounted for 15% of adrenal CS. Primary tumors in patients with EAS comprised both benign and malignant process. Almost half of primary tumors (45%) originated from thorax (Table 1).

3.2. *Clinical Features.* Weight gain was the most common presentation (Table 2). Moon face and/or supraclavicular fullness were present in most patients, while more specific features of CS (facial plethora, wide purplish striae, easy bruising, or proximal muscle weakness) were documented in less than half of patients. Of the 12 CD patients with available data on sex hormones prior to surgery, 4 patients had hypogonadotrophic hypogonadism. There were no CD patients with preoperative central hypothyroidism; 32 patients had normal thyroid function tests, and none had preoperative thyroid hormone supplement. The median age, ACTH, and UFC concentrations were significantly different among 3 subtypes of CS. These parameters were highest among patients with EAS. Duration between onset of symptoms to the diagnosis of CS and follow-up time was shortest among EAS, but was not significantly different compared with CD and adrenal CS (Table 3). ACTH concentrations were highest in the EAS group (Figure 1). The median ACTH concentrations were 68.9 (IQR 14.8–133.7), 15.0 (IQR 10.8–26.0) pmol/L in patients with EAS and CD, respectively. Most patients (62%) with adrenal CS had ACTH level below 2.2 pmol/L. Four patients with ACTH level greater than 4.4 pmol/L had apparent adrenal diseases and developed postoperative adrenal insufficiency.

3.3. *Treatment.* In CD, an overall remission rate after initial transsphenoidal surgeries was 62% (Table 4). ACTH-positive adenomas were confirmed in 31 patients, while Crooke's hyaline changes were documented in 3 patients. Normal pituitary tissue was documented in 9 patients, and 7 of them had an initial remission after TSS. Patients with pituitary microadenomas had better remission rates which were 68%, compared to 45% in patients with macroadenomas. The median time to recurrence was 23 months (range 12–39 months), with an overall recurrence rate after an initial remission of 13%. The median time to recovery of the HPA axis after TSS was 14 months (IQR 6–24); 10 months (range 6–17 months) in patients with recurrence, and 18 months (IQR 7–27) in the patients without recurrence). In patients with recurrence or persistent CD, 12 patients underwent repeat TSS. Medications were used prior to the subsequent TSS in 8 patients, which were ketoconazole, pasireotide, and mitotane. Nonfatal hepatitis occurred in 1 patient using ketoconazole. Bilateral adrenalectomy was done in 2 patients. There was no report of Nelson's syndrome in both patients during an 80-month follow-up time. Postoperative complications of TSS were found in 30 patients (67%); the most common complications were hypopituitarism (46%), diabetes insipidus (42%), and cerebrospinal fluid leakage (27%). These complications occurred after the first TSS in 25 patients. There was neither report of adrenal crisis nor venous thromboembolism.

All patients with unilateral cortisol-producing, aldosterone- and cortisol-cosecreting and ACC had postoperative adrenal insufficiency, while 3 out of 4 patients with either PPNAD or PBMAH underwent second contralateral adrenal surgery within 1 year after the first surgery due to

Table 1: Subtypes of CS.

Etiology	*n* (%)
CD	45 (55)
Pituitary microadenoma	34
Pituitary macroadenoma	11
Adrenal CS	26 (32)
Cortisol-producing adenoma	16
ACC	4
Aldosterone-and cortisol-cosecreting adenoma	2
PBMAH	2
PPNAD	2
EAS	11 (13)
Pulmonary	6
Small cell lung cancer	2
Carcinoid (bronchial and thymic)	3
Neuroendocrine tumor, unspecified	1
Abdomen	2
Pancreatic neuroendocrine tumor	1
Pheochromocytoma	1
MTC	1
Uncertain	2

CS, Cushing's syndrome; CD, Cushing's disease; ACC, adrenocortical carcinoma; PBMAH, primary bilateral macronodular adrenal hyperplasia; PPNAD, primary pigmented nodular adrenocortical disease; EAS, ectopic ACTH syndrome; and MTC, medullary thyroid carcinoma.

Table 2: Clinical features of CS.

Features	Frequency (%)
Overweight and obesity	67
Weight gain	63
BMI <23 kg/m^2	33
Amenorrhea	30
Moon face	72
Supraclavicular fullness	54
Dorsocervical fat pad	43
Wide purplish striae	37
Proximal muscle weakness	24
Facial plethora	21
Easy bruising	21
Dyslipidemia	73
Hypertension	68
DM	29
IFG	11
Osteoporosis/fracture	9
Low bone mass/osteopenia	6

BMI, body mass index; DM, diabetes mellitus; IFG, impair fasting glucose.

TABLE 3: Clinical characteristics of patients according to different subtypes of CS.

Features	CD ($n = 45$)	Adrenal CS ($n = 26$)	EAS ($n = 11$)	p value
Age (years)	33 (28–43)	40 (29–53)	48 (45–64)	0.003
Female (n, %)	37 (82)	22 (85)	7 (64)	0.308
Onset of symptoms (months)	12 (7–24)	12 (5–24)	7 (3–12)	0.427
Hypertension (n, %)	29 (64)	20 (77)	7 (64)	0.519
DM (n, %)	14 (31)	7 (27)	3 (27)	0.921
VTE (n, %)	1 (2)	1 (4)	2 (18)	0.085
Hypokalemia (n, %)	9 (20)	9 (35)	5 (45)	0.149
Morning cortisol (nmol/L)	690 (497–828)	690 (469–745)	1269 (1131–1738)	0.052
UFC (nmol/day)	1593 (759–2616)	378 (113–1673)	3003 (2089–13794)	0.013
Follow-up time (months)	42 (18–75)	32 (11–57)	5 (2–65)	0.174

Data were expressed in median (interquartile range). CS, Cushing's syndrome; CD, Cushing's disease; EAS, ectopic ACTH syndrome; DM, diabetes mellitus; VTE, venous thromboembolism; UFC, urinary free cortisol.

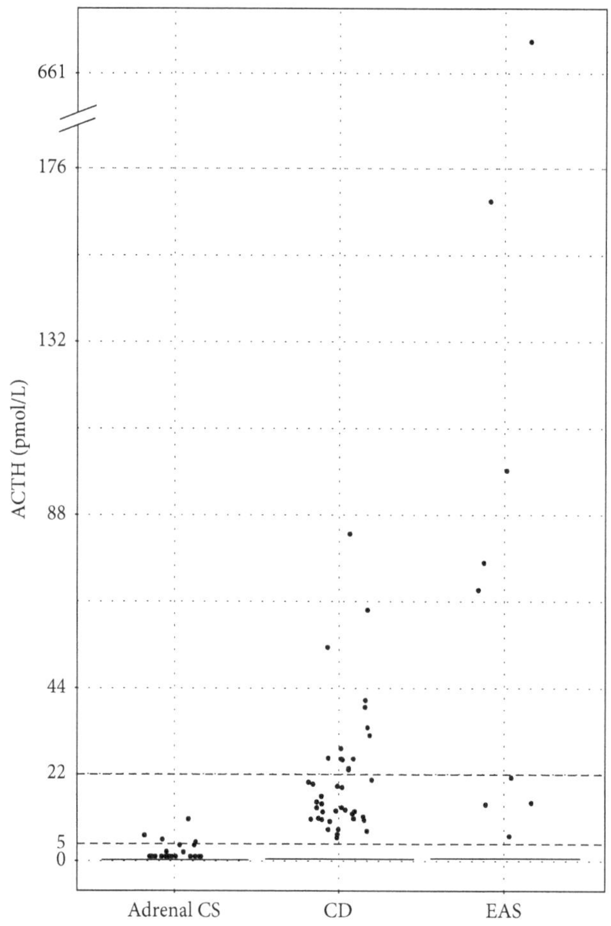

FIGURE 1: Scatter plots of the median ACTH concentrations. ACTH, adrenocorticotropic hormone; CS, Cushing's syndrome; CD, Cushing's disease; and EAS, ectopic ACTH syndrome.

TABLE 4: Treatment outcome in patients with CD.

	Outcome after initial TSS with selective adenomectomy			Remission after multiple surgeries and/or radiation (n)
	Remission (n)	Recurrent (n)	Persistent (n)	
Microadenomas ($n = 34$)	23	4	11	6
Macroadenomas ($n = 11$)	5	2	5	1

CD, Cushing's disease; TSS, transsphenoidal surgery.

TABLE 5: Clinical characteristics and treatment outcome in patients with ectopic ACTH syndrome.

No.	Age	Sex	Primary site	Metastasis	MRI	IPSS	CT	Medication	Outcome	Follow-up (months)
1	77	F	NA	—	—	+	—	Ketoconazole	Bilateral ADX	65
2	46	F	NA	—	+	+	—	Ketoconazole	Failure	2
3	47	F	Bronchial carcinoid	—	—	+	+	Ketoconazole	Cured	124
4	39	F	Thymic carcinoid	—		+	—	—	Bilateral ADX	125
5	35	F	Pancreatic NET	Liver	+	+	+	—	NA	5
6	51	M	Small cell lung cancer	Liver, adrenal		NA	—	Ketoconazole	Bilateral ADX	33
7	48	M	Medullary thyroid carcinoma	Liver, lung		—	—	Ketoconazole	Bilateral ADX	1
8	44	M	Small cell lung cancer	Liver		—	+	—	Death	3
9	75	M	NET, unspecified	Liver		—	—	—	Death	NA
10	52	F	Bronchial carcinoid	—	+	—	+	Ketoconazole	Death	NA
11	77	F	Pheochromocytoma	—		—	—	Etomidate	Death	1

F, female; M, male; NA, nonspecified; MRI, magnetic resonance imaging; IPSS, inferior petrosal sinus sampling; CT, computed tomography; ADX, adrenalectomy; AI, adrenal insufficiency; NET, neuroendocrine tumor.

persistent CS. Among patients with postoperative adrenal insufficiency, 8 patients had been followed up at our institute, and the median time to recovery of the HPA axis was 18 months (IQR 12–25). In patients with EAS, CS remission was achieved in 5 patients (45%), mostly from bilateral adrenalectomy (Table 5). There was only 1 patient who was cured after bronchial carcinoid resection. During a median follow-up of 5 months, 4 patients (36%) died, and 5 patients (45%) lost follow-up while having persistent CS.

4. Discussion

We reported a large and comprehensive study on CS in Southeast Asia. The most common subtypes of CS were CD, followed by adrenal CS and EAS. It was more common in female (80%). Usual presentations of the syndrome were weight gain and metabolic complications regarding hypertension and dyslipidemia. The median age, ACTH, and UFC concentrations were significantly different among 3 different subtypes of CS, all of which were highest in patients with EAS.

Consistent with previous studies, the female was predominant in every subtype of CS, with more proportion of male in patients with EAS as in previous reports [15, 16]. Regarding the distribution of CS, proportions of adrenal CS were comparable with studies from Philippines and China, but not as high as studies from Japan and Taiwan (Table 6) [8–12]. It supports a higher prevalence of ACTH-independent CS compared with data from other continents [17–19]. Adrenal adenomas were the most common etiology of adrenal CS in most studies, including ours. Although Ammini et al. reported a higher number of patients with ACC than adrenal adenomas from a single center in India, the author discussed that referral bias might have explained the findings [8]. With an increase in number of abdominal imaging performed these days, an incidentally-discovered adrenal mass was another presentation of adrenal CS, especially in patients with mild CS. However, all of our patients with adrenal CS had obvious clinical manifestations of cortisol excess.

Compared to other studies, weight gain was also a usual presentation, but 33% of our patients still had normal BMI even by Asian standard according to WHO classification [10, 16, 19, 20]. Therefore, being normal weight was not uncommon for CS in Thailand. Hypertension and dyslipidemia were the most common metabolic derangements. Frequency of these comorbidities was comparable with the previous study [8, 16]. Prevalence of DM in this study was less than previous reports which could have been from different testing procedure [8, 9, 16]. Since we did not perform OGTT in every patient, the number of patients with DM might have been underestimated. Only 20–40% of patients were documented having clinical features with more discriminant index of CS which include facial plethora, easy bruising, proximal muscle weakness, and wide purplish striae. Earlier study reported these signs in 56–88% of patients [20]. We could explain this frequency from incomplete documentation and failure to identify these signs from physical examinations. Asian skin could hardly explain this due to inconsistent results from the Philippines showing the percentage of patients having these clinical signs of 50–80% [10]. Hyperpigmentation, which was reported in around 20% of patients with EAS, was also not reported in our series [15, 21].

Regarding the study in by Reynolds et al., cortisol levels in Asians were lower than Europeans with CS [22]. The median serum cortisol level in our study was 717 nmol/L (IQR 500–1081), and the median urinary free cortisol was 1593 nmol/day (IQR 544–2616). Cortisol levels in our patients were higher than Asians' levels in the mentioned study. However, other studies in Asia, e.g., Ammini et al. and Edward N. Lo et al. demonstrated comparable levels of cortisol to our study.

In adrenal CS, there were 4 patients with ACTH concentrations of greater than 4.4 pmol/L. One patient was diagnosed with carcinoma while having an ACTH level of 10.6 pmol/L before undergoing adrenal surgery. Since adrenal insufficiency occurred after unilateral adrenalectomy in all patients with detectable ACTH. ACTH assay interference is the most likely explanation for this finding.

The median remission rate after an initial TSS in CD was 79% (range 25–100%) from a systematic review which included 6869 patients from different countries, including the studies from Japan and Korea [23, 24]. Higher initial remission and lower recurrence were more common in microadenoma than the macroadenoma subgroup.

Table 6: Subtypes of CS and gender distribution: comparison with published studies.

Studies	Number of patients	Female (*n*, %)	CD (*n*, %)	Adrenal CS (*n*, %)	EAS (*n*, %)	Uncertain (*n*, %)
Orth [17] (USA, 1995)	630	NA	428 (68)	120 (19)	76 (12)	—
Imai et al. [11] (Japan, 1996)	122	99 (79)	30 (25)	88 (72)	4 (3)	—
Invitti et al. [18] (Italy, 1999)	426	345 (76)	288 (67)	113 (26)	25 (6)	—
Valassi et al. [19] (European registry, 2011)	481	390 (81)	317 (66)	130 (27)	24 (5)	10 (2)
Lo et al. [10] (Philipines, 2013)	19	17 (89)	8 (42)	7 (37)	4 (21)	—
Tung et al. [12] (Taiwan, 2013)	84	62 (78)	18 (21)	63 (75)	3 (4)	—
Ammini et al. [8] (India, 2018)	364	250 (69)	215 (59)	71 (20)	22 (6)	56 (15)
Zhou et al. [9] (China, 2019)	1652	1289 (78)	1040 (63)	494 (30)	98 (6)	20 (1)
This study	82	65 (79)	45 (55)	26 (32)	11 (13)	—

CS, Cushing's syndrome; CD, Cushing's disease; EAS, ectopic ACTH syndrome.

Compared to studies from Japan and Korea, our remission rate was lower, but had higher proportion of macroadenomas [24, 25]. There was no report of Nelson's syndrome as this specific condition increases with longer follow-up time. Treatment outcome in adrenal CS was better than other subtypes of CS, with most patients had remission after their first surgeries. The median time to recovery of the HPA axis in CD and adrenal CS in our study were comparable with the previous study [26]. Adrenal function in CD patients with recurrence after initial remission recovered earlier than in patients without recurrence. For EAS, 36% of our patients underwent bilateral adrenalectomy. Ilias et al. also reported the same rate of bilateral adrenalectomy of 36% in patients with EAS in the National Institutes of Health (NIH) cohort [15]. Mortality rates were highest among this subtype of CS. It might have been higher since a number of patients were lost to follow-up before cured.

This was the largest study done in the region of Southeast Asia. Our study demonstrated clinical profiles and treatment outcomes in all subtypes of CS. Limitations were due to study design which was retrospective in nature. Moreover, referral bias might have occurred because this study was done in a single tertiary care setting. Characteristics of patients may differ from those in the national study. This requires a further national cohort.

5. Conclusions

In conclusion, this study reported clinical characteristics and treatment outcomes of CS in a tertiary referral center in Thailand. The distribution of CS subtypes was the same as previous studies in Asia, with more proportions of patients with ACTH-independent CS. Common presentations were weight gain, hypertension, and dyslipidemia. Most patients were obese, but a number of patients still had normal body weight. Remission rate was highest in patients with adrenal CS, compared to CD and EAS. Patients with EAS had the highest mortality rate and proportions of having bilateral adrenalectomy to alleviate severe hypercortisolism. However, a multicenter study is needed to better understand the natural history and treatment outcomes of CS in Thailand.

Acknowledgments

The authors would like to thank all the colleagues in the Division of Endocrinology and Metabolism, Department of Medicine, Faculty of Medicine, Chulalongkorn University, for all the support.

References

[1] C. Steffensen, A. M. Bak, K. Z. Rubeck, and J. O. L. Jørgensen, "Epidemiology of cushing's syndrome," *Neuroendocrinology*, vol. 92, no. 1, pp. 1–5, 2010.

[2] R. Pivonello, M. C. De Martino, M. De Leo, G. Lombardi, and A. Colao, "Cushing's syndrome," *Endocrinology and Metabolism Clinics of North America*, vol. 37, no. 1, pp. 135–149, 2008.

[3] J. Newell-Price, X. Bertagna, A. B. Grossman, and L. K. Nieman, "Cushing's syndrome," *The Lancet*, vol. 367, no. 9522, pp. 1605–1617, 2006.

[4] L. K. Nieman, B. M. K. Biller, J. W. Findling et al., "Treatment of cushing's syndrome: an endocrine society clinical practice guideline," *The Journal of Clinical Endocrinology & Metabolism*, vol. 100, no. 8, pp. 2807–2831, 2015.

[5] R. Pivonello, A. M. Isidori, M. C. De Martino, J. Newell-Price, B. M. K. Biller, and A. Colao, "Complications of cushing's syndrome: state of the art," *The Lancet Diabetes & Endocrinology*, vol. 4, no. 7, pp. 611–629, 2016.

[6] C. M. Plotz, A. I. Knowlton, and C. Ragan, "The natural history of cushing's syndrome," *The American Journal of Medicine*, vol. 13, no. 5, pp. 597–614, 1952.

[7] P. R. Cooper and W. A. Shucart, "Treatment of cushing's disease with o, p'-DDD," *The New England Journal of Medicine*, vol. 301, no. 1, pp. 48-49, 1979.

[8] A. Ammini, M. Barua, S. Bhattacarya et al., "Etiology and clinical profile of patients with cushing's syndrome: a single center experience," *Indian Journal of Endocrinology and Metabolism*, vol. 18, no. 1, pp. 99–105, 2014.

[9] J. Zhou, M. Zhang, and X. Bai, "Demographic characteristics, etiology, and comorbidities of patients with cushing's syndrome: a 10-year retrospective study at a large general hospital in China," *International Journal of Endocrinology*, vol. 2019, Article ID 7159696, 10 pages, 2019.

[10] T. E. N. Lo, J. M. Cabradilla, S. A. Lim, and C. A. Jimeno, "Endogenous cushing's syndrome: the Phillippine general hospital experience," *Journal of Solid Tumors*, vol. 4, no. 1, 2014.

[11] T. Imai, H. Funahashi, Y. Tanaka et al., "Adrenalectomy for treatment of cushing syndrome: results in 122 patients and long-term follow-up studies," *World Journal of Surgery*, vol. 20, no. 7, pp. 781–787, 1996.
[12] S. C. Tung, P. W. Wang, R. T. Liu et al., "Clinical characteristics of endogenous cushing's syndrome at a medical center in southern Taiwan," *International Journal of Endocrinology*, vol. 2013, Article ID 685375, 7 pages, 2013.
[13] L. K. Nieman, B. M. K. Biller, J. W. Findling et al., "The diagnosis of cushing's syndrome: an endocrine society clinical practice guideline," *The Journal of Clinical Endocrinology & Metabolism*, vol. 93, no. 5, pp. 1526–1540, 2008.
[14] American Diabetes Association, "2. Classification and diagnosis of diabetes: standards of medical care in diabetes-2019," *Diabetes Care*, vol. 42, no. Supplement 1, pp. S13–S28, 2019.
[15] I. Ilias, D. J. Torpy, K. Pacak, N. Mullen, R. A. Wesley, and L. K. Nieman, "Cushing's syndrome due to ectopic corticotropin secretion: twenty years' experience at the National Institutes of Health," *The Journal of Clinical Endocrinology & Metabolism*, vol. 90, no. 8, pp. 4955–4962, 2005.
[16] E. Ross and D. C. Linch, "Cushing's syndrome? Killing disease: discriminatory value of signs and symptoms aiding early diagnosis," *The Lancet*, vol. 320, no. 8299, pp. 646–649, 1982.
[17] D. N. Orth, "Cushing's syndrome," *New England Journal of Medicine*, vol. 332, no. 12, pp. 791–803, 1995.
[18] C. Invitti, F. Pecori Giraldi, and M. De Martin, "Diagnosis and management of cushing's syndrome: results of an Italian multicentre study," *Journal of Clinical Endocrinology & Metabolism*, vol. 84, no. 2, pp. 440–448, 1999.
[19] E. Valassi, A. Santos, M. Yaneva et al., "The European registry on cushing's syndrome: 2-year experience. Baseline demographic and clinical characteristics," *European Journal of Endocrinology*, vol. 165, no. 3, pp. 383–392, 2011.
[20] J. Newell-Price, P. Trainer, M. Besser, and A. Grossman, "The diagnosis and differential diagnosis of cushing's syndrome and pseudo-cushing's states," *Endocrine Reviews*, vol. 19, no. 5, pp. 647–672, 1998.
[21] K. I. Alexandraki and A. B. Grossman, "The ectopic ACTH syndrome," *Reviews in Endocrine and Metabolic Disorders*, vol. 11, no. 2, pp. 117–126, 2010.
[22] R. M. Reynolds, C. Fischbacher, R. Bhopal et al., "Differences in cortisol concentrations in South Asian and European men living in the United Kingdom," *Clinical Endocrinology*, vol. 64, no. 5, pp. 530–534, 2006.
[23] R. Pivonello, M. De Leo, A. Cozzolino, and A. Colao, "The treatment of cushing's disease," *Endocrine Reviews*, vol. 36, no. 4, pp. 385–486, 2015.
[24] T. Nakane, A. Kuwayama, M. Watanabe et al., "Long term results of transsphenoidal adenomectomy in patients with cushing's disease," *Neurosurgery*, vol. 21, no. 2, pp. 218–222, 1987.
[25] J. H. Kim, C. S. Shin, S. H. Paek, H. W. Jung, S. W. Kim, and S. Y. Kim, "Recurrence of cushing's disease after primary transsphenoidal surgery in a university hospital in Korea," *Endocrine Journal*, vol. 59, no. 10, pp. 881–888, 2012.
[26] C. M. Berr, G. Di Dalmazi, A. Osswald et al., "Time to recovery of adrenal function after curative surgery for cushing's syndrome depends on etiology," *The Journal of Clinical Endocrinology & Metabolism*, vol. 100, no. 4, pp. 1300–1308, 2015.

12

Co-Occurrence of Exogenous and Endogenous Cushing's Syndromes—Dilemma in Diagnosis

Chin Voon Tong [1] **and Subashini Rajoo** [2]

[1]Department of Medicine, Malacca Hospital, 75400, Malaysia
[2]Department of Medicine, Kuala Lumpur Hospital, 50586, Malaysia

Correspondence should be addressed to Chin Voon Tong; tchinvoon@yahoo.com

Academic Editor: Michael P. Kane

Approach to patients who manifest with features of Cushing's syndrome often begin with exclusion of exposure to excessive exogenous source of glucocorticoids (GC). Most guidelines advocate no further assessment if excessive exogenous GC use is present. We present a case of a 66-year-old lady who was noted to have typical features of Cushing's syndrome. As she gave a very clear history of ingesting exogenous GC for a year, no further work up was undertaken. Despite cessation of GC for a year, she continued to have thin skin and easy bruising. Upon admission for hypertensive emergency, her clinician took note of her changes and investigated her for endogenous Cushing's syndrome. Her cortisol post overnight dexamethasone suppression test was 707 nmol/l. Post low dose dexamethasone suppression test yielded a cortisol of 1133.2 nmol/l. 24 hours urine cortisol was 432.2 nmol/l. Plasma ACTH was 1.1 pmol/l, indicating an ACTH independent Cushing's syndrome. We proceeded with Computed tomography scan (CT scan) of adrenals which revealed a right adrenal adenoma measuring 4.4 × 3.4 × 4.0 cm. Right retroperiteneoscopic adrenalectomy was done. Histopathology examination was consistent with adrenal cortical adenoma with foci of myelolipoma. Post adrenalectomy she developed hypocortisolism secondary to contralateral adrenal suppression which lasted up to the present date. Her cutaneous and musculoskeletal manifestations improved substantially. Co-occurrence of endogenous and exogenous Cushing's syndromes is uncommon but should be considered in patients whose Cushingnoid features do not resolve after cessation of exogenous GC.

1. Introduction

While endogenous Cushing's syndrome is rare, with reported incidence of 2–3 per 1 million inhabitants per year [1], the actual incidence of exogenous or iatrogenic Cushing's syndrome is not known. The source of exogenous GC also varies from those being used in clinical setting to unknowing ingestion from traditional treatments. A local study found that 82% of older adults consume traditional medications. Samples of traditional medications used in this study were analysed and more than half (61.8%) contained steroids [2]. Traditional Chinese medications (TCM) are also popular among local population, including non-Chinese. While not all herbal TCM products contain steroids, adulteration of these products with exogenous steroids has been detected [3]. We report herein a patient who had both endogenous and exogenous Cushing's syndromes which contributed to a delay and dilemma in diagnosis.

2. Materials and Methods

Patient's file was retrieved and reviewed retrospectively.

3. Results

3.1. History. Our patient is a 66-year-old housewife whose daughter is a dentist and was able to give accurate medical history. She was noted to be Cushingnoid in 2009 by her attending physician. She had thin skin with easy bruising, truncal obesity, and proximal myopathy. At that time, she gave a clear history of ingesting TCM which was known to contain GC for a year. The medications were taken for general well-being. She was seen at another hospital and we were not able to trace her baseline cortisol taken then. She was advised to, and subsequently stopped taking it. After cessation of the exogenous

TABLE 1: Hormonal work up for Cushing's syndrome.

Parameters	Results
Morning cortisol (nmol/l)	841.2
Cortisol post overnight dexamethasone suppression test (nmol/l)	707.3
Cortisol post low dose dexamethasone suppression test (nmol/l)	1133.2
Plasma adrenocorticotropic hormone (pmol/l)	1.1
24 hours urine cortisol (nmol/L)	432.2

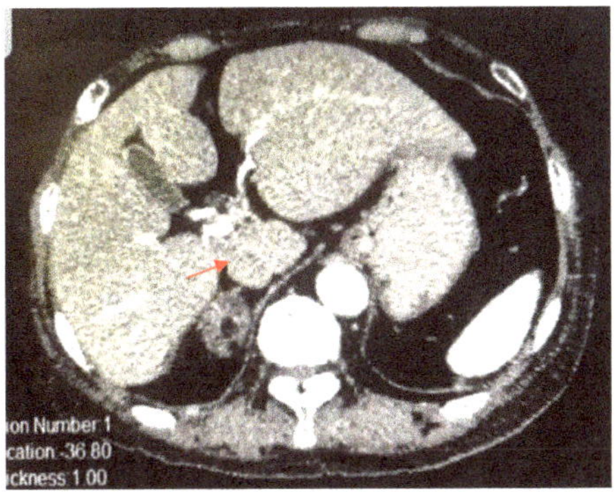

FIGURE 1: CT scan adrenal showing right adrenal adenoma.

GC, there was slight improvement in her Cushing's features, but they became more noticeable again in 2017. She then developed hypertension in 2010, diabetes mellitus in 2016, and had an osteoporotic fracture in 2011. During an admission for hypertensive crisis in 2017, a physician noticed her features and worked her up. During this admission, she had severe hypokalemia as well as hyponatremia. She was, however, on Indapamide for her hypertension prior to that.

3.2. Investigations. Her hormonal profile was consistent with ACTH independent Cushing's syndrome. Her results are summarized in Table 1.

Computed tomography (CT) scan of adrenal showed a right adrenal adenoma measuring 4.4 × 3.4 × 4.0 cm. Contralateral adrenal was normal (Figure 1). 24 hours metanephrines were not elevated.

3.3. Management. She underwent right retroperiteneoscopic adrenalectomy. Prior to surgery, she was given ketoconazole to control her cortisol excess. She required four anti hypertensives and one glucose lowering medications. Intraoperatively, a right adrenal adenoma measuring 4 × 4 cm was found. Post surgery, she required inotropic support for 24 hours despite being given hydrocortisone cover peri-operatively. Histopathology examination was consistent with adrenal cortical adenoma with foci of myelolipoma. She is currently into her 13th month post adrenalectomy. Her cutaneous manifestations have improved markedly. She now requires a single anti-hypertensive but is euglycemic without any glucose lowering therapies. Her cortisol remained suppressed with a pre dose cortisol of <13 nmol/l. She is now taking a physiological dose of oral hydrocortisone of 10 mg in the morning and 5 mg in the afternoon.

4. Discussion

Co-occurrence of both endogenous and exogenous Cushing's syndromes is rare, though its true incidence is not known. Both share similar clinical presentations. Some authors have reported certain differences in the two. Exogenous Cushing's syndrome tends to have more striking clinical features, relatively less hypertension and hypokalemia as well as increased incidence of glaucoma [4]. However, in our experience, it is often difficult to differentiate both based on clinical features. In our local setting, a thorough and repeated history taking is important to establish intake of exogenous GC, especially from alternative sources. Patients are often reluctant to reveal this. The exact dose or amount of corticosteroids taken that will lead to iatrogenic Cushing's syndrome is not known as multiple factors such as formulations used, pharmacokinetics, biologic potency, affinity for glucocorticoid activity and duration of action play a role in causing Cushingnoid features [4].

Prolonged exposure to exogenous GC can potentially lead to secondary adrenal insufficiency caused by suppression of the hypothalamic–pituitary–adrenal (HPA) axis. The amount, duration and mode of delivery of exogenous GC that causes secondary adrenal suppression varies between individual and is difficult to predict. Schlaghecke et al. who studied more than 200 patients receiving daily GC therapies concluded that pituitary-adrenal function in these patients cannot be accurately estimated from the dose of GC, the duration of therapy, or the basal cortisol concentration [5]. In terms of mode of delivery, even inhaled GC which were thought to be safe in the past, and unusual mode such as rectal GC have also been reported to cause adrenal crisis upon its withdrawal [6, 7].

Work up for a patient who presents with Cushing's syndrome should include assessment for adrenal insufficiency in those whose cause is deemed to be from an exogenous source. Bearing in mind that both can coexist, further follow up is still necessary for patients who are thought to have exogenous Cushing's syndrome and still have intact HPA axis. Our suggested approach to a patient presenting with features of Cushing's syndrome is depicted in Figure 2.

If exogenous GC use has been excluded, the work up is done for endogenous Cushing's syndrome [1]. In the event that there is use of exogenous GC, the use is continued if medically indicated. However if there is no clear indication, the GC is either ceased or switched to a morning dose of hydrocortisone. A prehydrocortisone morning cortisol is then measured. A level of <100 nmol/l indicates adrenal insufficiency and replacement is initiated. If the am cortisol ranges between 100 and 500 nmol/l, a short synacthen test is performed. Am cortisol of >500 nmol/l is an indication of intact HPA axis [8]. Clinicians should also be aware that GC like dexamethasone suppresses cortisol levels and others such as hydrocortisone are measurable in cortisol assays. We suggest further follow up for patients with intact HPA axis to assess for improvement of Cushingnoid features after cessation of GC. Persistence of symptoms warrants a further workup for concurrent endogenous cause.

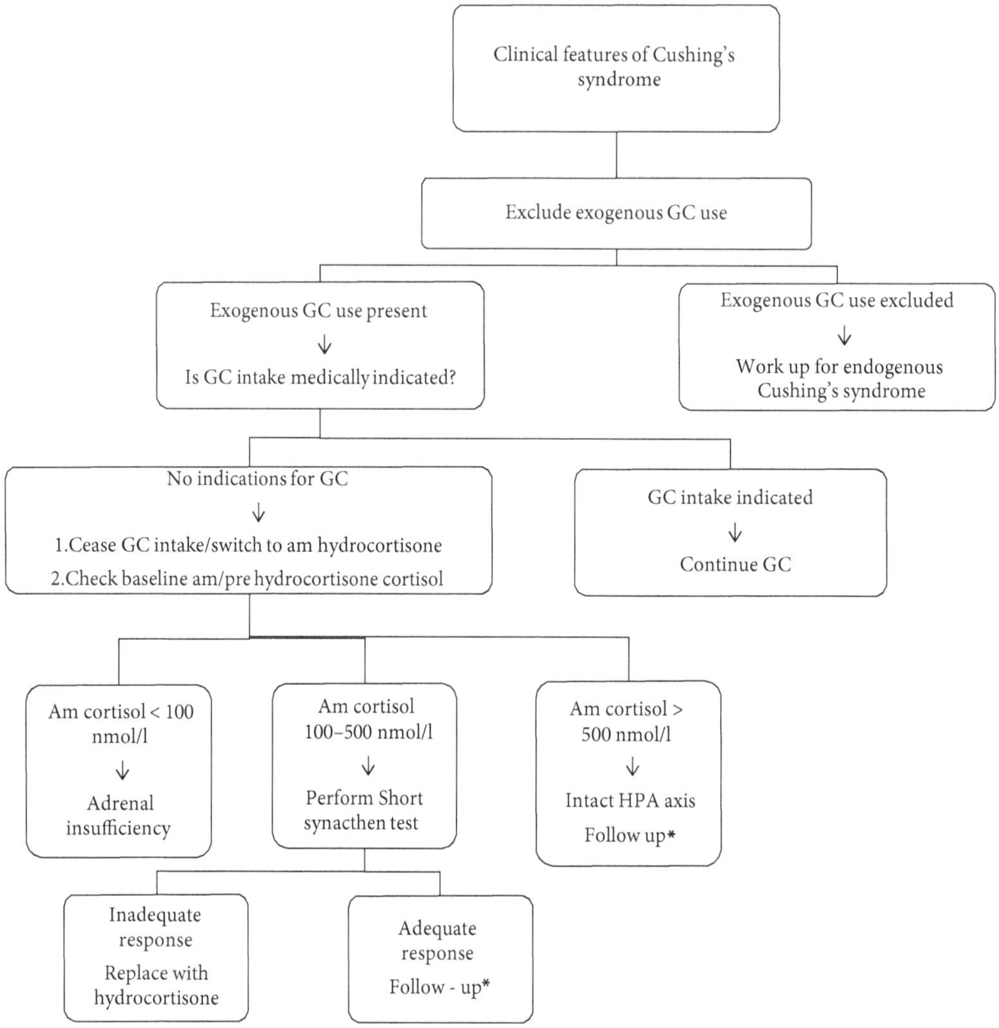

FIGURE 2: Algorithm for workup of a patient with exogenous Cushing's syndrome. *Glucocorticoids tapered and off. Patients are followed up and assessed for resolution of Cushingnoid features. If features persist, to consider concurrent endogenous Cushing's syndrome.

5. Conclusion

In conclusion, co-occurrence of endogenous and exogenous Cushing's syndromes is uncommon but should be considered in patients whose Cushingnoid features do not resolve after cessation of exogenous glucocorticoids.

References

[1] L. K. Nieman, B. M. K. Biller, J. W. Findling et al., "The diagnosis of Cushing's syndrome: an endocrine society clinical practice guideline," *The Journal of Clinical Endocrinology & Metabolism*, vol. 93, no. 5, pp. 1526–1540, 2008.

[2] Z. Ismail, R. Mohamed, M. H. Mohd Hassan, and S. K. Wan, "Usage of traditional medicines among elderly and the prevalence of prednisolone contamination," *Malaysian Journal of Medical Sciences*, vol. 12, no. 2, pp. 50–55, 2005.

[3] F. Y. Fung and Y. C. Linn, "Steroids in traditional Chinese medicine: what is the evidence?," *Singapore Medical Journal*, vol. 58, no. 3, pp. 115–120, 2017.

[4] R. L. Hopkins and M. C. Leinung, "Exogenous Cushing's syndrome and glucocorticoid withdrawal," *Endocrinology & Metabolism Clinics of North America*, vol. 34, no. 2, pp. 371–384.

[5] R. Schlaghecke, E. Kornely, R. T. Santen, and P. Ridderskamp, "The effect of long-term glucocorticoid therapy on pituitary–adrenal responses to exogenous corticotropin-releasing hormone," *New England Journal of Medicine*, vol. 326, no. 4, pp. 226–230, 1992.

[6] G. R. Todd, C. L. Acerini, R. Ross-Russell, S. Zahra, J. T. Warner, and D. McCance, "Survey of adrenal crisis associated with inhaled corticosteroids in the United Kingdom," *Archives of Disease in Childhood*, vol. 87, no. 6, pp. 457–461, 2002.

[7] A. D. Barlow, G. A. Clarke, and M. J. Kelly, "Acute adrenal crisis in a patient treated with rectal steroids," *Colorectal Disease*, vol. 6, no. 1, pp. 62–64, 2004.

[8] C. W. Le Roux, K. Meeran, and J. Alaghband-Zadeh, "Is a 0900-h serum cortisol useful prior to a short synacthen test in outpatient assessment?," *Annals of Clinical Biochemistry*, vol. 39, no. 2, pp. 148–150, 2002.

13

Addison's Disease Presenting as Acute Renal Failure and Hyperkalemic Paralysis: A Rare Presentation

Kundan Jana, Kalyana Janga, Sheldon Greenberg, and Amit Gulati

Division of Nephrology and Hypertension, Maimonides Medical Center, Brooklyn, NY 11219, USA

Correspondence should be addressed to Kundan Jana; kundanraja.j@gmail.com

Academic Editor: Toshihiro Kita

Hyperkalemic paralysis in the setting of acute renal failure can lead to a missed or delayed diagnosis of adrenal insufficiency as the raised potassium can be attributed to the renal failure. Acute kidney injury as the presenting manifestation in an adrenal crisis due to Addison's disease has been rarely reported in the literature. Here, we present the case of a young 37-year-old male who came with hyperkalemic paralysis and acute renal failure needing emergent hemodialysis. He had no past medical history and no medication history. His hyponatremia, hypotension, and hyperkalemia pointed to a picture of adrenal insufficiency confirmed by undetectable serum cortisol, elevated ACTH, renin, and low aldosterone levels and imaging. Replacement steroid therapy was given, and the patient made a steady recovery. He was advised on the importance of compliance to treatment at discharge to prevent another crisis event. Acute renal failure with hyperkalemia as a presenting manifestation of Addison's disease can be very misleading. It is especially important to be vigilant of adrenal insufficiency in such patients as the hyperkalemia is resistant to standard therapy of insulin dextrose and can precipitate fatal arrhythmia if treatment is delayed.

1. Introduction

Primary adrenal insufficiency is a rare disorder with low incidence and is usually a challenging diagnosis to make due to the vagueness of the symptoms patients present with. Patients with chronic Addison's disease present with weakness, fatigue, anorexia, skin hyperpigmentation, or acute adrenal crisis. Commonly encountered electrolyte abnormalities include hyponatremia and hyperkalemia. Hyperkalemic paralysis with acute renal failure can be a very misleading presentation of Addison's disease as the life-threatening hyperkalemia can be misdiagnosed as a consequence of the kidney injury. Very few cases in the literature have so far been reported where acute renal failure was the presenting manifestation of primary adrenal insufficiency [1–3]. Here, we present such a case of a young 37-year-old male who came in with acute flaccid paralysis secondary to life-threatening hyperkalemia and acute renal failure.

2. Case Report

A 37-year-old presented with acute weakness and inability to move his limbs after waking up from sleep. He experienced similar symptoms of weakness in the past after a prolonged period of rest, but none of them were as severe. There was no history of recent medication or drug use and no history of diarrhea, infections, or trauma. He had no other significant past medical history. On arrival to the Emergency Department, the patient was hypotensive with a blood pressure of 98/50 and a heart rate of 84 per minute. The patient endorsed some improvement in weakness on the way to the emergency department (ED). However, physical examination was still significant for weakness in all four limbs with intact sensations and no fecal or urinary incontinence. The patient also complained of inability to walk. While taking history and drawing his labs, the patient went into cardiac arrest. ECG showed sinus rhythm with PR interval prolongation and QRS widening (Figure 1). He was intubated and resuscitated with return of spontaneous circulation after 6 minutes. His blood work taken prior to the cardiac arrest was significant for acute hyperkalemia of 8.8 mmol/l (normal 3.5–5 mmol/l), hyponatremia of 124 mmol/l (normal 135–145 mmol/l), and acute kidney injury with serum creatinine of 1.7 mg/dl (normal 0.5–1.3 mg/dl) (Table 1).

The patient underwent emergent renal replacement therapy (RRT) for life-threatening hyperkalemia and was transferred subsequently to the intensive care unit. To exclude CNS causes of paralysis, brain and cervical spine MRI were done and they were unremarkable. Viral causes were excluded with nasopharyngeal swab for the respiratory pathogen panel, including enteroviruses, and serology for HIV and CMV. Thyroid dysfunction, as a cause for paralysis, was excluded with normal serum thyroid stimulating hormone (TSH) and negative thyroid peroxidase antibodies. Urine tox screen was also negative. Autoimmune serology for vasculitis including ANCA, ANA, rheumatoid factor, anti-SSA, anti-SSB, anti-SCL-70, and double-stranded DNA were all negative. Obstructive uropathy as a cause of the hyperkalemia and acute renal failure was ruled out with a draining Foley catheter, and imaging showed no signs of retention. Normal creatinine phosphokinase (CPK) and myoglobin levels in pre-cardiac arrest labs ruled out rhabdomyolysis as a cause of the acute kidney injury (AKI). Hyponatremia, hyperkalemia, and hypotension pointed to a differential diagnosis of probable adrenal insufficiency. Accordingly, serum cortisol levels, ACTH levels, plasma renin activity, and aldosterone levels were obtained. Our patient had undetectable cortisol levels of <0.4 μg/dl, elevated ACTH level, elevated renin level, and low aldosterone levels (Table 1). The trans-tubular potassium gradient (TTKG) was calculated to be less than 5. A diagnosis of primary adrenal insufficiency was made and further confirmed by imaging which showed bilateral atrophic adrenal glands. Further workup revealed the presence of adrenal antibodies suggestive of autoimmune adrenal insufficiency. The patient was diagnosed with Addison's disease presenting in adrenal crisis.

After the first emergent session of hemodialysis, the patient remained in oligoanuric renal failure with hemodynamic instability and underwent continuous renal replacement therapy (CRRT) over the next 4 days. His potassium levels gradually came back to normal levels on CRRT (Figure 2). He made a steady recovery and was off RRT and extubated on the fourth day of hospitalisation. By this time, his weakness had completely resolved. The patient was finally discharged on maintenance of hydrocortisone 10 mg twice daily and fludrocortisone 0.1 mg/day with instructions for stress-dose hydrocortisone three times the usual dose in case of febrile illness and use of emergency injectable vial of hydrocortisone in case of vomiting and inability to take pills.

3. Discussion

Addison's disease is a rare endocrinological disorder with an estimated prevalence of 35–140 cases per million and incidence of 4 per million [4]. Tuberculosis (TB) was the most common cause of Addison's disease. However, with the advent of effective medication for TB, autoimmune causes are currently considered to be the most common etiology [3]. Adrenal insufficiency does not manifest until 90% of the gland has been destroyed or atrophied as seen in imaging. It is notoriously difficult to diagnose with vague and varied presentations. A study showed that up to 60% of patients were needed to be evaluated by at least 2 physicians with a median duration of diagnosis of up to 2 years, attesting to the insidious nature of the disease [5]. Presenting signs and symptoms of Addison's disease include weakness, fatigue, anorexia, and skin pigmentation with hypotension, hyponatremia, and hyperkalemia.

Acute adrenal crisis is a life-threatening presentation of Addison's disease seen in as many as 25% of the patients [3]. Acute renal failure as a presenting symptom is extremely rare with an incidence of 6% reported in the literature [3]. Oftentimes, such a presentation can lead to a missed or delayed diagnosis of adrenal insufficiency as the electrolyte disturbances of hyperkalemia and hyponatremia can be explained by the renal failure. Our patient presented with life-threatening hyperkalemia which could have been attributed to the acute renal failure. However, no discernable cause of the kidney injury provided a clue to another underlying disease pathology. Many pathophysiological mechanisms have been hypothesized on the cause for AKI in patients with adrenal insufficiency. Mineralocorticoid deficiency-induced intravascular volume depletion leading to decreased renal perfusion causing reduction in glomerular filtration rate was the likely cause of AKI in our patient [1].

Paralysis is a rare and reversible complication of hyperkalemia that can be categorized into primary and secondary forms. Primary hyperkalemic periodic paralysis is due to a congenital defect in the *SCN4A* gene affecting the sodium channel in muscles [6]. Secondary hyperkalemic paralysis can be due to acute or chronic renal failure, adrenal insufficiency, excessive ingestion of potassium, rhabdomyolysis, and various drugs like angiotensin converting enzyme inhibitors (ACEis), potassium-sparing diuretics, and cotrimoxazole, with renal failure being the most common cause [7, 8]. Hyperkalemic paralysis due to primary adrenal insufficiency is rare and can lead to fatal arrhythmias if not diagnosed early. A high index of suspicion should be maintained, especially in young patients, even when the picture is complicated by AKI, as seen in this patient.

Prompt institution of resuscitative and steroid replacement therapy is absolutely necessary in patients with acute adrenal crisis. Life-threatening hyperkalemia in such patients, as seen in our case, is resistant to the standard therapy of insulin dextrose. In fact, insulin dextrose can be detrimental in such patients for the danger of precipitating hypoglycemia as the patients are predisposed due to low glucocorticoid levels [1]. Renal replacement therapy was emergently administered in our patient to bring down the potassium levels and control fatal arrhythmias. Subsequently, the patient was stabilized and counselled upon discharge on the need for religious adherence to steroid therapy, the importance of stress-dose steroid replacement as warranted, and the need to carry a Medical Alert ID.

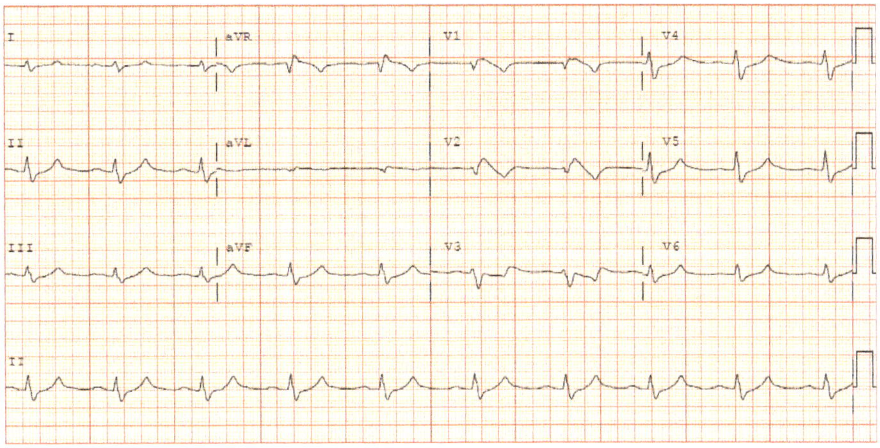

Figure 1: Pre-cardiac arrest ECG.

Table 1: Laboratory values.

Test	At admission	Day 3	Day 5	At discharge	6-month follow-up	Normal reference values
Glucose (mg/dl)	76	143	109	97	99	59–140
BUN (mg/dl)	32	25	28	23	14	7–21
Creatinine (mg/dl)	1.7	1.5	1.1	1	1.22	0.5–1.3
Serum sodium (mmol/l)	124	132	138	135	137	135–145
Serum potassium (mmol/l)	8.8	5.3	4	3.8	4.5	3.5–5
Serum chloride (mmol/l)	99	99	103	99	100	93–105
Serum CPK (IU/l)	280	1318				59–367
Serum osmolality (mosm/kg)	289					275–295
Renin (direct) (pg/ml)	>1500				47.1	<33
Plasma ACTH (pg/ml)	261		91.9			7.2–63.3
Serum cortisol (μg/dl)	<0.4					6.7–27.6
Serum aldosterone (ng/dl)	2.8					<23
Serum TSH (mIU/l)	3.7					0.4–4
Urine osmolality (mosm/kg)	445			628		500–800
Urine sodium (mmol/l)	97			62		
Urine potassium (mmol/l)	19			50		

BUN: blood urea nitrogen; CPK: creatinine phosphokinase; units are given in parentheses.

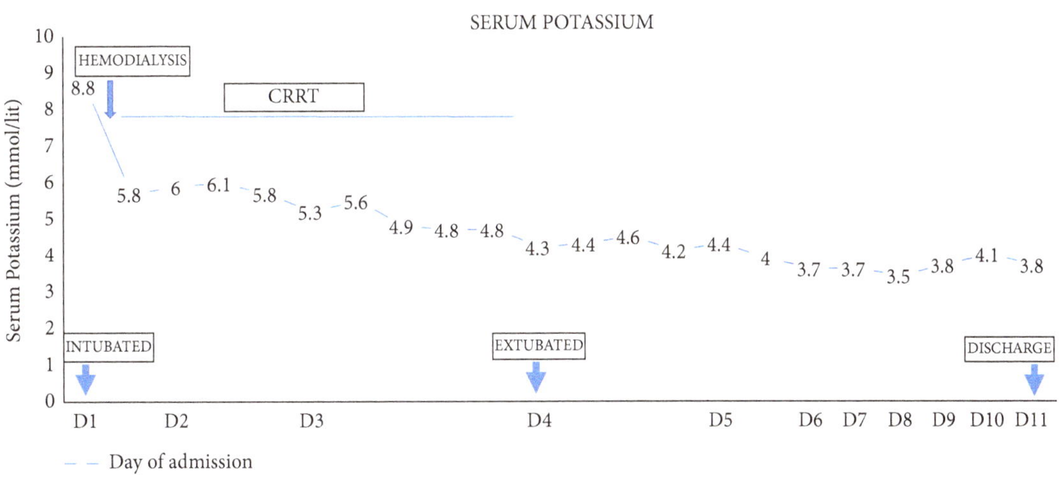

Figure 2: Course of hospitalisation with serum potassium levels.

4. Conclusion

Acute adrenal crisis due to Addison's disease presenting as acute renal failure with hyperkalemic paralysis is extremely rare and can lead to delayed diagnosis. Physicians should include adrenal insufficiency in their differential in such cases as hyperkalemia in such patients is resistant to standard therapy and can precipitate arrhythmias if diagnosis is delayed.

References

[1] A. Connor, S. Care, and J. Taylor, "Addison's disease presenting with acute kidney injury," *Clinical Medicine*, vol. 10, no. 5, pp. 515-516, 2010.

[2] S. Maki, C. Kramarz, P. Maria Heister, and K. Pasha, "First presentation of Addison's disease as hyperkalaemia in acute kidney injury," *BMJ Case Reports*, Article ID bcr2015213375, 2016.

[3] C. Fofi, B. Maresca, S. Altieri, P. Menè, and F. Festuccia, "Renal involvement in adrenal insufficiency (Addison disease): can we always recognize it?" *Internal and Emergency Medicine*, vol. 15, no. 1, pp. 23–31, 2020.

[4] A. Michels and N. Michels, "Addison disease: early detection and treatment principles," *American Family Physician*, vol. 89, no. 7, pp. 563–568, 2014.

[5] W. Arlt and B. Allolio, "Adrenal insufficiency," *Lancet*, vol. 361, no. 9372, pp. 1881–1893, 2003.

[6] S. C. Cannon, "Sodium channelopathies of skeletal muscle," *Voltage-gated Sodium Channels: Structure, Function and Channelopathies*, vol. 246, pp. 309–330, 2017.

[7] K. H. D. T. Hemachandra, M. B. K. Chandimal Dayasiri, and T. Kannangara, "Acute ascending flaccid paralysis secondary to multiple trigger factor induced hyperkalemia," *Case Reports in Neurological Medicine*, vol. 2018, pp. 1–4, 2018.

[8] K. Panichpisal, S. Gandhi, K. Nugent, and Y. Anziska, "Acute quadriplegia from hyperkalemia," *The Neurologist*, vol. 16, no. 6, pp. 390–393, 2010.

14

Vitamin D Intoxication and Nephrocalcinosis in a Young Breastfed Infant

Abdullah Al-Kandari,[1] **Hussain Sadeq**,[1] **Rita Alfattal,**[1] **Maryam AlRashid,**[2] **and Mayra Alsaeid**[3]

[1]*Department of Pediatrics, Al-Amiri Hospital, General Pediatrics Unit, Kuwait city, Kuwait*
[2]*Department of Pediatrics, Al-Amiri Hospital, Pediatric Endocrine Unit, Kuwait city, Kuwait*
[3]*Department of Pediatrics, Faculty of Medicine, Kuwait University, Kuwait city, Kuwait*

Correspondence should be addressed to Abdullah Al-Kandari; af.alkandari@hotmail.com

Academic Editor: Michaël R. Laurent

Numerous studies were performed assessing the benefits and side effects of vitamin D. Vitamin D helps in regulating the calcium and phosphate metabolism leading to a healthy mineral and bone development. Vitamin D intoxication is an uncommon event that leads to hypercalcemia which can be associated with both immediate and late morbidities that can cause severe renal complications. Here, we present a case of a 4-month-old girl with a history of decreased feed and activity due hypercalcemia and high vitamin D level, which led to nephrocalcinosis. The patient received IV fluids, IV diuretics, methylprednisolone, and bisphosphonate in order to normalize the calcium level in blood. With clear verbal and written instructions for the dosage and administration of vitamin D supplements, as well as clear warnings of the potential risks of overdose, vitamin D intoxication could be an easily avoidable condition.

1. Introduction

In the past decade, several studies focusing on the benefits of vitamin D have been reported [1–5]. Vitamin D is an essential hormone in the human body that regulates calcium homeostasis and prevents the development of rickets [6–8]. Vitamin D intoxication is an uncommon event that leads to hypercalcemia, which is associated with both immediate and late morbidities that can cause severe renal complications [9–15]. Recently, there have been several case reports of vitamin D toxicity in very young infants due to vitamin D overdose [10, 12]. The present case study reports an infant who developed acute hypercalcemia and nephrocalcinosis after prolonged administration of an overdose of over-the-counter vitamin D supplements by the mother. Over-the-counter drugs are safe when used properly as directed by the pharmacist; however, misuse or miscommunication can lead to a rare devastating consequence, such as our report.

2. Case Presentation

A 4-month-old girl was brought to the emergency department with a history of lethargy, decreased feeding, and constipation for more than a month. On examination, the patient exhibited signs of moderate dehydration such as dry skin, poor skin turgor, and decreased urine output although initial vital signs were within normal limit (heart rate was 122 beats per minute, respiratory rate was 38 respiration per minute, and blood pressure was 90/60 mmHg). Routine investigations performed in the emergency department identified a high corrected calcium level (5.60 mmol/L; normal range: 2.25–2.75). Upon further questioning of the parents, it became apparent that the girl had been receiving an excessive dose of vitamin D supplementation. The patient had been receiving a full 1 mL dropper of an over-the-counter vitamin D supplement (1 mL dose equal to 5000 IU) three times a day on a daily basis, for a one-month period, instead of the intended dose of three drops once per day

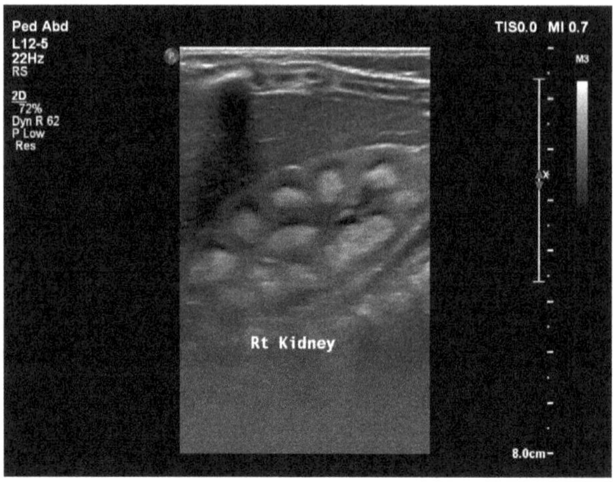

FIGURE 1: Ultrasound image of patient's right kidney showing echogenic medullary pyramids suggestive of nephrocalcinosis.

(three drops dose equals to 400 IU). Parents are highly educated with excellent socioeconomic status; however, miscommunication with the pharmacist regarding the dosage led to this mistake. This unfortunate event led the patient to present with vitamin D intoxication, with the blood test for vitamin 25-hydroxyvitamin D (25(OH)D) levels showing a level of 350 nmol/L (critical level: >250 nmol/L).

The infant was admitted to a general pediatric ward for further management of calcium and vitamin D levels. She was put on intravenous (IV) fluids containing normal saline and dextrose at rate of 28 ml/hour, which equals to 150 ml/kg/day. She also received 1 mg/kg furosemide IV divided into three doses per day along with the 3-day IV course of 0.3 mg/kg methylprednisolone once daily. Furthermore, the patient was fed with low calcium formula milk (Nutricia™ Kindergen).

As part of the routine assessment of hypercalcemia and vitamin D toxicity, various laboratory and radiological investigations were performed to assess the extent of the toxicity on the patient's renal system. Both serum creatinine and urea were normal upon admission, 32 umol/L (normal range: 11–34 umol/L) and 5.9 mmol/L (normal range: 1.8–6.4 mmol/L), respectively. Urine analysis was performed as well and showed no abnormal parameters. However, urine calcium (mmol/L) to urine creatinine (mmol/L) ratio was significantly abnormal (6.17; normal range: 0.08–0.57). Additionally, an abdominal ultrasound was performed, showing evidence of nephrocalcinosis (Figure 1).

Furosemide (1 mg/kg/dose three times per day) was replaced with thiazide (1 mg/kg/dose twice per day) on day 3 of admission, and potassium citrate (1 mmol dose three times per day) was administered to reduce the risk of exacerbating the existing nephrocalcinosis.

The rate of reduction of the corrected calcium level was unsatisfactory, as on day 4 of admission, the level remained high at 4.17 mmol/L. At this point, bisphosphonate therapy was initiated, with two doses given (first dose of 0.5 mg/kg and second dose of 1 mg/kg).

On day 9 of admission, the corrected calcium level was 3.44 mmol/L, and the clinical condition of the patient had improved in terms of feeding and physical activity level. At the point of discharge after 10 days in the hospital, the patient's corrected calcium level had reduced to 2.96 mmol/L. The patient was discharged with a prescription of low calcium milk formula and potassium citrate (0.5 mmol three times per day). Furthermore, follow-up appointments with an endocrinologist and nephrologist were also given. Summary of daily laboratory results is gathered and presented in Table 1.

3. Discussion

Although breastfeeding remains the best source of infant nutrition, breast milk can lack adequate amounts of vitamin D [10, 16]. The American Academy of Pediatrics (AAP) recommends the provision of vitamin D supplements to any breastfed infant to avoid the risk of developing nutritional vitamin D deficiency, also known as nutritional rickets [10]. Guidelines issued by the AAP and the National Academy of Sciences indicate that all breastfeeding and nonbreastfeeding infants who drink <500 ml per day should receive 20 IU of vitamin D supplement per day [17]. Over-the-counter vitamin D supplements are easily and readily available [18]. The inappropriate administration of high doses of vitamin D in infants are typically provided by families for complaints such as delayed teething, late walking, and knock-knee gait [9]. Without appropriate instructions on dosing and administration, a significant risk of vitamin D toxicity exists [13, 18]. The Endocrine Society states that vitamin D toxicity is defined as 25(OH)D concentrations exceeding 375 nmol/L [19], with levels above this toxic threshold associated with the onset of hypercalcemia [19–21]. Signs and symptoms of vitamin D intoxication are directly related to the effects of hypercalcemia [17, 20, 22], including decreased oral intake, nausea, vomiting, constipation, weakness, lethargy, and generalized malaise [17, 20, 21]. Hypercalcemia and vitamin D toxicity can lead to serious complications including renal failure, hypertension, and nephrocalcinosis [17, 23, 24]. Medullary nephrocalcinosis can be detected by ultrasound [9]. Nephrocalcinosis is a common

Table 1: Summary of daily laboratory results during patient's hospital stay.

Day/ lab.	Ca (mmol/L), NR: 2.25–2.75	PO_4 (mmol/L), NR: 0.81–2.26	BUN (mmol/L), NR: 1.8–6.4	Cr (umol/L), NR: 11–34	Urine Ca : Cr ratio, NR: 0.08–0.57
Day 1	5.60	1.28	5.9	32	6.17
Day 2	4.69	1.23	4.8	28	9.83
Day 3	4.42	1.05	2.9	29	—
Day 4	4.17	1.28	2.2	29	—
Day 5	4.33	1.22	1.9	33	2.58
Day 6	3.92	1.20	1.6	30	—
Day 7	4.19	1.30	2.6	31	—
Day 8	4.14	1.12	2.8	31	—
Day 9	3.44	0.85	1.0	24	2.71
Day 10	2.96	0.84	<0.8	26	—

*NR, normal range.

pathological condition, characterized by hypercalciuria and/or hypercalcemia, with only 10% of cases caused by vitamin D intoxication [9]. Treatment for vitamin D toxicity usually involves removal of the exogenous source, intravenous fluid hydration, diuretics, a low-calcium diet, the administration of steroids, bisphosphonate therapy, and sometimes, renal dialysis [6, 23–25].

4. Conclusions and Recommendations

With clear verbal and written instructions for the dosage and administration of vitamin D supplements, as well as clear warnings of the potential risks of overdose, vitamin D intoxication could be an easily avoidable condition. Parents should also be advised to carefully read the instructions provided for any over-the-counter vitamin D supplements. Moreover, the inclusion of proper medication reconciliation with each visit to a pediatric clinic could help parents to avoid this type of mistake.

Acknowledgments

The authors' thank and convey their best regards to the Pediatrics Department of Amiri Hospital's nurses and to the parents of the patient.

References

[1] M. G. Vogiatzi, E. Jacobson-Dickman, and M. D. DeBoer, "Vitamin D supplementation and risk of toxicity in pediatrics: a review of current literature," *The Journal of Clinical Endocrinology and Metabolism*, vol. 99, no. 4, pp. 1132–1141, 2014.

[2] S. Kimball, G. E.-H. Fuleihan, and R. Vieth, "Vitamin D: a growing perspective," *Critical Reviews in Clinical Laboratory Sciences*, vol. 45, no. 4, pp. 339–414, 2008.

[3] M. F. Holick, "The D-lightful vitamin D for child health," *JPEN. Journal of Parenteral and Enteral Nutrition*, vol. 36, no. 1 Suppl, pp. 9s–19s, 2012.

[4] F. Alshahrani and N. Aljohani, "Vitamin D: deficiency, sufficiency and toxicity," *Nutrients*, vol. 5, no. 9, pp. 3605–3616, 2013.

[5] K. K. Pandita, S. Razdan, R. P. Kudyar, A. Beigh, S. Kuchay, and T. Banday, ""Excess good can be dangerous". A case series of iatrogenic symptomatic hypercalcemia due to hypervitaminosis D," *Clinical Cases in Mineral and Bone Metabolism*, vol. 9, no. 2, p. 118, 2012.

[6] M. Chatterjee and P. W. Speiser, "Pamidronate treatment of hypercalcemia caused by vitamin D toxicity," *Journal of Pediatric Endocrinology and Metabolism*, vol. 20, no. 11, pp. 1241–1248, 2007.

[7] M. Jazayeri, Y. Moradi, A. Rasti, M. Nakhjavani, M. Kamali, and H. R. Baradaran, "Prevalence of vitamin D deficiency in healthy Iranian children: a systematic review and meta-analysis," *Medical Journal of the Islamic Republic of Iran*, vol. 32, p. 83, 2018.

[8] S. Makariou, E. N. Liberopoulos, M. Elisaf, and A. Challa, "Novel roles of vitamin D in disease: what is new in 2011?" *European Journal of Internal Medicine*, vol. 22, no. 4, pp. 355–362, 2011.

[9] V. Talarico, M Barreca, R Galiano, M. C Galati, and G Raiola, "Vitamin D and risk for vitamin A intoxication in an 18-month-old boy," *Case Reports in Pediatrics*, vol. 2016, Article ID 1395718, 2016.

[10] N. A. Bilbao, "Vitamin D toxicity in young breastfed infants: report of 2 cases," *Global Pediatric Health*, vol. 4, Article ID 2333794x17731695, 2017.

[11] S. Kaptein, A. J. Risselada, E. C. Boerma, P. H. M. Egbers, and P. Nieboer, "Life-threatening complications of vitamin D intoxication due to over-the-counter supplements," *Clinical Toxicology*, vol. 48, no. 5, pp. 460–462, 2010.

[12] T. Araki, M. F. Holick, B. D. Alfonso et al., "Vitamin D intoxication with severe hypercalcemia due to manufacturing and labeling errors of two dietary supplements made in the United States," *The Journal of Clinical Endocrinology & Metabolism*, vol. 96, no. 12, pp. 3603–3608, 2011.

[13] A. Anık, G. Çatlı, A. Abacı, C. Dizdarer, and E. Böber, "Acute vitamin D intoxication possibly due to faulty production of a multivitamin preparation," *Journal of Clinical Research in Pediatric Endocrinology*, vol. 5, no. 2, pp. 136–9, 2013.

[14] P. Kaur, S. K. Mishra, and A. Mithal, "Vitamin D toxicity resulting from overzealous correction of vitamin D deficiency," *Clinical Endocrinology*, vol. 83, no. 3, pp. 327–331, 2015.

[15] D. A. Bell, M. J. Crooke, N. Hay, and P. Glendenning, "Prolonged vitamin D intoxication: presentation, pathogenesis and progress," *Internal Medicine Journal*, vol. 43, no. 10, pp. 1148–1150, 2013.

[16] A. Dawodu and R. C. Tsang, "Maternal vitamin D status: effect on milk vitamin D content and vitamin D status of

breastfeeding infants," *Advances in Nutrition*, vol. 3, no. 3, pp. 353–361, 2012.
[17] F. Barrueto, "Acute vitamin D intoxication in a child," *Pediatrics*, vol. 116, no. 3, pp. e453–e456, 2005.
[18] P. N. Taylor and J. S. Davies, "A review of the growing risk of vitamin D toxicity from inappropriate practice," *British Journal of Clinical Pharmacology*, vol. 84, no. 6, pp. 1121–1127, 2018.
[19] M. F. Holick, N. C. Binkley, H. A. Bischoff-Ferrari et al., "Evaluation, treatment, and prevention of vitamin D deficiency: an Endocrine Society clinical practice guideline," *The Journal of Clinical Endocrinology and Metabolism*, vol. 96, no. 7, pp. 1911–1930, 2011.
[20] E. Marcinowska-Suchowierska, M. Kupisz-Urbańska, J. Łukaszkiewicz, P. Płudowski, and G. Jones, "Vitamin D toxicity-A clinical perspective," *Frontiers in Endocrinology*, vol. 9, p. 550, 2018.
[21] N. E. Cusano, S. Thys-Jacobs, and J. P. Bilezikian, "Hypercalcemia due to vitamin D toxicity," *Vitamin D*, pp. 507–526, Elsevier, 2018.
[22] V. Guerra, O. M. Vieira Neto, A. F. Laurindo, F. J. Paula, and M. Moysés Neto, "Hypercalcemia and renal function impairment associated with vitamin D toxicity: case report," *Jornal brasileiro de nefrologia : 'orgao oficial de Sociedades Brasileira e Latino-Americana de Nefrologia*, vol. 38, no. 4, pp. 466–469, 2016.
[23] M. Nimesh, "An unsuspected pharmacological vitamin D toxicity in a child and its brief review of literature," *Toxicol Int*, vol. 22, pp. 167–169, 2015.
[24] A. Çağlar and H. Tuğçe Çağlar, "Vitamin D intoxication due to misuse: 5 year experience," *Archives de pediatrie : organe officiel de la Societe francaise de pediatrie*, vol. 28, no. 3, pp. 222–225, 2021.
[25] G. Conti, V Chirico, A Lacquaniti et al., "Vitamin D intoxication in two brothers: be careful with dietary supplements," *Journal of Pediatric Endocrinology & Metabolism : JPEM*, vol. 27, no. 7-8, pp. 763–767, 2014.

15

Primary Hypothyroidism with Pituitary Hyperplasia in an Omani Girl

Wafa Abdallah Fadle,[1] Ali Al Reesi,[2] Saud Al-Shabibi,[3] and Maryam Khamis Al-Badi[1]

[1]*Department of Pediatric Endocrinology, National Diabetes and Endocrine Center, Royal Hospital, Muscat, Oman*
[2]*Department of Internal Medicine, Sohar Hospital, Sohar, Oman*
[3]*Department of Radiology, Royal Hospital, Muscat, Oman*

Correspondence should be addressed to Maryam Khamis Al-Badi; talbadi20@hotmail.com

Academic Editor: Wayne V. Moore

Pituitary hyperplasia secondary to primary hypothyroidism (PHPH) is uncommon in children and is reversible with thyroxine therapy. We report an Omani girl who presented at the age of 13 years and 6 months with profound primary hypothyroidism due to Hashimoto's thyroiditis and secondary pituitary hyperplasia and hyperprolactinemia. Pituitary magnetic resonance imaging confirmed the presence of pituitary hyperplasia which regressed during follow-up after the administration of thyroxine therapy. The diagnosis of PHPH is very important in both children and adults in order to avoid unnecessary brain surgery or medical treatment for a presumed pituitary mass or adenoma. To our knowledge, this patient represents the first case of an Omani child presenting with PHPH.

1. Background

Primary hypothyroidism is a common endocrine disorder in children [1]. Hashimoto's thyroiditis is the most common cause of hypothyroidism in children; according to recent epidemiological data, the prevalence of primary hypothyroidism (autoimmune thyroiditis) is 0% among children aged 1–6 years, 1.2% among children aged 6–12 years, and 3.2% among children aged 12–16 years [2]. Long-standing primary hypothyroidism in children with high serum levels of thyroid-stimulating hormone (TSH), and the subsequent proliferation of TSH-releasing cells, may lead to pituitary hyperplasia, causing what is known as pituitary hyperplasia secondary to primary hypothyroidism (PHPH) [1]. PHPH was first reported in adults by Niepce in 1851, with similar cases reported thereafter [3–5]. However, PHPH is rarely reported in children; a recent review identified only 18 cases of pediatric PHPH in the literature [1]. Here, we present an interesting case of an Omani female adolescent who presented with a history of severe headache and short stature at the age of 13 years and 6 months and who was subsequently found to have an enlarged pituitary gland secondary to profound primary hypothyroidism.

2. Case Report

2.1. Patient History. An Omani girl aged 13 years and 6 months presented to a local hospital with a history of headache and was seen by an endocrinologist. She was found to have abnormal thyroid function test findings indicative of primary hypothyroidism and high prolactin levels; accordingly, she was started on thyroxine therapy and referred to the National Diabetes and Endocrine Center, Muscat, Oman. Her initial symptoms consisted of a two-year history of edema of the face, hands, and feet associated with cold intolerance and poor academic performance. In addition, she complained of recurrent headaches over the preceding 6 months. There were no symptoms of vomiting, blurred vision, seizure, changes in bowel habits, dysphagia, dysphonia, hair loss, or chest symptoms; however, she suffered from fatigue throughout the day. There was no family history of similar issues, short stature, or autoimmune disorders.

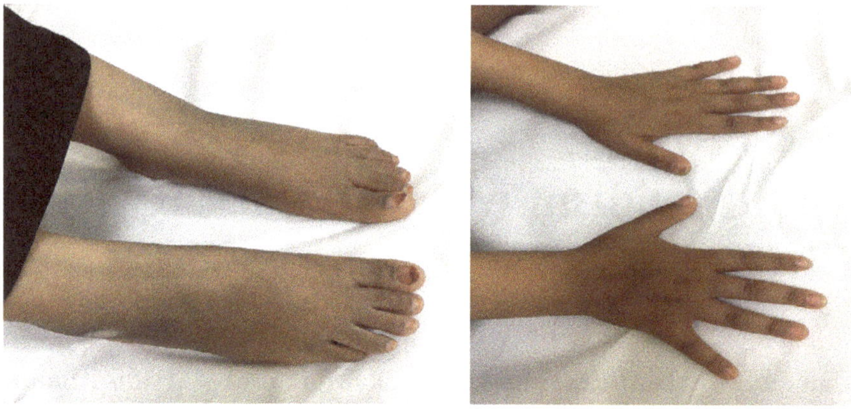

FIGURE 1: Photographs showing edema of both hands and feet.

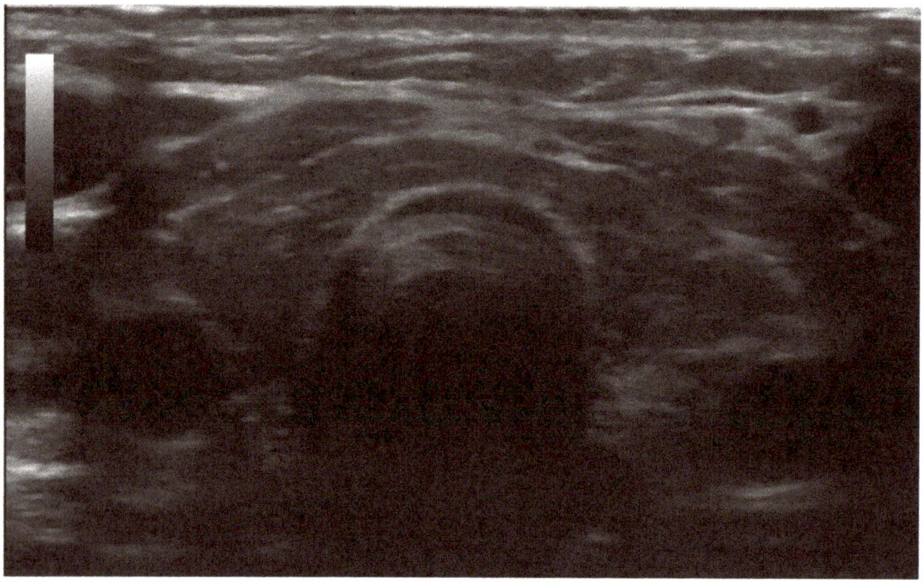

FIGURE 2: Thyroid ultrasound showing the relatively small size of the lobes and isthmus, diffuse coarse, heterogenous parenchymal echotexture with multiple fibrous echogenic lines, and no focal nodule.

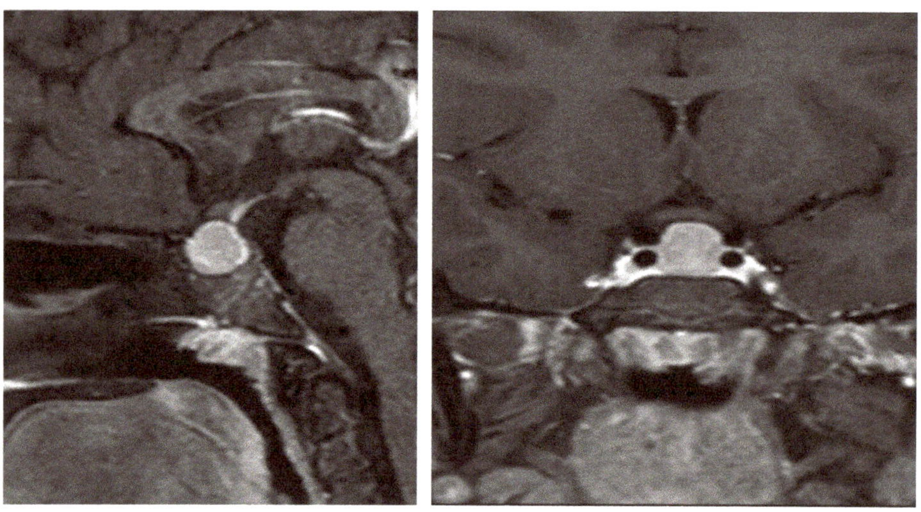

FIGURE 3: Sagittal and coronal contrast-enhanced T1-weighted magnetic resonance images taken at presentation. The images showed a homogenously enhancing solid mass arising from the pituitary gland with a superior concave border abutting the optic chiasm. There was no cystic/necrotic, haemorrhagic, or calcific component.

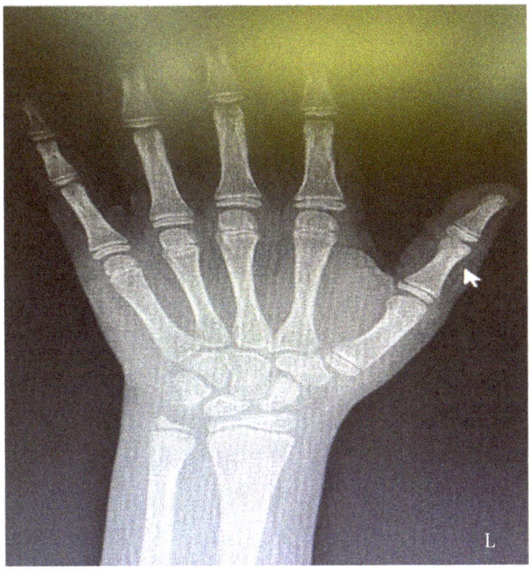

FIGURE 4: Left wrist X-ray showing a bone age of 10 years in contrast to chronological age of 13.6 years. Bone age was determined using Greulich and Pyle's radiographic atlas of skeletal development of the hand and wrist [6].

Her developmental history was normal. There was no history of surgery and she was not currently taking any long-term medications.

2.2. Physical Examination. The patient was 127 cm in height, had a body weight of 33.9 kg, and had a midparental height of 145 cm. Based on the criteria of the World Health Organization, she was below the 3rd percentile for both height (−4.8 cm SD below the mean) and midparental height (4.1 cm SD below the mean) and within the 3rd percentile for body weight. Her body mass index was 21.01 kg/m^2, conforming to the 95th centile. Her pulse rate was 77 beats per minutes, and her blood pressure was 100/63 mmHg. During the physical examination, the patient was found to have a small, diffuse, palpable thyroid gland with no palpable nodules or lymph nodes. There was visual evidence of facial puffiness and edema in both hands and feet (Figure 1), without calf muscle hypertrophy. In terms of sexual development, the patient had breasts and pubic hair (Tanner stage 3) but had no axillary hair and had not yet attained menarche. There was normal speech and limb activity. A neurological examination was normal. She was also seen by an ophthalmologist who confirmed that there was no papilledema.

2.3. Laboratory Findings. Basic biochemical findings indicated low free thyroxine (FT4) levels (<0.8 pmol/L; normal range: 8.5–22.5 pmol/L), high TSH levels (>100 mIU/mL; normal range: 0.35–5 mIU/L), high thyroglobulin antibody levels (76.1 IU/mL; normal range: <0.4 IU/mL), and high anti-thyroid peroxidase antibody levels (560.8 IU/mL; normal range: <6 IU/mL). In addition, her prolactin level was high initially (3,173 IU/mL; normal range: 102–496 IU/mL). Levels of insulin-like growth factor (IGF)-1 (21.8 nmol/L; normal range: 18.6–68.8 nmol/L) and IGF-binding protein 3 (3.9 mg/L; normal range: 3.1–9.5 mg/L) were in the low end of normal range. All other laboratory investigations including liver function test, renal function test, bone profile, and cortisol levels were normal, apart from a lipid profile which showed high levels of low-density lipoprotein cholesterol (4.49 mmol; normal range: <2.7 mmol) and total cholesterol (5.82 mmol; normal range: 3.2–5.18 mmol), with normal levels of high-density lipoprotein cholesterol. The patient was also investigated for puberty markers, including luteinizing hormone, follicle-stimulating hormone, and estradiol levels, all of which were found to be in the normal pubertal range.

2.4. Radiological Examination. An ultrasound of the thyroid showed that both lobes and isthmus were relatively small in size, with diffuse, coarse, heterogenous parenchymal echotexture with multiple fibrous echogenic lines and no focal nodule (Figure 2). As the patient complained of severe headaches, pituitary magnetic resonance imaging (MRI) was performed, revealing a large, nearly homogenous lesion replacing the pituitary glands, with an isointense signal on T1- and T2-weighted images with widening of the *sella turcica* and superior displacement of the pituitary stalk (Figure 3). The lesion measured approximately 1.3 × 1.4 × 1.4 cm (anteroposterior x transverse x coronal). The T1-weighted images showed high signal intensity of the posterior pituitary glands. There was no significant evidence of necrosis or hemorrhage within the lesion. The radiological examination of the rest of the brain was unremarkable. Despite the child's chronological age being 13 years and 6 months, her bone age was estimated to be 10 years (Figure 4), as per Greulich and Pyle's radiographic atlas of skeletal development of the hand and wrist [6]. A repeated left wrist X-ray at the age of 16 years and 2 months showed a delayed bone age of 13 years.

2.5. Treatment. The patient was started on 25 μg of thyroxine once daily which was increased gradually according to her thyroid function test results (Table 1). Following the administration of thyroxine, her prolactin levels decreased until they normalized. Due to the patient's short stature, a growth hormone stimulation test was performed once her thyroid function results normalized. Both glucagon and clonidine showed poor response (Tables 2 and 3). The patient was started on growth hormone (GH) therapy at 30 μg/kg/day and showed good response, with a growth velocity of 8 cm/year in the first year. She received GH therapy for two years, before stopping for one month. During this time, a repeated GH stimulation test using glucagon on her last follow-up visit at the age of 16 years and 2 months showed poor response, with a peak of 6.33 mIU/L (normal range: >20 mIU/L). The GH therapy was therefore reinitiated.

2.6. Follow-Up. The patient was followed up every three months and continued taking thyroxine in combination with GH therapy, demonstrating good clinical and

Table 1: Biochemical and radiological findings and thyroid hormone doses at diagnosis and during follow-up.

Variable	Time interval					
	At diagnosis	3 m	6 m	9 m	18 m	Last visit
Age	13 y 6 m	13 y 9 m	14 y	14 y 3 m	15 y	16 y 2 m
TSH (mIU/L)*	>100	4.96	3.08	2.1	0.755	0.854
FT4 (pmol/L)**	0.8	12.4	10.8	10.8	15.4	12.7
LDL (mmol/L)†	5.7	3.3	3.5	2.8	2.8	2.8
Prolactin (mIU/mL)‡	3,173	444	—	—	261	—
Thyroxine treatment	25 μg	50 μg	75 μg for 4 days/50 μg for 3 days	-	75 μg for 4 days/50 μg for 3 days	75 μg for 4 days/50 μg for 3 days
Wrist X-ray	Bone age of 10 years as per Greulich and Pyle [6]	—	—	—	—	Bone age of 13 years as per Greulich and Pyle [6]
Pituitary MRI	Mass in the sellar and suprasellar region measuring 1.3 × 1.4 × 1.4 cm	—	Mass in the sellar and suprasellar region measuring 1.2 × 0.7 × 1.1 cm	—	—	Significant improvement of the mass in terms of size and appearance

y = year; m = month; TSH = thyroid-stimulating hormone; FT4 = free thyroxine; LDL = low-density lipoprotein; MRI = magnetic resonance imaging. *Normal range: 0.35–5 mIU/L. **Normal range: 8.5–22.5 pmol/L. †Normal range: <2.7 mmol. ‡Normal range: 102–496 IU/mL.

Table 2: Growth hormone stimulation test findings following clonidine intake.

	Time after clonidine intake (minutes)				
	0	30	60	90	120
GH (mIU/L)*	0.94	0.89	6.53	3.00	1.3

GH = growth hormone. *Normal range: >20 mIU/L.

Table 3: Growth hormone stimulation test findings following glucagon intake.

	Time after glucagon intake (minutes)						
	0	30	60	90	120	150	180
GH (mIU/L)*	0.9	0.57	1.19	4.09	1.28	4.31	6.96

GH = growth hormone. *Normal range: >20 mIU/L.

biochemical response with regards to thyroid function, lipid profile, and prolactin levels (Table 1). Follow-up contrast-enhanced pituitary MRI was performed 6 months after the initiation of thyroxine therapy. The comparison sagittal and coronal T1-weighted images demonstrated a moderate interval reduction in the size of the pituitary mass (now measuring 1.2 × 0.7 × 1.1 cm) (Figure 5). Moreover, at 18 months, follow-up sagittal and coronal contrast-enhanced T1 weighted images showed significant improvement of the pituitary mass with a marked reduction in size and returning to normal appearance (Figure 6). At her last consultation, the patient was aged 16 years and 2 months, her height was 144.8 cm, her midparental height was 145.4 cm, and she was found to be at stage 3 of puberty. She was clinically well and demonstrated normal biochemical features.

3. Discussion

Prolonged primary hypothyroidism can lead to pituitary hyperplasia due to the loss of negative feedback caused by a lack of FT4 and triiodothyronine (T3), which leads to excessive secretion of thyrotropin-releasing hormone (TRH) from the hypothalamus [4]. In addition, long-standing stimulation of TRH can promote the proliferation of prolactin-releasing cells, leading to the oversecretion of prolactin [7]. In this case report, we describe a female adolescent with PHPH who presented with a history of headaches and hand and facial edema of almost one year in duration. To our knowledge, this is the first report of an Omani pediatric patient with PHPH in the literature.

The binding of the thyroid hormone to the nuclear receptor stimulates the synthesis of GH. As such, children with PHPH typically exhibit low or no secretion of GH from the pituitary gland after stimulation [8, 9]. A recent literature review identified 18 cases of PHPH in children, of which 13 were found to have elevated prolactin levels and four with decreased GH levels [1]. In the present case, our patient had a high prolactin level which normalized after introducing thyroxine therapy. She also showed low peak GH levels following stimulation tests performed with clonidine and glucagon even, once her thyroid function test results had normalized.

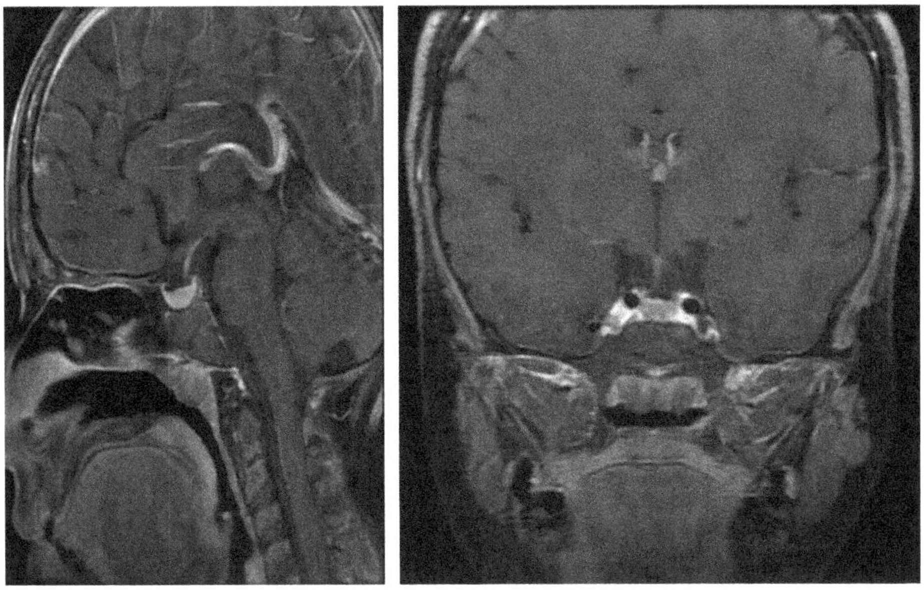

Figure 5: Sagittal and coronal contrast-enhanced T1-weighted magnetic resonance images taken at follow-up after 6 months of thyroid hormone replacement therapy. The images showed a moderate interval reduction in the size of the pituitary mass.

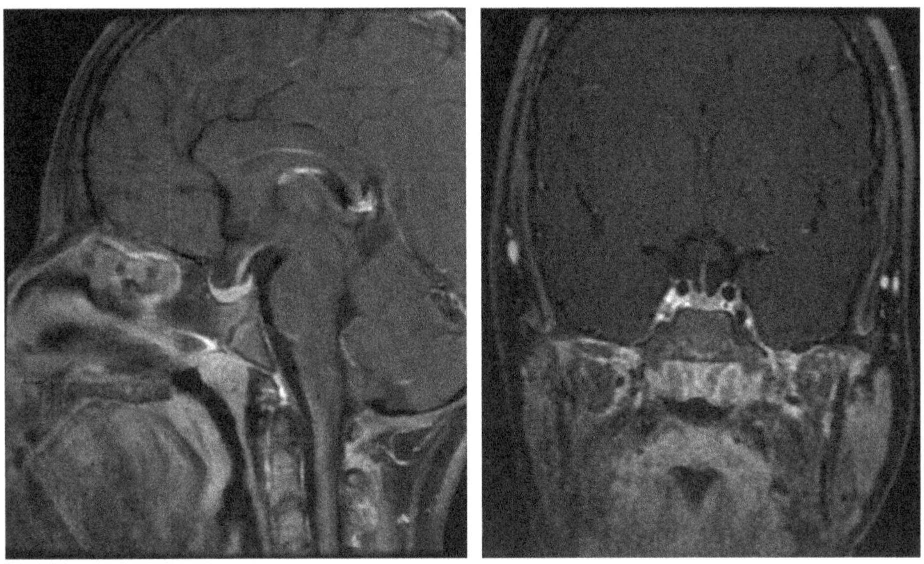

Figure 6: Sagittal and coronal contrast-enhanced T1-weighted magnetic resonance images taken after two years of follow-up. The images showed significant improvement of the pituitary mass as demonstrated by the marked reduction in size, returning to a normal appearance.

The prevalence of isolated growth hormone deficiency (GHD) in Hashimoto's thyroiditis in adults was found to be 5% according to two studies [10, 11]. Another Dutch study in adults showed the prevalence of GHD in Hashimoto's thyroiditis to be much lower (0.4%) [12]. Our patient was investigated for GHD as she was significantly short in stature, with a height SD of −4.8 cm below the mean. She was started on a small dose of 30 μg/kg/day of GH therapy, resulting in some response in her growth velocity, although this could also have been related to the introduction of thyroxine treatment. However, a repeated GH stimulation test showed poor response; hence, the GH therapy was continued.

Laboratory findings in our patient were similar to those reported in the literature, with high TSH levels and low T4 and T3 levels. She was started on low-dose thyroxine treatment with gradual incrementation; as a result, her symptoms improved dramatically. Her pituitary MRI showed an enlarged pituitary gland with marked regression in size within six months of treatment with biochemical improvement. Based on the literature, regression of a pituitary mass to normal size usually occurs over 2–4 months, ranging from 1 to 18 months [13, 14].

In conclusion, it can be challenging to differentiate PHPH from pituitary adenomas based on the initial clinical presentation and MRI findings. Thyrotropin (TSH)-

secreting pituitary adenomas (TSH-omas) are a rare cause of hyperthyroidism. In this situation, TSH secretion is autonomous and refractory to the negative feedback of thyroid hormones (inappropriate TSH secretion), and TSH itself is responsible for the hyperstimulation of the thyroid gland and the consequent hypersecretion of T4 and T3 [15,16] .However, a definitive diagnosis is crucial as treatment varies widely. Pituitary adenomas usually require surgical resection or medical treatment, whereas thyroid hormone replacement therapy is the principal means of treatment of PHPH. As such, an understanding of the differences between these conditions is essential to avoid irreversible complications arising from unnecessary surgical or medical intervention. Repeated brain MRI 6 months after thyroxine therapy can be useful to confirm the diagnosis of PHPH. There is an urgent need for further research to assess the true incidence and prevalence of PHPH in children with Hashimoto's thyroiditis as it is likely that this condition is underdiagnosed.

References

[1] J. Cao, T. Lei, F. Chen, C. Zhang, C. Ma, and H. Huang, "Primary hypothyroidism in a child leads to pituitary hyperplasia: a case report and literature review," *Medicine*, vol. 97, no. 42, Article ID e12703, 2018.

[2] E. García-García, M. Á. Vázquez-López, E. García-Fuentes et al., "Iodine intake and prevalence of thyroid autoimmunity and autoimmune thyroiditis in children and adolescents aged between 1 and 16 years," *European Journal of Endocrinology*, vol. 167, no. 3, pp. 387-392, 2012.

[3] V. H. Nguyen-Michel, N. Schwald, S. Hubert, A. Chahwakilian, and S. Debray-Meignan, "Central hypothyroidism allows discovery of a pituitary disorder in older people," *Journal of the American Geriatrics Society*, vol. 55, no. 4, pp. 630-631, 2007.

[4] L. Han, J. Wang, K. Shu, and T. Lei, "Pituitary tumorous hyperplasia due to primary hypothyroidism," *Acta Neurochirurgica*, vol. 154, no. 8, pp. 1489-1492, 2012.

[5] A. Moumen, A. Meftah, H. El Jadi, S. Elmoussaoui, and G. Belmejdoub, "An unusual pituitary mass revealing a primary hypothyroidism," *Clinical Practice*, vol. 5, no. 1, p. 733, 2015.

[6] W. W. Greulich and S. I. Pyle, *Radiographic Atlas of Skeletal Development of the Hand and Wrist*, Stanford University Press, Redwood city, CA, USA, 1999.

[7] E. Horvath, "Pituitary hyperplasia," *Pathology, Research & Practice*, vol. 183, no. 5, pp. 623-625, 1988.

[8] C. Y. Lee, H. H. Hsu, H. Y. Lai, and S. T. Lee, "Rapid progression of hypothyroidism-related pituitary hyperplasia," *Journal of Neurosurgery: Pediatrics*, vol. 2, no. 3, pp. 212-214, 2008.

[9] M. Kocova, S. Netkov, and E. Sukarova-Angelovska, "Pituitary pseudotumor with unusual presentation reversed shortly after the introduction of thyroxine replacement therapy," *Journal of Pediatric Endocrinology & Metabolism*, vol. 14, no. 9, pp. 1665-1669, 2001.

[10] A. De Bellis, A. Bizzarro, M. Conte et al., "Antipituitary antibodies in adults with apparently idiopathic growth hormone deficiency and in adults with autoimmune endocrine diseases," *Journal of Clinical Endocrinology & Metabolism*, vol. 88, no. 2, pp. 650-654, 2003.

[11] L. Manetti, I. Lupi, L. L. Morselli et al., "Prevalence and functional significance of antipituitary antibodies in patients with autoimmune and non-autoimmune thyroid diseases," *Journal of Clinical Endocrinology & Metabolism*, vol. 92, no. 6, pp. 2176-2181, 2007.

[12] S. A. Eskes, E. Endert, E. Fliers, and W. M. Wiersinga, "Prevalence of growth hormone deficiency in Hashimoto's thyroiditis," *Journal of Clinical Endocrinology & Metabolism*, vol. 95, no. 5, pp. 2266-2270, 2010.

[13] W. W. Ashley Jr., J. G. Ojemann, T. S. Park, and F. J. Wippold, "Primary hypothyroidism in a 12-year-old girl with a suprasellar pituitary mass: rapid regression after thyroid replacement therapy: case report," *Journal of Neurosurgery: Pediatrics*, vol. 102, no. 4, pp. 413-416, 2005.

[14] R. Franceschi, U. Rozzanigo, R. Failo, M. Bellizzi, and A. Di Palma, "Pituitary hyperplasia secondary to acquired hypothyroidism: case report," *Italian Journal of Pediatrics*, vol. 37, no. 1, p. 15, 2011.

[15] P. Beck-Peccoz, F. Brucker-Davis, L. Persani, R. C. Smallridge, and B. D. Weintraub, "Thyrotropin-secreting pituitary tumors," *Endocrine Reviews*, vol. 17, no. 6, pp. 610-638, 1996.

[16] *TSH-producing adenomas: in Endocrinology, Adult and Pediatric*, Sauderns Elsevier, Amsterdam, Netherlands, 7th edition, 2015.

16

A New MEN2 Syndrome with Clinical Features of Both MEN2A and MEN2B Associated with a New *RET* Germline Deletion

Carlotta Giani ,[1] Teresa Ramone,[1] Cristina Romei,[1] Raffaele Ciampi,[1] Alessia Tacito,[1] Laura Valerio,[1] Laura Agate,[1] Clara Ugolini,[2] Michele Marinò,[1] Fulvio Basolo,[2] Alessandro Franchi,[3] Simona Borsari,[1] Angela Michelucci ,[4] Cesare Selli,[5] Gabriele Materazzi,[6] Filomena Cetani,[1] and Rossella Elisei [1]

[1]*Endocrine Unit, Department of Clinical and Experimental Medicine, University Hospital of Pisa, 56124 Pisa, Italy*
[2]*Pathology Unit, Department of Surgical and Medical Pathology, University Hospital of Pisa, 56124 Pisa, Italy*
[3]*Pathology Unit, Department of Translational Research and New Technologies in Medicine and Surgery, University Hospital of Pisa, 56124 Pisa, Italy*
[4]*Unit of Molecular Genetics, Department of Laboratory Medicine, University Hospital of Pisa, 56126 Pisa, Italy*
[5]*Division of Urology, Department of Translational Research and New Technologies in Medicine and Surgery, University Hospital of Pisa, 56124 Pisa, Italy*
[6]*Surgery Unit, Department of Surgical and Medical Pathology, University Hospital of Pisa, 56124 Pisa, Italy*

Correspondence should be addressed to Rossella Elisei; rossella.elisei@med.unipi.it

Academic Editor: Mihail A. Boyanov

Background. Multiple endocrine neoplasia type 2 (MEN2) is a hereditary cancer syndrome caused by *RET* proto-oncogene mutation. Two different clinical variants of MEN2 are known (MEN2A and MEN2B): medullary thyroid carcinoma (MTC) almost always present and associated with pheochromocytoma (Pheo), and primary hyperparathyroidism (HPTH) in MEN2A and with Pheo and other nonendocrine diseases in MEN2B. *Case Report.* A 7-year-old girl, previously treated for a pelvic plexiform neurofibroma, arrived at our observation with a peculiar MEN2B syndrome and with HPTH. The neck ultrasound showed bilateral thyroid nodules, local lymph node lesions, and a suspicious left hyperplastic parathyroid. The CT scan showed a megacolon and described the persistence of the pelvic tumor. A new *RET* germline deletion in exon 11 (c.1892_1899delCGAGCT; p.Glu632_Leu633del) was found. She underwent total thyroidectomy, central compartment and latero-cervical lymph node dissection, and neck exploration for primary HPTH. The histology confirmed bilateral MTC, multiple lymph node metastases, a hyperplastic parathyroid, and a parathyroid adenoma. *Conclusions.* This is the first case of a complex syndrome characterized by peculiar features of MEN2B, without Pheo but with a pelvic plexiform neurofibroma and with HPTH, which is typical of MEN2A. A "de novo" new germline *RET* deletion located in exon 11 was found.

1. Introduction

Multiple endocrine neoplasia type 2 (MEN2) is an autosomal dominant hereditary cancer syndrome caused by missense gain-of-function mutations in the *RET* proto-oncogene [1]. Medullary thyroid carcinoma (MTC) is highly penetrant in MEN2 (100% of cases), and it can be associated with pheochromocytoma (Pheo) and primary hyperparathyroidism (HPTH) [2]. Two different clinical variants of MEN2 are known: MEN2A and MEN2B. In MEN2A, approximately 50% of patients develop Pheo and less frequently (25%) develop HPTH [3]. The only nonendocrine disease that is present in 15–20% of MEN2A patients is interscapular cutaneous lichen amyloidosis (CLA) [4]. The vast majority of MEN2B patients have a marfanoid habitus, thick blueberry lips, corneal nerve thickening, and cutaneous and mucosal neuromas [5, 6].

Another very common disorder in MEN2B is gastrointestinal syndrome, varying from different degrees of constipation or, rarely, diarrhea, abdominal discomfort, and megacolon. The incidence of this disorder in MEN2B is 61–90% [7] and is due to intestinal ganglioneuromatosis, which is histologically characterized by hypertrophy of ganglion cells, supportive cells, and nerve fibers in all layers of the intestinal wall [8]. Pheo is present in approximately 50% of MEN2B cases, while HPTH has never been reported so far [6].

MEN2 syndromes are characterized by a strong genotype-phenotype correlation [1, 9]. Numerous *RET* point mutations, duplications, insertions, and deletions have been identified in patients with MEN2A, but the Cys634Arg mutation in exon 11 remains the most common mutation associated with the classic MEN2A syndrome characterized by the association of MTC with Pheo and HPTH [10]. In contrast, only two *RET* mutations (mainly M918T and, rarely, A883F) have been identified in patients with MEN2B [11]. This is the first report describing a complex syndrome in a young girl affected by MEN2B and MEN2A symptoms and carrying a *RET* deletion never described thus far in association with MEN2 syndrome (http://www.arup.utah.edu/database/MEN2/MEN2_welcome.php). Both the patient's parents and the local ethical committee gave their consent for the report of this case.

2. Case Presentation

A 7-year-old girl was referred to the Oncology Section of the Endocrine Unit of the University Hospital of Pisa, Italy, for suspected MTC based on the presence of both thyroid nodules and elevated serum levels of calcitonin (Ct).

The medical history of the child showed that she was born after a caesarean section at 38 weeks with a weight of 2400 g as well as with newborn jaundice and biliary vomiting. Because of the failure to pass meconium, congenital intestinal dysganglionoses or cystic fibrosis was hypothesized, but at that time, both were ruled out by a rectal biopsy and sweat test, respectively. The patient continued to experience biliary vomiting and failure to thrive; for this reason, she was fed using a nasogastric tube for a long period of time. When she was 2 years old, pyloric stenosis was suspected, and the girl underwent digestive system scintigraphy that demonstrated slowed gastric emptying. On the basis of this test, the patient underwent dilatation of the pylorus but did not achieve any clinical benefit. During gastroscopy, an irregular and small duodenum associated with esophagitis was documented. Magnetic resonance imaging (MRI) demonstrated an abdominal solid massive and expansive lesion (14 cm at the largest diameter) that extended down to the pubic region and surrounded the urethra and the bladder, without any cleavage plans, thus causing mild hydronephrosis. She underwent laparotomy with debulking of the lesion since it was unresectable. The histology described a ganglioneuroma. Over the years, she developed vesicoureteral reflux and recurrent pyelonephritis due to an increasing pressure of the pelvic mass on the bladder that forced her to practice intermittent catheterizations. At 6 years of age, urological control demonstrated high-grade (grade III) vesicoureteral reflux with markedly decreased excretive functioning bilaterally.

At 7 years of age, a serum calcium level of 11.3 mg/dl with a serum parathyroid hormone (PTH) level of 49 pg/ml was found. A neck ultrasound documented bilateral solid hypoechoic thyroid micronodules, a left roundish hypoechoic lesion of 9 mm outside the thyroid gland suspected of lymphadenopathy or hyperplastic parathyroid, and other suspected left latero-cervical lymphadenopathies. A high serum level of Ct was found (665 pg/ml Ct) with normal thyroid function. Fine-needle aspiration of the extrathyroid lesion of 9 mm was suspicious for hyperplastic parathyroid with very high levels of PTH in the wash-out of the needle used for aspiration. The fine-needle aspiration cytology (FNAC) of a left latero-cervical lymphadenopathy was diagnosed as lymph node metastasis of MTC.

The patient arrived for observation in June 2018 for the management of MTC. Upon presentation, she had an evident marfanoid habitus (Figure 1(a)), and bilateral mucosal neuromas of the mouth (Figure 1(b)) that were completely overlooked until that moment.

The laboratory assessments confirmed high levels of Ct (496 ng/L; normal value <18 ng/L), normal thyroid function, hypercalcemia (11.2 mg/dL; normal range: 8.6–10.2 mg/dL), and high levels of PTH (51 ng/L; normal range: 8–40 ng/L). Moreover, an increase in bone-specific alkaline phosphatase isoenzymes (B-ALP 127 μg/L; normal range: 4.7–27.1 μg/L) and osteocalcin (98.7 μg/L; normal range: 10.4–45.6 μg/L) was found to be associated with a mild/low 25-hydroxyvitamin D level (21 μg/L; normal value >30 μg/L).

The neck ultrasound showed three bilateral micronodules and, in particular, a suspicious left solid hypoechoic nodule with an irregular margin of 11 mm. Below the left thyroid lobe, the hypoechoic nodular lesion of 9 mm suspicious for hyperplastic parathyroid was confirmed. In the jugular and left latero-cervical regions, multiple micro-lymphadenopathies were described. The total body computed tomography (CT) scan excluded the presence of distant metastases and clearly revealed the presence of a megacolon (Figure 1(c)). Examination of the pelvic mass by MRI confirmed the presence of a large pelvic lesion (Figure 1(d)) that was substantially stable with respect to the previous radiological exam.

After an accurate evaluation and the exclusion of the presence of Pheo (i.e., negative adrenal gland imaging and normal values of metanephrines), she underwent total thyroidectomy, central compartment and left latero-cervical dissection, and bilateral neck exploration for primary HPTH. Moreover, during surgery, the mucosal neuromas of the mouth were biopsied for a more accurate diagnosis. The histological results described a multifocal, bilateral MTC (Figure 2, panels A and A_1) associated with C cell hyperplasia. In particular, four different microfoci of MTC, three in the left lobe and one in the right lobe, were found; the biggest one (approximately 1 cm) was found in the left lobe, which was the only microfoci detected by neck ultrasound. A strong positive immunoreactivity to anticalcitonin (Figure 2, panel A_2) and negative immunoreactivity to

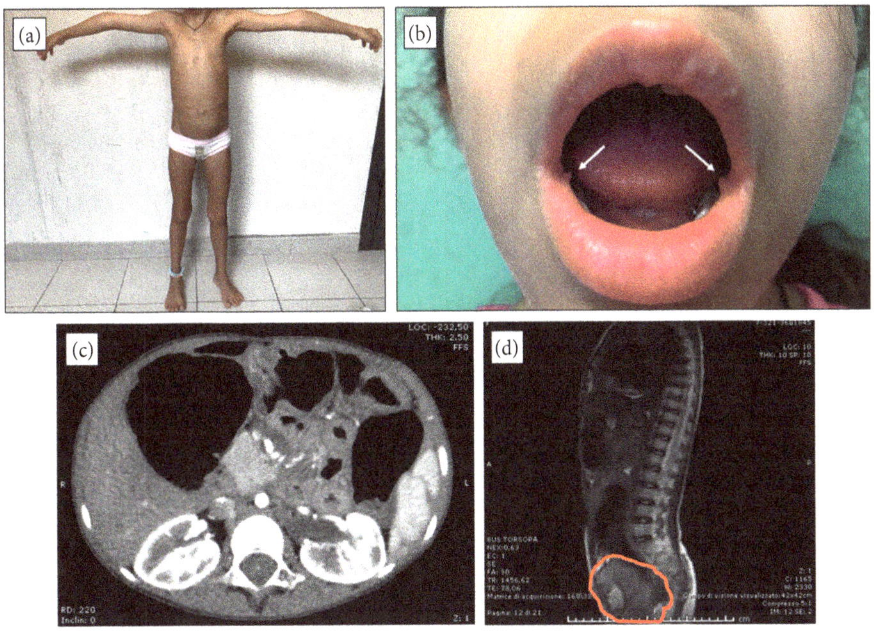

FIGURE 1: Nonendocrine features present in our patient. (a) Marfanoid habitus with long arms and long legs with respect to the trunk and skeletal abnormalities. (b) Bilateral mucosal neuromas of the mouth as indicated by the 2 arrows. (c) CT cross section of the abdomen showing the megacolon. (d) MRI sagittal section of the pelvic plexiform neurofibroma.

antithyroglobulin (Figure 2, panel A_3) antibodies of the MTC tissue were shown. The largest microfocus of the tumor invaded the perithyroid soft tissue (Figure 2, panels B and B_1), and extensive neoplastic lymphangiosis and vascular embolization (Figure 2, panel C) were present. In the perithyroid soft tissue, numerous neoplastic vascular emboli and tumoral deposits infiltrating an adjacent ganglioneuromatosis lesion were found (Figure 2, panels B and B_1). Multiple central compartment (5/10) and left laterocervical (5/32) lymph nodes that were removed were confirmed to be metastases from MTC (Figure 2, panel D). The pathologic tumor stage according to the VIII AJCC/TNM staging [12] was pT1a(m)N1bM0. Moreover, the histology report confirmed the presence of hyperplastic parathyroid (6 mm) and parathyroid adenoma (8 mm). The histology report of the mucosal neuromas of the mouth described the presence of diffuse ganglioneuromatosis (Figure 2, panel E). Histopathologic revision of the pelvic lesion, which had been partially removed at 2 years of age in another center, revealed plexiform neurofibroma associated with ganglioneuromatosis involving the bladder wall (Figure 2, panels F_1, F_2, and F_3). The plexiform neurofibroma component consisted of multiple nodules, often delimited by residual perineural sheaths (Figure 2, panel F_1), formed by a proliferation of uniform bland spindle cells with scant cytoplasm and wavy nuclei, and set within fibrillary collagenous matrix with myxoid areas (Figure 2, panel F_2). The ganglioneuromatosis component consisted mainly of large ganglion cells with a basophilic cytoplasm, vesicular nucleus, and prominent nucleolus (Figure 2, panel F_3). Both components were closely related to the smooth muscle fascicles of the bladder wall. Immunohistochemical analysis revealed diffuse strong S100 positivity in the plexiform neurofibroma, whereas ganglion-like cells were positive for synaptophysin and neuron specific enolase (NSE). Epithelial membrane antigen- (EMA-) positive perineurial cells were present around the neurofibromatous fascicles.

Two months after surgery, our patient still had high levels of Ct (52 ng/L), normal calcium levels on calcitriol therapy 0.25 μg/die (calcium 9.5 mg/dl; normal range: 8.6–10.2 mg/dl), normal PTH values (21 ng/L; normal range: 8–40 ng/L), and better values of both B-ALP and osteocalcin (75 μg/L and 79.4 μg/L, respectively). Moreover, no images suspicious for local disease recurrence were described by neck ultrasound. Eight months after surgery, the CT scan and abdominal MRI confirmed the absence of metastatic lesions and the stability of the pelvic mass. Serum Ct and CEA serum levels were also stable.

3. Genetic Analysis

The parents of the patient gave written informed consent for a detailed genetic examination and for the reporting of the case for scientific and/or teaching purposes. Genomic DNA was extracted from blood, amplified by PCR and sequenced as previously described [13]. A *RET* germline deletion in exon 11 involving codons 631–633 (i.e., c.1893_1898delCGAGCT; p. Asp631_Leu633delinsGlu) was found (Figure 3(a)). The deletion involved the third nucleotide (i.e., C nucleotide) of codon 631, the entire codon 632, and the first two nucleotides of codon 633 (i.e., C and T nucleotides). With this deletion, codon 631 returned in frame with the third nucleotide of codon 633 (G nucleotide), changing codon 631 from aspartate (Asp) to glutamic acid (Glu) (Figure 3(b)). An NGS approach [14] was used to analyze the MTC primary tumor, neck lymph node metastasis, and

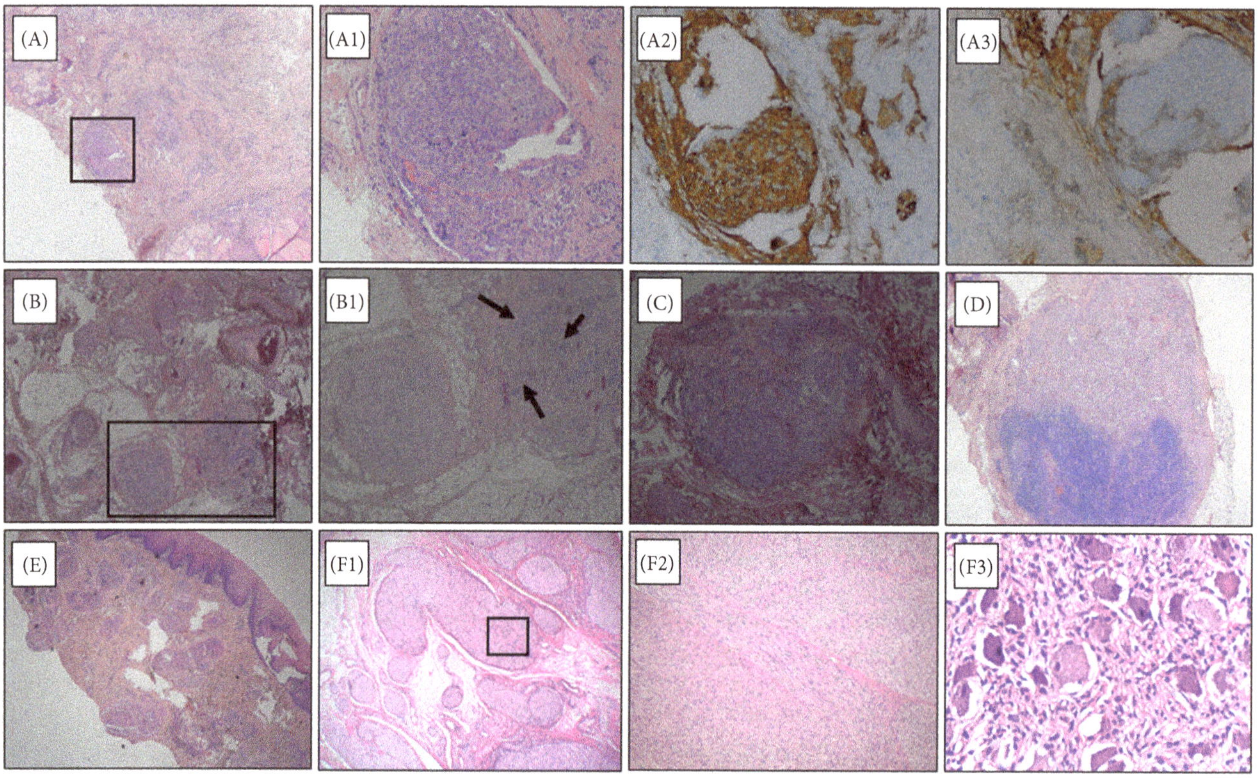

FIGURE 2: Histology of MTC and other lesions. Panels A and A_1: MTC hematoxylin/eosin staining, magnification 2X and 10X, respectively. Panels A_2 and A_3: positive anticalcitonin immunostaining (10X) and negative antithyroglobulin immunostaining (10X) confirming the diagnosis of MTC. Panels B and B_1: MTC infiltrating the perithyroid gangliar tissue, as indicated by the arrows (panel B, 2X, panel B1, 4X). Panel C: MTC vascular invasion with a neoplastic embolus (4X). Panel D: central compartment lymph node metastasis (2X). Panel E: hematoxylin/eosin staining of ganglioneuromatosis in the mucosal neuromas of the mouth excised during surgery (2X). Panel F_1: low-power view of the pelvic plexiform neurofibroma. Panel F_2: at higher power, the neurofibroma component consists of a uniform population of bland spindle cells with wavy elongated nuclei set in a fibrillary matrix. Panel F_3: the ganglioneuromatosis elements, which consist of large ganglion-like neurons.

plexiform neurofibroma; no additional somatic mutations were found in the 3 tissues. Due to the complexity of the syndrome and in order to exclude the association with other genetic syndromes, such as MEN1, MEN4, neurofibromatosis 1, Cowden's disease, Marfan syndrome, and pure mucosal neuroma syndrome, we looked for mutations in the *menin*, *CDKN1B*, *NF1*, *PTEN*, *FBN1*, and *SOS1* genes, but no other variants were found.

The *RET* germline deletion was not detected in the blood of the patient's parents and brother, thus showing its "de novo" origin.

4. Discussion

MEN2B is a very rare syndrome in which the combination of MTC, Pheo, and some peculiar features, such as marfanoid habitus, mucosal neurinomas, and bumpy lips, are commonly associated [5]. To our knowledge, no cases of MEN2B associated with HPTH have been reported, even in large series [6]. In terms of the variance, HPTH is present in approximately 25% of MEN2A cases, but in this syndrome, the only "nonendocrine" associated disease is CLA [4]. Our patient was affected by a very peculiar syndrome characterized by the presence of the most common features of MEN2B with the simultaneous presence of HPTH, which is indeed a peculiar feature of MEN2A. Interestingly, the young patient was not affected by Pheo but by a pelvic plexiform neurofibroma with diffuse ganglioneuromatosis. Neurofibromatosis of the genitourinary tract is rare; less than 70 cases of bladder involvement, which is the most frequent site involved, have been described thus far. Among these cases, only 25 occurred in the pediatric population [15]. Plexiform neurofibroma is a benign tumor that is pathognomonic for neurofibromatosis type 1 (NF1), and it occurs in approximately 25% of people with this syndrome. To our knowledge, there are only 2 cases of reported plexiform neurofibroma with diffuse ganglioneuromatosis of the bladder in infants with NF1 [16, 17], but no cases of plexiform neurofibroma have been reported in patients with MEN2A or MEN2B.

Ganglioneuromatosis, consisting of hypertrophy of the diffuse autonomic plexus of the alimentary tract, is usually present in MEN2B and is responsible for the loss of bowel tone, distension, segmental dilation, and ultimately megacolon associated with typical gastrointestinal symptoms of MEN2B patients; however, to the best of our knowledge, no cases of ganglioneuromatosis in the urinary tract have been described in individuals with MEN2B [6]. Thus far, only two

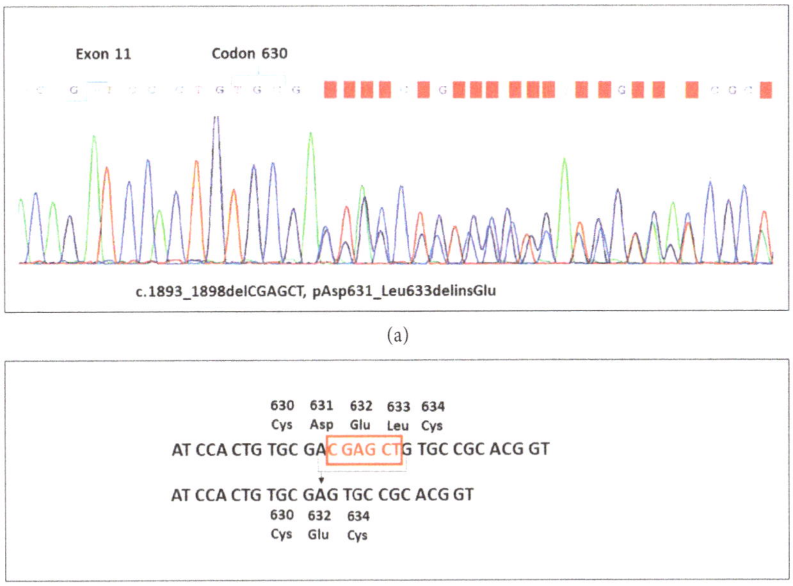

(a)

(b)

Figure 3: The *RET* germline deletion in exon 11 of our patient. (a) Sanger sequence analysis of the constitutive DNA showing the heterozygous germline deletion of 6 nucleotides (C GAG CT) that determined an "in frame" deletion of the *RET* gene at the level of codons 631–633 in exon 11. (b) The deletion involved the third nucleotide (i.e., C nucleotide) of codon 631, the entire codon 632, and the first two nucleotides of codon 633 (i.e., C and T nucleotides). With this deletion, codon 631 returned in frame with the third nucleotide of codon 633 (G nucleotide), changing codon 631 from aspartate (Asp) to glutamic acid (Glu).

cases of adrenal ganglioneuroma in children with MEN 2 have been reported [18]. In particular, the case of a 6-year-old girl with MEN2B and an 11-year-old boy with MEN2A as well as the association with a pure single adrenal ganglioneuroma have been described. In our patient, we found a plexiform neurofibroma with diffuse ganglioneuromatosis that was a different pathological and histological entity with respect to the abovementioned cases of adrenal ganglioneuroma [19, 20].

Although germline complex alterations have already been described and reported in the ARUP database [21], the *RET* mutation found in our case has never been reported in association with MEN syndromes. Nevertheless, this variant has been previously reported at the somatic level (COSM983) [22].

Interestingly, this alteration is very close to Cys634 in exon 11. In fact, codon 634 is commonly mutated in classic MEN2A; thus, we could better expect a typical MEN2A without marfanoid habitus and mucosal neuromas that were clinically (Figure 1) and histologically (Figure 2) confirmed in our patient. Moreover, the megacolon is also typical of MEN2B but has never been reported in MEN2A. It is of interest that this *RET* mutation was a "de novo" mutation, as demonstrated by the absence of the germline mutation in the DNA of the parents and brother of our patient. In this regard, it is relevant to recall that the vast majority of MEN2B syndromes are characterized by a "de novo" mutation [6], while although possible, this event is rather rare in MEN2A [23].

Another possibility to explain this peculiar case could be the combination of MEN2B with other genetic diseases such as MEN1 or MEN4 syndromes or neurofibromatosis as well as real Marfan syndrome, but the absence of mutations in all the specific genes involved in these syndromes excluded this hypothesis.

In conclusion, this is the first case reported thus far of a complex syndrome, MEN2B/MEN2A, characterized by some peculiar features of MEN2B (i.e., MTC, marfanoid habitus and mucosal neurinomas) as well as the absence of Pheo; however, it is associated with the presence of pelvic plexiform neurofibroma, diffuse ganglioneuromatosis, and HPTH, which is indeed more characteristic of MEN2A, and is determined by a "de novo" new germline *RET* deletion located in exon 11 that is more frequently characterized by mutations correlated to MEN2A.

Disclosure

This study was in part presented at the European Thyroid Congress that took place in Budapest on September 7–10, 2019.

Authors' Contributions

Carlotta Giani was involved in the clinical management of the patient and was involved in the preparation and submission of the manuscript. Ramone Teresa performed DNA extraction, prepared samples for NGS analysis, and performed *RET* screening and NGS analysis on the primary tumor tissue. Tacito Alessia performed *RET* genetic screening and identified the new *RET* mutation. Romei

Cristina and Ciampi Raffaele performed NGS analysis on the tumor tissues, supervised all molecular biology experiments, and were involved in the preparation of the manuscript. Valerio Laura and Agate Laura organized multidisciplinary meetings to discuss the clinical follow-up of the patient. Cetani Filomena and Marinò Michele were responsible for the management of primary hyperparathyroidism of the patient. Ugolini Clara and Basolo Fulvio were involved in the histological diagnosis of medullary thyroid cancer and primary hyperparathyroidism and revision of the slides. Franchi Alessandro was involved in the histological diagnosis and revision of the slides of the pelvic plexiform neurofibroma. Borsari Simona performed the germline analysis of menin and CDKN1B. Michelucci Angela performed the germline analysis of PTEN, FBN1, and SOS1. Materazzi Gabriele was involved in the surgical treatment of the patient. Selli Cesare was involved in the follow-up of the urological problem of the patient. Elisei Rossella was responsible of the clinical management of the patient and supervised both the experiments and manuscript preparation.

Acknowledgments

This study was supported by Associazione Italiana Ricerca sul Cancro (IG 2018, cod. 21790); Agenzia Italiana del Farmaco (cod. AIFA-2016-02365049); and PRA_2018_27 "Studio del profilo di progressione tumorale nei carcinomi midollari tiroidei e paratiroidei."

References

[1] C. Romei, R. Ciampi, and R. Elisei, "A comprehensive overview of the role of the RET proto-oncogene in thyroid carcinoma," *Nature Reviews Endocrinology*, vol. 12, no. 4, pp. 192–202, 2016.

[2] F. Raue and K. Frank-Raue, "Update multiple endocrine neoplasia type 2," *Familial Cancer*, vol. 9, no. 3, pp. 449–457, 2010.

[3] D. Viola and R. Elisei, "Management of medullary thyroid cancer," *Endocrinology and Metabolism Clinics of North America*, vol. 48, no. 1, pp. 285–301, 2019.

[4] C. Romei, E. Pardi, F. Cetani, and R. Elisei, "Genetic and clinical features of multiple endocrine neoplasia types 1 and 2," *Journal of Oncology*, vol. 2012, Article ID 705036, 15 pages, 2012.

[5] R. Elisei, A. Matrone, L. Valerio et al., "Fifty years after the first description, MEN 2B syndrome diagnosis is still late: descriptions of two recent cases," *The Journal of Clinical Endocrinology & Metabolism*, vol. 104, no. 7, pp. 2520–2526, 2018.

[6] F. Castinetti, S. G. Waguespack, A. Machens et al., "Natural history, treatment, and long-term follow up of patients with multiple endocrine neoplasia type 2B: an international, multicentre, retrospective study," *The Lancet Diabetes & Endocrinology*, vol. 7, no. 3, pp. 213–220, 2019.

[7] M. Brauckhoff, O. Gimm, C.-L. Weiss et al., "Multiple endocrine neoplasia 2B syndrome due to codon 918 mutation: clinical manifestation and course in early and late onset disease," *World Journal of Surgery*, vol. 28, no. 12, pp. 1305–1311, 2004.

[8] D. Gibbons, M. Camilleri, A. D. Nelson, and D. Eckert, "Characteristics of chronic megacolon among patients diagnosed with multiple endocrine neoplasia type 2B," *United European Gastroenterology Journal*, vol. 4, no. 3, pp. 449–454, 2016.

[9] F. Raue and K. Frank-Raue, "Update on multiple endocrine neoplasia type 2: focus on medullary thyroid carcinoma," *Journal of the Endocrine Society*, vol. 2, no. 8, pp. 933–943, 2018.

[10] C. Eng, D. Clayton, I. Schuffenecker et al., "The relationship between specific RET proto-oncogene mutations and disease phenotype in multiple endocrine neoplasia type 2. International RET mutation consortium analysis," *JAMA: The Journal of the American Medical Association*, vol. 276, no. 19, pp. 1575–1579, 1996.

[11] S. A. Wells, F. Pacini, B. G. Robinson, and M. Santoro, "Multiple endocrine neoplasia type 2 and familial medullary thyroid carcinoma: an update," *The Journal of Clinical Endocrinology & Metabolism*, vol. 98, no. 8, pp. 3149–3164, 2013.

[12] J. D. Brierley, M. K. Gospodarowicz, and C. Wittekind, *TNM Classification of Malignant Tumours*, Union for International Cancer Control, Geneva, Switzerland, 8th edition, 2016.

[13] C. Romei, A. Tacito, E. Molinaro et al., "Twenty years of lesson learning: how does theRETgenetic screening test impact the clinical management of medullary thyroid cancer?" *Clinical Endocrinology*, vol. 82, no. 6, pp. 892–899, 2015.

[14] R. Ciampi, C. Romei, T. Ramone et al., "Genetic landscape of somatic mutations in a large cohort of sporadic medullary thyroid carcinomas studied by next-generation targeted sequencing," *iScience*, vol. 20, pp. 324–336, 2019.

[15] L. Cheng, B. W. Scheithauer, B. C. Leibovich, D. M. Ramnani, J. C. Cheville, and D. G. Bostwick, "Neurofibroma of the urinary bladder," *Cancer*, vol. 86, no. 3, pp. 505–513, 1999.

[16] B. W. Scheithauer, M. Santi, E. R. Richter, B. Belman, and E. J. Rushing, "Diffuse ganglioneuromatosis and plexiform neurofibroma of the urinary bladder: report of a pediatric example and literature review," *Human Pathology*, vol. 39, no. 11, pp. 1708–1712, 2008.

[17] M. Salvitti, F. Celestino, S. Gerocarni Nappo, and P. Caione, "Diffuse ganglioneuromatosis and plexiform neurofibroma of the urinary bladder: an uncommon cause of severe urological disease in an infant," *Journal of Pediatric Urology*, vol. 9, no. 3, pp. e131–e133, 2013.

[18] M. S. Lora, S. G. Waguespack, J. F. Moley, and E. C. Walvoord, "Adrenal ganglioneuromas in children with multiple endocrine neoplasia type 2: a report of two cases," *The Journal of Clinical Endocrinology & Metabolism*, vol. 90, no. 7, pp. 4383–4387, 2005.

[19] V. Y. Jo and C. D. M. Fletcher, "WHO classification of soft tissue tumours: an update based on the 2013 4th edition," *Pathology*, vol. 46, no. 2, pp. 95–104, 2014.

[20] M. Peuchmaur, E. S. G. d'Amore, V. V. Joshi et al., "Revision of the international neuroblastoma pathology classification: confirmation of favorable and unfavorable prognostic subsets in ganglioneuroblastoma, nodular," *Cancer*, vol. 98, no. 10, pp. 2274–2281, 2003.

[21] R. L. Margraf, D. K. Crockett, P. M. F. Krautscheid et al., "Multiple endocrine neoplasia type 2RETprotooncogene database: repository of MEN2-associatedRETsequence variation and reference for genotype/phenotype correlations," *Human Mutation*, vol. 30, no. 4, pp. 548–556, 2009.

[22] G. Pennelli, F. Galuppini, S. Barollo et al., "The PDCD4/miR-21 pathway in medullary thyroid carcinoma," *Human Pathology*, vol. 46, no. 1, pp. 50–57, 2015.
[23] R. Elisei, A. Tacito, T. Ramone et al., "Twenty-five years experience on RET genetic screening on hereditary MTC: an update on the prevalence of germline RET mutations," *Genes*, vol. 10, no. 9, p. 698, 2019.

17

Malignant Insulinoma with Multiple Liver Metastases and Hypercalcitoninemia in a Patient with Type 2 Diabetes Mellitus Presenting as Recurrent Episodes of Diaphoresis due to Severe Hypoglycemia

Marco Ciacciarelli,[1] Gianluca Caruso,[2] Marco Rengo,[3] Piero Maceroni,[3] Carmen Misurale,[1] Eleonora D'Armiento,[1] Alessandro Polidoro,[1] Cristina Napoli,[1] Alberto Lombardini,[1] Umberto Ceratti,[1] Ruben Manuel Luciano Colunga Biancatelli,[1] Leonardo Calvosa,[1] Romina Milanese,[1] Sonia Ferri,[1] Teresa Massaro,[1] Andrea Lorusso,[1] Veronica Sorrentino,[2] Vincenzo Petrozza,[2] and Luigi Iuliano[1]

[1]*Department of Medico-Surgical Sciences and Biotechnologies, Internal Medicine Unit, ICOT Hospital, "Sapienza" University of Rome, Via Franco Faggiana 1668, Latina 04100, Italy*
[2]*Department of Medico-Surgical Sciences and Biotechnologies, Pathology Unit, ICOT Hospital, "Sapienza" University of Rome, Via Franco Faggiana 1668, Latina 04100, Italy*
[3]*Department of Radiological Sciences, Oncology and Pathology, ICOT Hospital, "Sapienza" University of Rome, Via Franco Faggiana 1668, Latina 04100, Italy*

Correspondence should be addressed to Marco Ciacciarelli; marco.ciacciarelli@uniroma1.it

Academic Editor: Mihail A. Boyanov

Insulinoma is an insulin-producing pancreatic neuroendocrine tumor that can be malignant in about 10% of cases. Locoregional invasion, lymph node metastases, or remote metastases are the main criteria of malignant insulinoma. Its incidence in patients with pre-existing diabetes mellitus (DM) is exceptionally rare. In this report, we describe a 66-year-old man with long-standing type 2 DM who presented with recurrent episodes of diaphoresis due to severe hypoglycemia despite the withdrawal of insulin therapy, hypercalcitoninemia, and biochemical and radiological findings suggestive of metastatic malignant insulinoma. Unfortunately, after few days of diazoxide treatment, edema, hypotension, oliguria, and water retention were observed, patient's clinical status deteriorated rapidly, and he died in our department from acute renal failure.

1. Introduction

Insulinoma is an insulin-producing pancreatic neuroendocrine tumor (PNET) that can be malignant in about 10% of cases [1]. Locoregional invasion, lymph node metastases, or remote metastases are the main criteria of malignant insulinoma. The incidence of insulinoma, especially the malignant type, in patients with diabetes mellitus (DM) is extremely rare, and the diagnosis can be challenging due to concomitant glucose-lowering drugs, mistaken as the cause of hypoglycemia. Here, we report the case of a 66-year-old man with a medical history of long-standing type 2 DM diagnosed with malignant metastatic insulinoma, presented as recurrent episodes of diaphoresis. Furthermore, we discuss its relevance within the contest of PNETs and similar cases described in the literature, to aware physician of this, yet rare but dramatic and challenging disease that could affect the diabetic population.

2. Case

A 66-year-old man was admitted to our internal medicine department for recurrent episodes of severe hypoglycemia.

Type 2 DM was diagnosed when he was 31 years old and initially treated with oral antihyperglycemic agents. The patient discontinued oral antidiabetic agents and started insulin therapy 4 years before admission. At that time, he was treated with long-acting insulin glargine and insulin aspart. This insulin regimen was switched to insulin degludec/liraglutide 3 months before admission. While he was on insulin degludec/liraglutide, his home blood glucose monitoring ranged from 110 to 70 mg/dL. Five days before admission, while on insulin degludec/liraglutide in a dose of 18 IU daily, the patient started having recurrent episodes of diaphoresis. During those episodes, usually in the early morning before breakfast, his blood glucose levels were below 50 mg/dL. The patient suffered from several further episodes despite insulin dosage tapering and even after discontinuation. His past medical history was notable for heart failure with reduced ejection fraction, acute coronary syndrome, and osteomyelitis of the left foot. His family medical history included atrial fibrillation and DM. In addition to insulin, his therapy consisted in acetylsalicylic acid, bisoprolol, furosemide, ramipril, and atorvastatin. He denied oral antihyperglycemic agents. He had no known drug allergies, he was a former smoker, and he did not drink alcohol or use illicit drugs.

On admission, the patient's blood pressure was 130/80 mmHg, heart rate was 71 beats per minute, respiratory rate was 14 breaths per minute, and oxygen saturation was 98%, while he was breathing ambient air. The patient's body mass index was 26.7 kg/m^2 (height: 173 cm; weight: 80 kg), and the physical examination was unremarkable. Laboratory data on admission showed glucose 50 mg/dl, HbA1c 50 mmol/mol, normocytic anemia (hemoglobin 11.9 g/dL, hematocrit 34.8%, and mean corpuscular volume 85 fl), a normal white cell and platelet count, aspartate aminotransferase (AST) 87 IU/L (normal range: 17–59), alanine aminotransferase (ALT) 62 IU/l (normal range: 21–72), gamma glutamyl-transferase 545 IU/l (normal range: 15–73), alkaline phosphatase 177 IU/l (normal range: 38–126), total bilirubin 0.47 mg/dL (normal range: 0.20–1.30), lactate dehydrogenase 1021 IU/L (normal range: 313–618), albumin 3.5 g/dL (normal range: 3.6–5.5), INR 1.18, C-reactive protein 7.5 mg/dl (normal range: 0-1), erythrocyte sedimentation rate 90 mm/h (normal range: 0–15), fibrinogen 621 mg/dl (normal range: 170–410), iron 37 μg/dl (normal range: 49–181), and ferritin 776 ng/ml (normal range: 20–325). Viral markers for hepatitis B and C were negative.

Further blood tests were ordered to rule out endogenous hyperinsulinism: C-peptide was 4.2 ng/mL (normal range: 0.5–3), insulin 89 μIU/mL (normal range: 5–25), while the patient's glucose level was 40 mg/dL, and sulfonylurea screening test was negative, confirming endogenous hyperinsulinism. Markers of neuroendocrine tumors were severely increased: chromogranin A (CgA) was 1790 ng/ml (normal range: 0–100), and neuron-specific enolase (NSE) was 458 ng/ml (normal range: 0–11).

Given the high suspicion of insulinoma and the altered liver function tests on admission, a full-body CT scan was ordered. CT scan showed a 4.3 × 2.2 cm pancreatic tail mass containing calcifications with multiple regional lymphadenopathies (Figure 1). Multiple liver secondary lesions were found: the largest ones measuring 12 and 11 cm, respectively, in II-III and IVb-V segments. No lungs, bone, and brain metastases were detected. Additionally, a thyroid nodule of 2.6 cm was incidentally found. Hepatic metastases were highly suspected to be secondary to a malignant insulinoma, so ultrasound-guided percutaneous biopsies of the lesion in the II-III segments were performed (Figure 2). Histological findings of four core biopsies consisted of hepatocytes infiltrated by a poorly differentiated and focally necrotic proliferating tissue of medium-sized atypical epithelial cells with solid growth pattern (Figure 3). The cancer cells showed hyperchromatic nuclei with "salt and pepper" chromatin markedly Ki-67 positive, high mitotic index (10 figures × 10 HPF), and scant cytoplasm. Immunohistochemistry studies revealed the neuroendocrine nature and the partial insulin secreting activity of the lesion; CgA, synaptophysin, CD56, and CAM5.2 were diffusely positive; there was patchy (<5%) insulin expression. Ki-67 index was 40–50. These findings were consistent with the diagnosis of metastatic, poorly differentiated (G3), neuroendocrine carcinoma with morphology and immunophenotype favoring a pancreatic primary tumor. Thyroid ultrasound (Figure 4) showed a weakly hypoechoic solid nodule (2.8 × 3.2 × 1.3 cm) with a central cystic component and regular margins located in the isthmus and a markedly hypoechoic solid nodule (0.9 × 0.9 × 0.6 cm) adjacent to the lower pole of the left lobe. Calcifications and intranodular flow were absent in both nodules, and regional lymph nodes were not enlarged. The results of thyroid function tests were within normal limits (TSH 0.7 mUI/L, normal range: 0.46–4.68), as well as were parathormone (PTH) (80.1 pg/mL, normal range: 13.6–85.8), calcium (8.76 mg/dL, normal range: 8.4–10.2), and phosphorus (4.32 mg/dL, normal range: 2.5–4.5). Serum calcitonin was slightly raised (30 pg/mL, normal range: 0–6), but immunohistochemical staining of the liver lesions was negative for such markers.

The patient's hospital stay was characterized by different episodes of severe hypoglycemia (as low as 18 mg/dL) occurring especially at night and in the early morning, manifesting only with diaphoresis. During those episodes, the patient never lost consciousness or developed seizures and even never complained of confusion, amnesia, weakness, diplopia, blurred vision, palpitations, or hunger. In order to reduce the hypoglycemic events, we started a symptomatic treatment with diazoxide and IV infusion of 10% dextrose, while waiting for histopathological confirmation of the disease. Unfortunately, due to the severity of this malignancy, after 8 days of treatment edema, hypotension, oliguria, and weight gain of 10 kg were observed; the patient's clinical status deteriorated rapidly, and 3 days later, the patient died from acute renal failure. Postmortem examination was not carried out according to his family's request.

3. Discussion

PNETs are rare neuroendocrine malignancies that count only for the 2% of total pancreatic tumors. Their incidence is around 1 case per 100,000 people, and only about 10% of

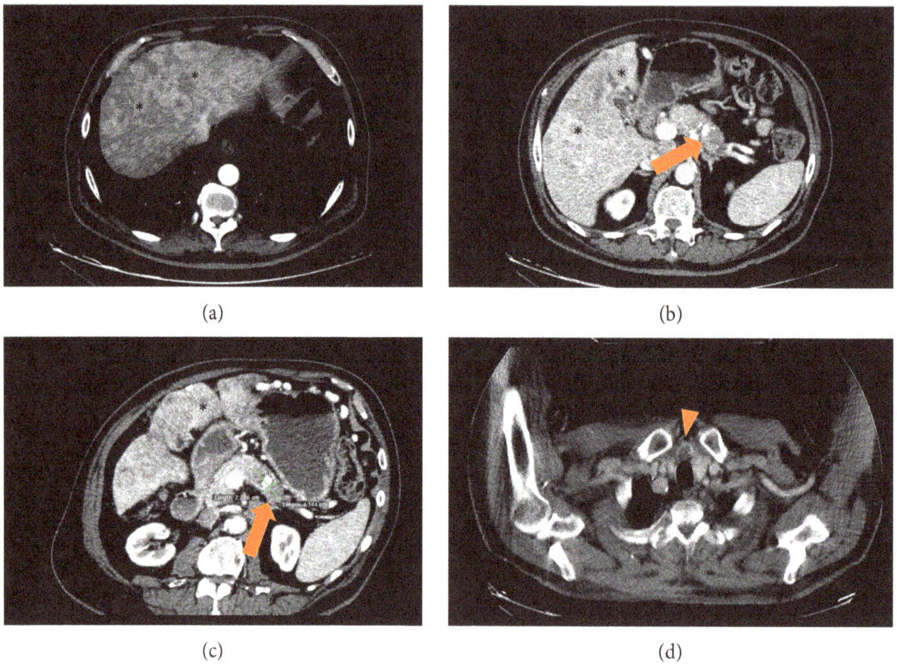

Figure 1: CT images (a)–(c) show multiple hypervascular liver metastases (∗) and a focal solid lesion of the pancreatic tail (arrow). A thyroid nodule (arrow head) was also detected (d).

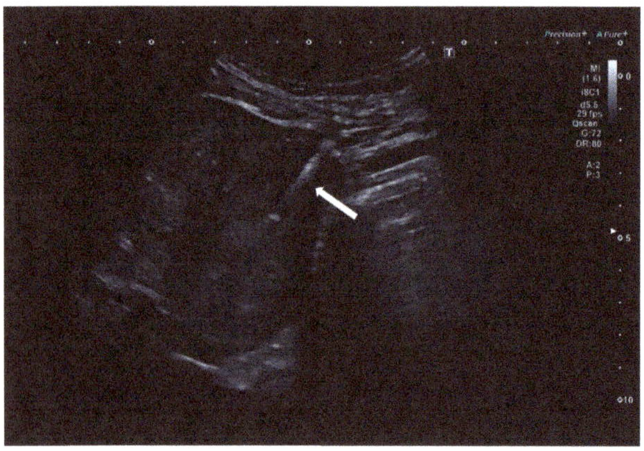

Figure 2: Ultrasound-guided percutaneous biopsies of the lesion located in the liver segments II-III. White arrow shows the needle penetrating in the subglissonian isoechoic/hypoechoic solid nodule with irregular margins (maximum diameter: 2.2 cm).

them are classified as functional, as they release hormones or peptides that cause specific symptoms and signs [2]. With an estimated incidence of 4 cases per 1 million person-years [3], insulinomas and insulin-producing tumors, are the most common functional PNETs, and unlike other PNETs, which are malignant in 50–100% of cases, they are malignant only in about 10% of cases [4].

Locoregional invasion, lymph node metastases, or remote metastases are the main criteria of malignant insulinoma. Most patients with malignant insulinoma have lymph node or liver metastases [5–7], and only rare metastases in other sites such as bones [8, 9], lungs [10], brain [11], ovaries [12, 13], and gallbladder [14]. Liver metastases at presentation count for almost 60% of the patients with PNETs [2].

In this report, we described a malignant insulinoma with multiple liver metastases in a 66-year-old man with longstanding type 2 DM. Although benign insulinoma occurs rarely in patients with pre-existing DM [15–17], malignant insulinoma in this population seems to be even rarer, and only sparse cases are described in the literature, in both type 2 [18–23] and type 1 DM [12, 24, 25]. However, despite the rare occurrence of insulinoma in diabetic population, clinicians should be aware of this possible differential diagnosis when managing diabetic patients with recurrent episodes of symptomatic hypoglycemia despite tapering and withdrawal of glucose-lowering drugs. We searched the PubMed database, and to the best of our knowledge, we collected the clinical, pathologic, and biochemical data of all previously reported cases of malignant insulinoma in patients with DM (Table 1). As reported by Yu et al. [26], short hypoglycemic symptoms duration before diagnosis of tumor seems to be common in patients with malignant insulinoma (median duration: 30 days). Furthermore, as shown in the same study, high proinsulin and CgA levels and a large proinsulin/insulin molar ratio should raise the suspicion of malignant insulinoma in patients with hyperinsulinemic hypoglycemia. In our case, similarly, hypoglycemic symptoms duration before diagnosis of malignant insulinoma was short (20 days), and CgA levels were markedly elevated (1790 ng/ml). Unfortunately, we could not measure proinsulin levels and calculate proinsulin/insulin molar ratio due to laboratory limitations.

Insulinoma is a pancreatic islet cell tumor which may be associated with multiple endocrine neoplasia type 1 (MEN-1). MEN-1 diagnosis was excluded because of age, a negative family medical history, and the absence of any clinical features of the most common endocrine and nonendocrine tumors associated with this rare syndrome. Primary

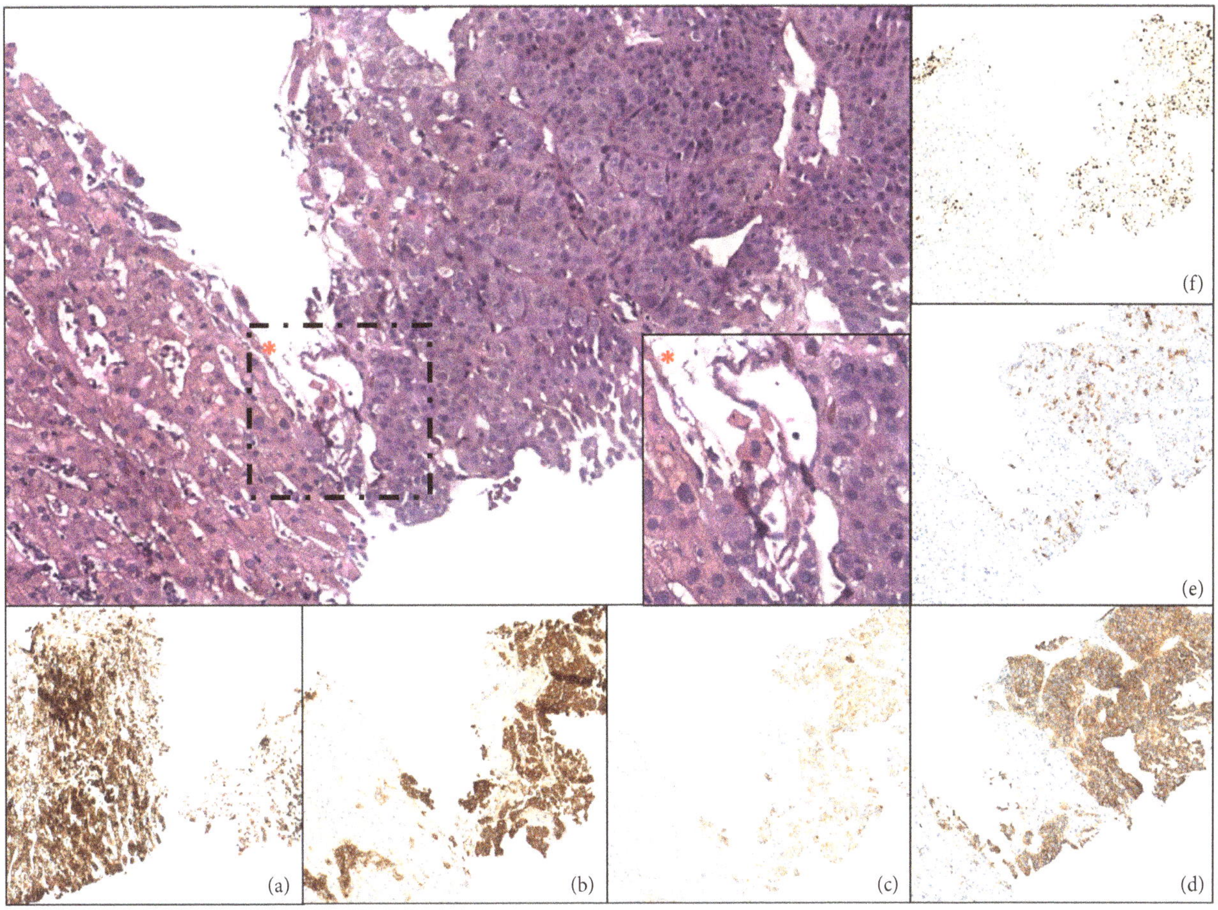

FIGURE 3: Poorly differentiated neuroendocrine carcinoma metastatic to the liver (H&E, magnification: 10x). The * box represents a detailed view of neoplasia (H&E, magnification: 40x). Immunohistochemical staining for CAM5.2 (a), synaptophysin (b), chromogranin A (c), CD56 (d), insulin (e), and Ki-67 proliferation index (f) (magnification: 10x).

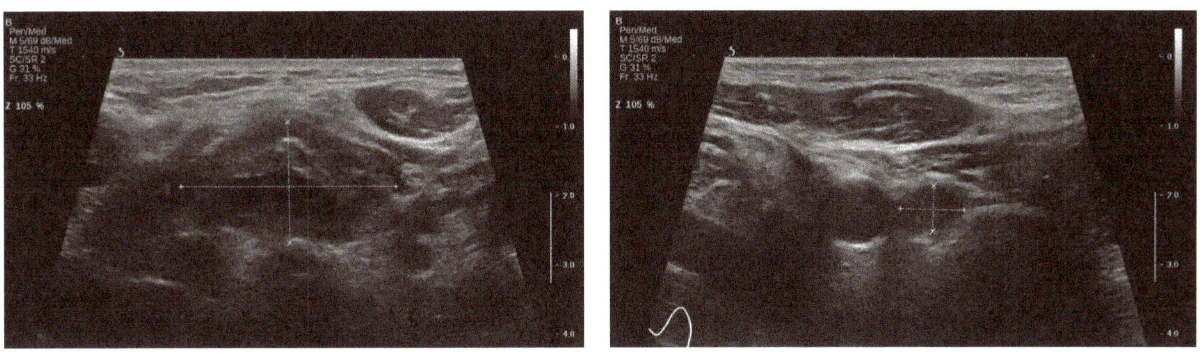

(a) (b)

FIGURE 4: Thyroid ultrasound. Weakly hypoechoic solid nodule ($2.8 \times 3.2 \times 1.3$ cm) with a central cystic component and regular margins located in the isthmus (a). Markedly hypoechoic solid nodule ($0.9 \times 0.9 \times 0.6$ cm) adjacent to the lower pole of the left lobe (b).

hyperparathyroidism is commonly associated with MEN-1, and at least 90% of patients develop it by the age of 50 years. The absence of history of osteoporosis or nephrolithiasis and normal serum calcium and PTH levels led us to rule out primary hyperparathyroidism. Since our patient had no symptoms or signs of a pituitary tumor, we did not order pituitary hormones (other than TSH) and pituitary MRI to rule out a pituitary tumor.

Metastatic insulinoma in our patient was extremely aggressive, and only progressively increased doses of diazoxide, up to 500 mg per day, were able to avoid severe hypoglycemic episodes. Unfortunately, as reported in other cases [19], our patient rapidly developed edema, hypotension, oliguria, and water retention secondary to diazoxide toxicity and died from acute renal failure. First-line chemotherapy regimen for poorly differentiated pancreatic

TABLE 1: Clinical, pathologic, and biochemical data of reported cases of malignant insulinoma in patients with diabetes mellitus.

Authors	Year	DM type	Age, sex	Site	Size (cm)	Metastases	Hypoglycemia symptoms	Insulin (μUI/ml)	C-peptide (ng/ml)	CgA (ng/ml)	Thyroid disease	Calcitonin (pg/ml)
Svartberg [12]	1996	1	33, F	Tail	Not reported	Liver Ovaries	Unconsciousness	86	8.4	Not reported	No	Not reported
Siraji [18]	2006	2	74, F	Tail, head	7.3 × 5.7 3 × 3 3.1 × 1.8	Liver	Diaphoresis Palpitations Confusion Seizures	39 (G: 28)	5.2	Not reported	No	Not reported
Schmitt [19]	2008	2	79, F	Body, tail	Not reported	Liver	Hunger Dizziness Tiredness	74 (G: 34)	9.7	↑ (404)	Hypothyroidism	Normal (<3)
FerrerGarcìa [20]	2011	2	78, M	Head	4.7 × 3	Liver	Not reported	23 (G: 35) (F)	4.6	↑ (834)	No	Not reported
Abbasakoor [21]	2011	2	67, F	Body	2.6 × 2 5-6	Liver Lymph nodes	Unconsciousness Anxiety Diaphoresis	91 (G: 19) (F)	8.2	Not reported	No	Not reported
Ademoglu [22]	2012	2	45, F	Head	0.8 × 0.7 0.9 × 1 0.7 × 0.7	Liver Lymph nodes	Confusion Diaphoresis	114 (G: 35) (F)	4.8	Not reported	No	Not reported
Lablanche [24]	2015	1	31, M	Head	6.3 × 5.6	Lymph nodes	Not reported	18 (G: 37) (F)	7.8	Not reported	Hashimoto thyroiditis	Not reported
Gjelberg [25]	2017	1	43, F	Tail	11 × 7	Liver Lymph nodes	Not reported	9 (G: 45) (F)	1.6	↑ (323)	Hypothyroidism	Normal
Our patient	2019	2	66, M	Tail	4.3 × 2.2	Liver	Diaphoresis	89 (G:40)	4.2	↑ (1790)	Thyroid nodules	↑ (30)

G: glucose (mg/dl); F: fasting.

neuroendocrine carcinoma consists with a combination of etoposide and either cisplatin or carboplatin. Unfortunately, when we obtained the report of histological analysis of liver biopsy, our patient was hemodynamically unstable and his renal function has worsened significantly, so we were not able to start chemotherapy with traditional regimen. Everolimus is an mTOR inhibitor with hyperglycemic and antitumoral effects indicated in treatment of malignant insulinoma. Given its toxicity, it is used as third-line treatment of recurrent episodes of hypoglycemia after failure of diazoxide and somatostatin analogs. The antitumoral effect of everolimus has been shown to improve progression-free survival of patients with well-differentiated PNETs. However, the antitumor efficacy of everolimus in poorly differentiated pancreatic neuroendocrine carcinoma remains to be determined.

Interestingly, our patient displayed increased serum calcitonin levels (30 pg/ml, normal range 0–6). Calcitonin is a peptide hormone secreted by C cells of the thyroid that acts as a physiologic antagonist to PTH, lowering blood calcium levels. Despite hypercalcitoninemia is a typical marker of medullary thyroid carcinoma (MTC), calcitonin can be found increased in several conditions: after exhausting physical activity, because of interfering drugs, in thyroid and non-thyroid diseases. These conditions should be always ruled out in cases with basal calcitonin values between 10 and 100 pg/mL [27], as observed in our patient.

He was sedentary, and at the time of blood sample analysis, he was not taking interfering drugs (e.g., omeprazole, glucocorticoids, or beta-blockers). In fact, bisoprolol was discontinued on admission in the attempt of increasing the adrenergic warning symptoms of hypoglycemia. Although glucagon-like peptide 1 analogs such as liraglutide are well known to cause slightly increases of calcitonin, we rejected this hypothesis because our patient discontinued liraglutide 22 days before calcitonin measurement.

Follicular and papillary thyroid carcinomas are thyroid diseases that may be associated to slightly raised calcitonin levels. Although the two thyroid nodules of our patient appeared benign and did not show any signs of malignancy (e.g., calcifications, intranodular flow, taller-than-wide shape, irregular margins, local invasion of surrounding structures, suspicious neck lymph nodes), we could not completely rule out any type of thyroid carcinoma, including MTC, as fine needle aspiration was not carried out due to severe worsening of the patient's clinical status. However, it is unlikely that ultrasound thyroid findings paired with thyroid malignancies and two different neuroendocrine tumors such as MTC and malignant insulinoma developed simultaneously.

Hypercalcitoninemia may also occur in nonthyroid diseases such as chronic renal failure, hyperparathyroidism-related hypercalcemia, and hypergastrinemia. Our patient had normal renal function, normal calcium levels, and no clinical features of conditions commonly associated with hypergastrinemia such as atrophic gastritis and gastrinoma; therefore, serum gastrin levels were not measured.

Hypercalcitoninemia due to ectopic calcitonin secretion by several types of PNETs, including insulinoma, has been described [28–33]; therefore, we measured calcitonin levels even if our patient had no family history of MTC or clinical and laboratory findings consistent with hyperparathyroidism or pheochromocytoma. Moreover, hypercalcitoninemia due to calcitonin-producing insulinoma has been documented in patients with benign thyroid nodules [31, 32].

Since a specific endocrine syndrome related to hypercalcitoninemia has not been identified yet, calcitonin-producing PNETs are currently classified as nonfunctional, unless they secrete "eutopic" biologically active hormones (insulin, glucagon, somatostatin, and pancreatic polypeptide). Interestingly, according to Uccella et al. [33], calcitonin expression is not related to either a more aggressive behavior or a worse prognosis, so it seems to not identify a separate subset of PNETs. The immunohistochemical detection of calcitonin in cells from pancreatic mass and the normalization of its value after tumor resection are important findings in confirming the diagnosis of calcitonin-producing insulinoma [29, 31, 32]. Due to the history of heart failure with reduced ejection fraction and the high suspicion of liver metastases, we performed a less-invasive diagnostic procedure such as liver biopsy rather than endoscopic ultrasound-guided biopsies of the pancreatic mass, as successfully reported in similar cases [5–7]. To the best of our knowledge, the few cases of calcitonin-producing insulinoma reported in the literature were not associated to metastases in liver or in other sites. In our case, immunohistochemistry of the liver lesion was negative for calcitonin; however, it should be noted that immunostaining of hepatic lesions secondary to calcitonin-producing PNETs may be negative for calcitonin probably because metastases can dedifferentiate and lose their secretory activity [34].

Despite the diagnosis of malignant insulinoma in our patient was made with biopsy of liver metastasis rather than biopsy of the pancreatic mass, in the absence of other apparent causes of hypercalcitoninemia, we hypothesized that cells of the pancreatic malignancy were able to produce calcitonin with following elevation of this serum marker.

4. Conclusion

In conclusion, although very rare, malignant insulinoma can occur in patients with both type 2 and type 1 DM. Most patients with malignant insulinoma have lymph node or liver metastases at presentation. Malignant insulinoma with liver metastases should always be considered as a cause of recurrent episodes of symptomatic hypoglycemia in diabetic patients with altered liver function tests, especially when severe hypoglycemia persists after withdrawal of glucose-lowering agents.

Furthermore, this case underlines that hypercalcitoninemia in patients with thyroid nodules is not necessarily due to MTC. Several physiologic and pathologic conditions other than MTC have been associated with increased calcitonin levels, including calcitonin-producing PNETs. Since the majority of PNETs are malignant, nonfunctional and hence represent a diagnostic challenge for physicians, all patients with raised calcitonin levels and thyroid nodules not clearly suggestive of MTC should be submitted to a careful investigation in order to rule out a calcitonin-producing PNET, a rare but recognized cause of hypercalcitoninemia.

References

[1] B. Hirshberg, C. Cochran, M. C. Skarulis et al., "Malignant insulinoma," *Cancer*, vol. 104, no. 2, pp. 264–272, 2005.

[2] A. Lewis, D. Li, J. Williams, and G. Singh, "Pancreatic neuroendocrine tumors: state-of-the-art diagnosis and management," *Oncology (Williston Park, NY)*, vol. 31, no. 10, pp. e1–12, 2017.

[3] F. J. Service, M. M. McMahon, P. C. O'brien, and D. J. Ballard, "Functioning insulinoma-incidence, recurrence, and long-term survival of patients: a 60-year study," *Mayo Clinic Proceedings*, vol. 66, no. 7, pp. 711–719, 1991.

[4] D. W. Lee, M. K. Kim, and H. G. Kim, "Diagnosis of pancreatic neuroendocrine tumors," *Clinical Endoscopy*, vol. 50, no. 6, pp. 537–545, 2017.

[5] C. Toyoda, K. Hosokawa, Y. Atsumi et al., "Malignant insulinoma with extensive liver metastases presenting as disturbance of consciousness," *Internal Medicine*, vol. 37, no. 5, pp. 476–479, 1998.

[6] R. Baldelli, G. Ettorre, G. Vennarecci et al., "Malignant insulinoma presenting as metastatic liver tumor. Case report and review of the literature," *Journal of Experimental & Clinical Cancer Research: CR*, vol. 26, no. 4, pp. 603–607, 2007.

[7] A. Barnabei, E. Askin, F. Kose et al., "Erratum to: rapidly progressing malignant insulinoma presented with multiple liver metastases: a case report," *Journal of Gastrointestinal Cancer*, vol. 41, no. 4, pp. 272–274, 2010.

[8] C. S. Hesdorffer, M. Stoopler, and J. Javitch, "Aggressive insulinoma with bone metastases," *American Journal of Clinical Oncology*, vol. 12, no. 6, pp. 498–501, 1989.

[9] A. Naganuma, H. Mayahara, C. Morizane et al., "Successful control of intractable hypoglycemia using radiopharmaceutical therapy with strontium-89 in a case with malignant insulinoma and bone metastases," *Japanese Journal of Clinical Oncology*, vol. 42, no. 7, pp. 640–645, 2012.

[10] A. Albu, A. Zirnea, O. Georgescu, D. Terzea, D. Jinga, and S. Fica, "Malignant insulinoma with hepatic and pulmonary metastases associated with primary hyperparathyroidism. Case report and review of the literature," *Journal of Medicine and Life*, vol. 1, no. 2, pp. 210–217, 2008.

[11] J. L. Frazier and J. D. Weingart, "Metastatic insulinoma to the brain," *Endocrinologist*, vol. 19, no. 1, p. 5, 2009.

[12] J. Svartberg, M. Stridsberg, E. Wilander, D. E. H. Andersson, and B. Eriksson, "Tumour-induced hypoglycaemia in a patient with insulin-dependent diabetes mellitus," *Journal of Internal Medicine*, vol. 239, no. 2, pp. 181–185, 1996.

[13] O. Bélissant Benesty, T. Cassou-Mounat, C. Vatier, J.-N. Talbot, and F. Montravers, "Tumor heterogeneity detected by 68Ga DOTATOC and 18F-FDG PET/CTs in one malignant insulinoma with involvement of the portal splenic confluence and ovarian metastases," *Clinical Nuclear Medicine*, vol. 41, no. 11, pp. 874–876, 2016.

[14] M. Imamura, E. Miyashita, K. Miyagawa, S. Matsuno, and T. Sato, "Malignant insulinoma with metastasis to gallbladder and bone, accompanied by past history of peptic ulcer and hyperthyroidism," *Digestive Diseases and Sciences*, vol. 32, no. 11, pp. 1319–1324, 1987.

[15] L. A. Kane, C. S. Grant, T. B. Nippoldt, and F. J. Service, "Insulinoma in a patient with NIDDM," *Diabetes Care*, vol. 16, no. 9, pp. 1298–1300, 1993.

[16] H. Ishii, T. Ito, S. Moriya, Y. Horie, and M. Tsuchiya, "Insulinoma—a statistical review of 443 cases in Japan," *Nippon Rinsho*, vol. 51, no. Suppl, pp. 199–206, 1993.

[17] W.-Y. Lei, T.-E. Wang, T.-L. Chen, W.-H. Chang, T.-L. Yang, and C.-Y. Wang, "Insulinoma causing hypoglycemia in a patient with type 2 diabetes," *Journal of the Formosan Medical Association*, vol. 106, no. 5, pp. 392–396, 2007.

[18] E. S. Siraj, G. Samuel, S. Saber, S. Samuel, A. H. Hamrahian, and S. S. K. Reddy, "Metastatic malignant insulinoma in a patient with type 2 diabetes mellitus: case presentation and literature review," *Endocrine Practice*, vol. 12, no. 4, pp. 411–416, 2006.

[19] J. Schmitt, S. Boullu-Sanchis, F. Moreau et al., "Association of malignant insulinoma and type 2 diabetes mellitus: a case report," *Annales d'Endocrinologie*, vol. 69, no. 1, pp. 69–72, 2008.

[20] J. Ferrer-García, M. Tolosa-Torréns, C. Hernando-Meliá, L. Arribas-Palomar, and C. Sánchez-Juan, "Everolimus resolving hypoglycemia, producing hyperglycemia, and necessitating insulin use in a patient with diabetes and nonresectable malignant insulinoma," *Endocrine Practice*, vol. 17, no. 2, pp. e17–e20, 2011.

[21] N. O. Abbasakoor, M. L. Healy, D. O'Shea et al., "Metastatic insulinoma in a patient with type 2 diabetes mellitus: case report and review of the literature," *International Journal of Endocrinology*, vol. 2011, Article ID 124078, 5 pages, 2011.

[22] E. Ademoğlu, U. Unlütürk, K. Ağbaht, A. Karabork, and D. Corapçioğlu, "Type 2 diabetes mellitus in a patient with malignant insulinoma manifesting following surgery," *Diabetic Medicine*, vol. 29, no. 7, pp. e133–137, 2012.

[23] V. I. Podzolkov, N. A. Dragomiretskaia, T. V. Koroleva, N. N. Kavtaradze, H. H. Iakovleva, and A. V. Podzolkov, "A rare case of hypoglycemia in an elderly patient with type 2 diabetes mellitus: malignant metastasizing insulinoma," *Klin Med (Mosk)*.vol. 92, no. 2, pp. 65–70, 2014.

[24] S. Lablanche, M. Chobert-Bakouline, O. Risse, M.-H. Laverrière, O. Chabre, and P.-Y. Benhamou, "Malignant insulinoma may arise during the course of type 1 diabetes mellitus: a case report," *Diabetes & Metabolism*, vol. 41, no. 3, pp. 258–261, 2015.

[25] H. K. Gjelberg, D. Hoem, C. S. Verbeke, J. Eide, J. G. Cooper, and A. Molven, "Hypoglycemia and decreased insulin requirement caused by malignant insulinoma in a type 1 diabetic patient: when the hoof beats are from a zebra, not a horse," *Clinical Case Reports*, vol. 5, no. 6, pp. 761–768, 2017.

[26] R. Yu, N. N. Nissen, A. Hendifar et al., "A clinicopathological study of malignant insulinoma in a contemporary series," *Pancreas*, vol. 46, no. 1, pp. 48–56, 2017.

[27] S. P. Fan, D. M. Lourenço, M. A. Santos, M. R. Tavares, R. A. Toledo, and J. E. de Menezes Correia-Deur, "Hypercalcitoninemia is not pathognomonic of medullary thyroid carcinoma," *Clinics (Sao Paulo)*.vol. 64, no. 7, pp. 699–706, 2009.

[28] A. Ooi, I. Nakanishi, T. Kameya, Y. Funaki, and K. Kobayashi, "Calcitonin-producing insulinoma: an immunohistochemical and electron microscopic study," *Pathology International*, vol. 36, no. 12, pp. 1897–1903, 1986.

[29] D. E. Price, S. R. Absalom, K. Davidson, A. Bolia, P. R. F. Bell, and T. A. Howlett, "A case of multiple endocrine neoplasia: hyperparathyroidism, insulinoma, GRF-OMA, hypercalcitoninaemia and intractable peptic ulceration," *Clinical Endocrinology*, vol. 37, no. 2, pp. 187-188, 1992.

[30] A. Gaulier, J. Cahen, J. L. Buisson, G. Périé, G. Vacher, and B. Poulet, "Pancreatic insulinoma, adenomatosis of the Wirsung's duct and chronic pancreatitis. Apropos of a case," *Archives d'anatomie et de cytologie pathologiques*, vol. 41, no. 5-6, pp. 245–250, 1993.

[31] M. J. G. M. Bugalho, L. Roque, L. G. Sobrinho et al., "Calcitonin-producing insulinoma: clinical, immunocytochemical and cytogenetical study," *Clinical Endocrinology*, vol. 41, no. 2, pp. 257–260, 1994.

[32] P. Pusztai, B. Sármán, G. Illyés et al., "Hypercalcitoninemia in a patient with a recurrent goitre and insulinoma: a case report," *Experimental and Clinical Endocrinology & Diabetes*, vol. 114, no. 05, pp. 217–221, 2006.

[33] S. Uccella, A. Blank, R. Maragliano, F. Sessa, A. Perren, and S. La Rosa, "Calcitonin-producing neuroendocrine neoplasms of the pancreas: clinicopathological study of 25 cases and review of the literature," *Endocrine Pathology*, vol. 28, no. 4, pp. 351–361, 2017.

[34] E. Giannetta, D. Gianfrilli, C. Pozza et al., "Extrathyroidal calcitonin secreting tumors," *Medicine*, vol. 95, no. 3, p. e2419, 2016.

18

Multifocal Multisystem Langerhans Cell Histiocytosis Involving Pituitary Masquerading as Crohn's Disease: A Case Report and Review of the Literature

Mohd. Ashraf Ganie,[1] Bhanu Malhotra,[2] Manpreet Saini,[3] Arshiya Dutta,[4] Atul Sharma,[1] Kim Vaiphie,[5] and Pinaki Dutta[2]

[1]*Department of Endocrinology, Sher-I-Kasmir Institute of Medical Sciences, Srinagar, India*
[2]*Department of Endocrinology, PGIMER, Chandigarh 160012, India*
[3]*Baba Farid University, Faridkot, Punjab, India*
[4]*MMC and Hospital, Solan, Himachal Pradesh, India*
[5]*Department of Histopathology, PGIMER, Chandigarh 160012, India*

Correspondence should be addressed to Pinaki Dutta; drpinakidutta12@gmail.com

Academic Editor: Osamu Isozaki

Background/Objective. We present a case of Langerhans cell histiocytosis (LCH) with gastrointestinal involvement masquerading as inflammatory bowel disease (IBD) in a patient who initially had features of central diabetes insipidus (CDI). *Case Report.* A 19-year-old male presented at 14 years of age with central diabetes insipidus. He subsequently developed panhypopituitarism and sellar-suprasellar mass, the biopsy of which was inconclusive. Secondary causes for hypophysitis were ruled out. Five years later, he developed perianal pus discharging sinuses, positive ASCA, and sacroiliitis. Rectal ulcer biopsy showed nonspecific inflammation and necrosis. Hence, he was managed as inflammatory bowel disease (IBD). Due to nonresponsiveness of symptoms, doubt about diagnosis was invoked and rectal ulcer biopsy was repeated, which then showed infiltration by Langerhans cells. Hence, he was diagnosed with LCH and showed resolution of symptoms on initiating steroids and vinblastine. *Discussion.* Gastrointestinal involvement by LCH is unusual and only rarely has represented a prominent clinical manifestation. In most cases, such involvement suggests widespread multisystem disease. Its distinctive morphologic and immunohistochemical features allow LCH to be distinguished from other inflammatory infiltrations found in mucosal biopsy specimens. *Conclusion.* Preceding CDI and hypopituitarism may predict LCH in patients with IBD-like diseases.

1. Introduction

Langerhans cell histiocytosis (LCH) is characterized by abnormal proliferation of Langerhans cells (antigen-presenting immune cells). The disease has characteristics of both an abnormal reactive and a neoplastic process. It is associated with mutations in BRAF V600E and MAPK pathway [1]. It may present as a rash or bony lesions or be disseminated and involve bone marrow, lungs, liver, spleen, lymph nodes, gastrointestinal (GI) tract, and the pituitary gland. Hypothalamic-pituitary region (HPR) infiltration is present in 5%–50% of the cases with LCH [2]. Central diabetes insipidus (CDI) and anterior pituitary deficiencies frequently develop in HPR-involved LCH. The most common hormone deficiency is growth hormone (GH) (53–67%) followed by gonadotropin (53–58%) and thyroid-stimulating hormone (3.9%) deficiency [3, 4]. Gastrointestinal involvement is rare in LCH (1–5%) [5]. It may be totally asymptomatic, incidentally found on colonoscopy or presented as haematochezia, diarrhoea, abdominal pain, and vomiting. Here, we present a case of LCH masquerading as IBD in a young male who initially had features of CDI.

2. Case Report

A 19-year-old male, presented at 14 years of age with polyuria and polydipsia for a duration of one year. There was no history of headache, visual disturbances, or pain abdomen at that time. He was obese and had gynaecomastia (Figure 1(a)). Evaluation at the time revealed CDI on the water deprivation test. MRI sella was abnormal for loss of posterior pituitary bright spot but a normal stalk and anterior pituitary (Figure 2(a)). Anterior pituitary hormonal profile was suggestive of central hypothyroidism with normal cortisol (Total T4 = 4.87 μg/dl (5–12 μg/dl), 8 am Cortisol-14.6 μg/dl (5–25 μg/dl), LH-0.24 (1.42–15.4 IU/L), FSH-0.13 (0.3–10 IU/L), Testosterone < 10 (100–300 ng/dl). He was prescribed oral desmopressin and levothyroxine but he defaulted on medication with poor compliance.

Three years later, he had presented with delayed puberty. Repeated investigations confirmed hypogonadotropic hypogonadism and CDI (water deprivation test was repeated) along with central hypothyroidism (Total T4-5.55 μg/dl (on thyroxine), 8am Cortisol-20.57 μg/dl (on prednisolone), testosterone-22.1 ng/dl, LH-0.37 mIU/ml, FSH-1.93 mIU/ml). Repeated MRI showed an enhancing lesion involving the suprasellar area (hypothalamus) and thickened stalk (Figure 2(b)). Tumor markers were negative and secondary causes for hypophysitis were ruled out (Table 1). The patient was subjected to biopsy via transsphenoidal approach. Intraoperative findings were reported as soft, suckable, yellowish, moderately vascular, and non-encapsulated supra-sellar mass (7 × 12 × 4 mm), and a crush biopsy revealed features suggestive of an inflammatory mass. Histopathological examination (HPE) revealed features of dense chronic inflammation. Immunostaining for CD1a was inconclusive probably due to nonrepresentative sample. Postoperatively, patient was continued on oral desmopressin, prednisolone, injectable testosterone, and levothyroxine therapy.

After two and half years, patient developed painful perianal ulcers with serosanguineous discharge (Figure 1(b)). Colonoscopy revealed multiple perianal fistulae with diffuse rectal erythema. Antisaccharomyces *cerevisiae* antibody (ASCA) titre was positive (61.7 units), P-ANCA was negative, and fecal calprotectin was not performed. (Table 1). Ulcer biopsy revealed necrotic bits with slough and granulation tissue. Culture of the discharge grew *Klebsiella* pneumonia. The patient then developed pain in bilateral hip region associated with low back ache. Contrast-enhanced computed tomography (CECT) pelvis suggested features of sacroiliitis and perirectal fat stranding. In view of proctitis, sacroiliitis, and positive ASCA, the patient was diagnosed and managed with inflammatory bowel disease (IBD).

Due to lack of improvement in his symptoms, a repeat biopsy was performed from the perianal lesion, which developed later in the course of illness. HPE showed sheets of epithelioid cells with abundant eosinophilic cytoplasm having pleomorphic round to oval nuclei with nuclear grooving. Immunohistochemical (IHC) studies showed atypical histiocytic cells which stained positively for CD1a, Langerin, and S-100, confirming the presence of Langerhans cells (Figure 3). After ruling out other diseases, the patient was diagnosed with LCH with pituitary and gastrointestinal involvement. He was treated with steroids and vinblastine which resulted in improvement of his symptoms. CDI was resolved and perianal ulcers were healed. Hormone replacement was still being continued.

3. Discussion

We present a case of a young male who had initially presented with CDI and subsequently developed panhypopituitarism, sellar-suprasellar mass lesion, and inconclusive sellar biopsy. Subsequent development of rectal ulcers with fistulae and positive ASCA suggested it to be a case of inflammatory bowel disease (IBD). ASCA seropositivity has been reported in Crohn's disease, ulcerative colitis, celiac disease, Behcet's disease, and hidradenitis suppurativa [6, 7]. It has been linked to common physiopathology such as inflammation of small intestine mucosa, loss of oral tolerance of alimentary antigen(s), altered gut permeability, and immune dysregulation (IL-23) [8]. Bilateral sacroiliitis also supported the diagnosis of IBD, though inflammatory involvement of sacroiliac joint and intervertebral disc can also occur in LCH [9]. Infundibulo-hypophysitis was assumed to be an extraintestinal manifestation of IBD. Previously, two cases of hypophysitis with CDI have been reported in IBD. Both the patients were middle-aged females (mean age-40 years) who developed sellar mass lesions several years after the diagnosis of IBD was made. While one patient had lymphocytic hypophysitis, the other had biopsy proven granulomatous hypophysitis which was refractory to steroids and responded to infliximab [10, 11].

LCH is a rare hematopoietic neoplastic disease, which can be diagnosed among all age groups; however, it is more common in children of 1–3 years of age. The incidence is three to five cases per million children, whereas in adults, it is one to two cases per million per year [12, 13]. The new disease classification has been simplified to single system LCH and multisystem LCH [14]. Multisystem LCH, seen in 45% of cases, involves two or more organs or systems. LCH has a particular predilection for involvement of the hypothalamic-pituitary axis. In a retrospective study by Kaltsas et al., out of 12 adults LCH with GI involvement, DI and anterior pituitary dysfunction were present in 3 and 4 patients, respectively, but only 1 had both at the onset. CDI can antedate, concur, or develop subsequent to the diagnosis of LCH, based on the presence of other lesions. CDI can be the initial presenting feature in about 1/3 of patients [15]. Pituitary stalk thickening can precede peripheral lesions by several months. During this early phase of the disease, a water deprivation test and possibly pituitary stalk biopsy may be helpful [16]. Among paediatric patients, multisystem disease and craniofacial involvement at diagnosis carry a significantly increased risk to develop DI during their course [17].

LCH involvement of the gastrointestinal tract (GI) is exceedingly rare. It occurs most commonly in the context of

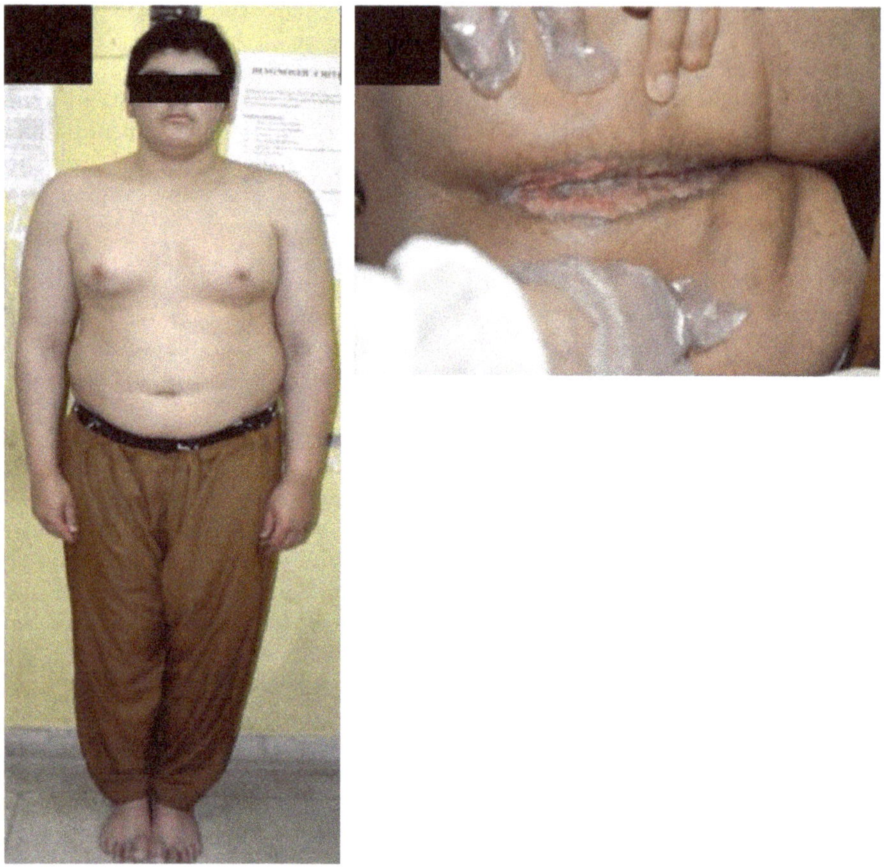

Figure 1: Clinical image of the patient showing (a) gynaecomastia and absent body and facial hair (b) perianal ulcers.

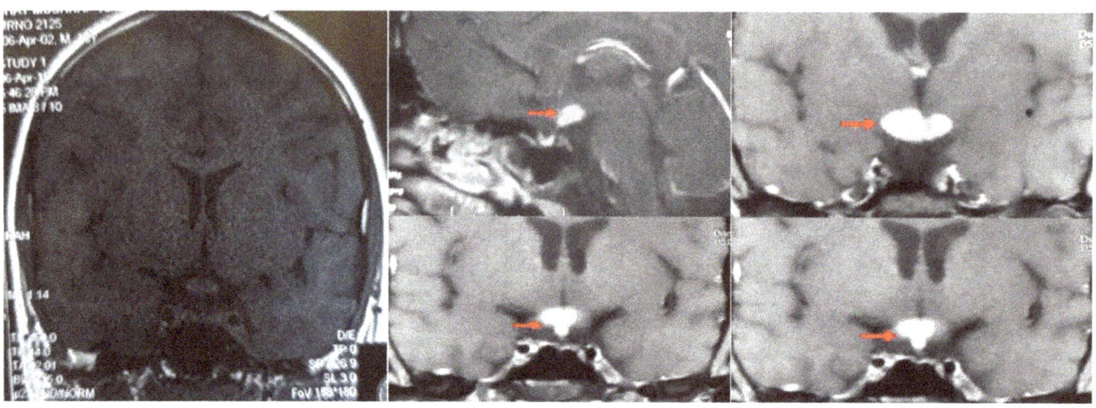

(a) (b)

Figure 2: MRI sella showing (a) enhancing lesion involving hypothalamus and infundibular stalk 14×8 mm, isointense on T1W and hypointense on T2W at 3 years after 1st presentation, and (b) increase in size of enhancing mass lesion in the upper part of stalk $20 \times 17 \times 15$ mm, 2 years after biopsy.

the multisystem disease. The GI manifestations could be confused with infectious, allergic, immunodeficiency, and inflammatory bowel diseases. GI-LCH is more common in children aged <2 years with a male preponderance (male : female = 2 : 1) and has poor prognosis [18]. LCH in the paediatric population classically presents with symptoms including diarrhoea, bloody stools, failure to thrive, abdominal pain, and vomiting [19]. In adults, LCH is reported as an isolated finding within the GI tract. It characteristically presents as an incidental polyp found on colonoscopy in asymptomatic individuals being evaluated for another reason [20]. Singhi et al. described 10 cases of adult LCH involving the GI tract. Five out of 10 adults were asymptomatic and the other five were presented with unrelated symptoms when the LCH was diagnosed during screening colonoscopy, and none had antecedent central diabetes insipidus.

TABLE 1: Diagnostic evaluation for etiology of secondary hypophysitis.

Laboratory test	Result	Reference range
ESR	37 mm/hr	0–9
ANA	Negative	
Serum alpha-fetoprotein (AFP)	1.2 ng/ml	0–8.5
Serum beta hCG	<0.01 IU/l	<25
CSF alpha-fetoprotein	0.09 IU/l	
CSF beta hCG	Undetectable	<0.4 ng/ml
Serum ACE	26.0 U/L	8–65
Anti-*Saccharomyces cerevisiae* (ASCA) IgG antibody	61.70 Units	0–20
Anti-myeloperoxidase antibodies (p-ANCA)	6.51 Units	<20

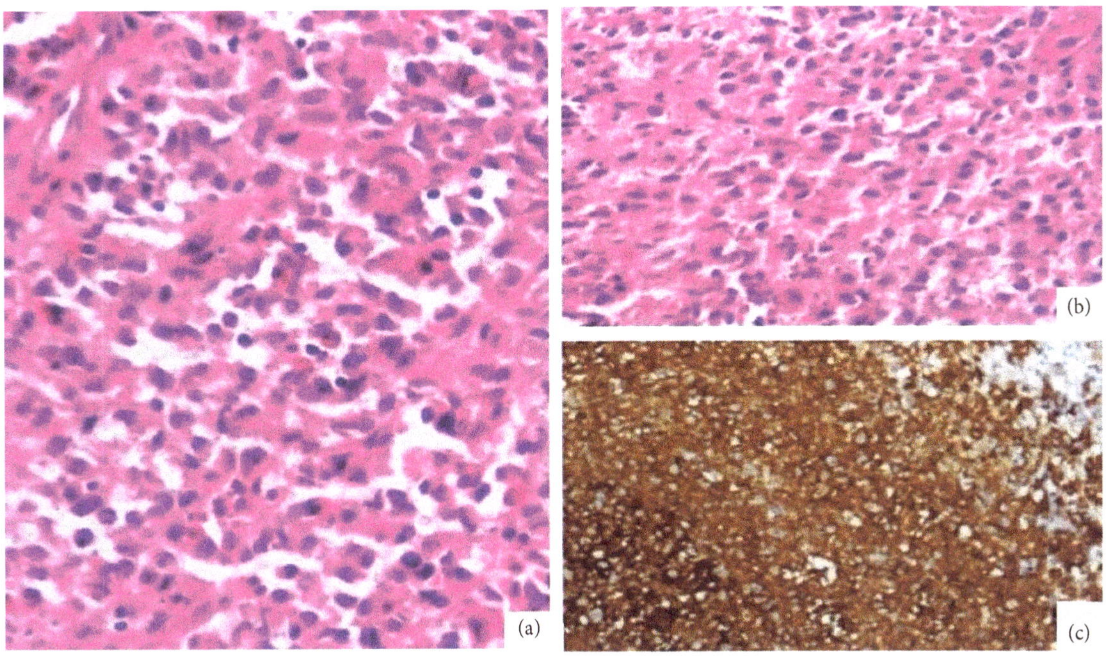

FIGURE 3: A panel of photomicrograph of perianal lesion showing sheets of epithelioid like cells with abundant amount of eosinophilic cytoplasm having mildly pleomorphic round to oval nuclei with nuclear grooving. Admixed with these cells are scattered eosinophils, lymphocytes, and plasma cells (a) (HE, x25). (b) The cell morphology is brought out better in high-power photomicrograph (HE, x400). (c) Immunohistochemical staining showing atypical histiocytic cells positive for CD1a, Langerin, and S-100 (not shown) confirming a diagnosis of Langerhans cell histiocytosis (by peroxidase anti-peroxidase, x500 on paraffin-embedded tissue sections).

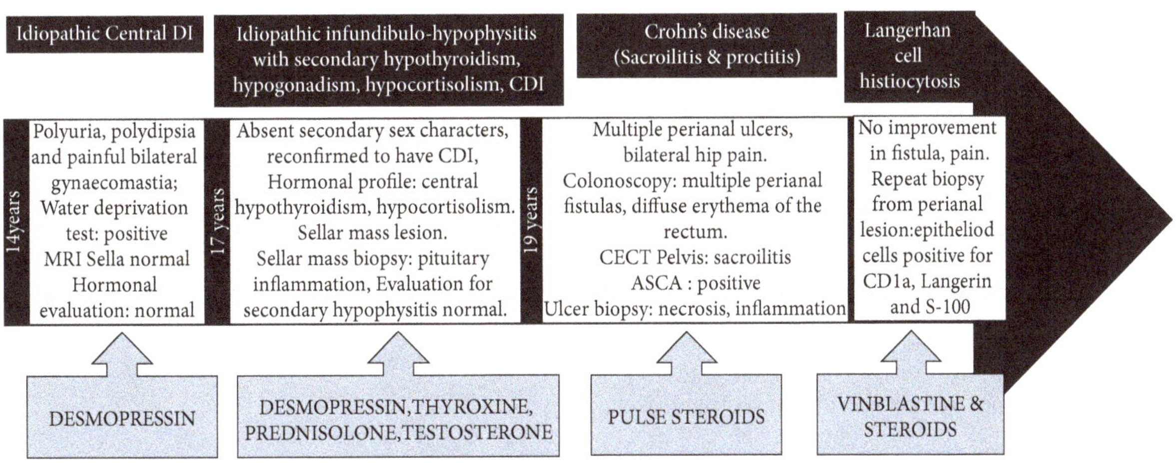

FIGURE 4: Flow chart showing the clinical course of the patient.

AndiónCatalán et al. [13] reported 2 paediatric patients of GI-LCH, of which one was a 12-year-old girl who was initially presented with diabetes insipidus, with subsequent development of panhypopituitarism. Further testing (colonoscopy) revealed LCH in gastrointestinal tract. Flow chart showing clinical course of the patient is shown in Figure 4.

This case highlights the varied manifestations of LCH that develop over a course of time. In this patient, it was the rectal involvement that gave insight into the disease pathology and clinched the diagnosis.

4. Conclusion

Preceding CDI and hypopituitarism may predict LCH in patients with IBD-like diseases.

Consent

The authors hereby declare that an informed consent has been taken from the patient for sharing his details in the manuscript, which includes both clinical data and the clinical images of the patient.

References

[1] G. Goyal, A. Tazi, R. S. Go et al., "International expert consensus recommendations for the diagnosis and treatment of Langerhans cell histiocytosis in adults," *Blood*, vol. 139, no. 17, pp. 2601–2621, 2022.

[2] E Vaiani, G. Felizzia, A Belgorosky et al., "Paediatric Paediatric Langerhans Cell Histiocytosis Disease: Long-Term Sequelae in the Hypothalamic Endocrine Systemangerhans cell histiocytosis disease: long-term sequelae in the hypothalamic endocrine system," *Horm Res Paediatr*, vol. 94, no. 1-2, pp. 9–17, 2021.

[3] E. Mittheisz, M. Wnorowski, H. Prosch et al., "Central nervous system-related permanent consequences in patients with Langerhans cell histiocytosis," *Pediatric Blood & Cancer*, vol. 48, no. 1, pp. 50–56, 2007.

[4] J. Donadieu, T. Genereau, D. Frappaz et al., "Endocrine involvement in pediatric-onset Langerhans' cell histiocytosis: a population-based study," *The Journal of Pediatrics*, vol. 144, no. 3, pp. 344–35050, 2004.

[5] S P. Yadav, G. Kharya, G. Kapoor et al., "Langerhans cell histiocytosis with digestive tract involvement," *Pediatric Blood & Cancer*, vol. 55, no. 4, pp. 748–753, 2010.

[6] S. Desplat-Jégo, C. Johanet, A. Escande et al., "Update on Anti-Saccharomyces cerevisiae antibodies, anti-nuclear associated anti-neutrophil antibodies and antibodies to exocrine pancreas detected by indirect immunofluorescence as biomarkers in chronic inflammatory bowel diseases: Results of a multicenter studyesults of a multicenter study," *World Journal of Gastroenterology*, vol. 13, no. 16, pp. 2312–2318, 2007, https://pubmed.ncbi.nlm.nih.gov/?term=Ballot+E&cauthor_id=17511029.

[7] J. W. Frew, "Anti-Saccharomyces cervisiae antibodies in hidradenitis suppurativa: Anti–Saccharomyces cervisiae antibodies in hidradenitis suppurativa: More than a gut feelingore than a gut feeling," *Journal of Allergy and Clinical Immunology*, vol. 146, no. 2, p. 458, 2020 Aug.

[8] E. Kvedaraite, F. Cohen-Aubart, J. Mitchell et al., "Patients with both Langerhans cell histiocytosis and Crohn's disease highlight a common role of interleukin-23," *Acta PaediatrActa Paediatrica*, vol. 110, no. 4, pp. 1315–1321, 2021 Apr.

[9] Z. Maraş Özdemir, A. Sagir Kahraman, C A. Gormeli et al., "Langerhans cell histiocytosis with atypical intervertebral disc and sacroiliac joint involvement mimicking osteoarticular tuberculosis in an adult," *Balkan Medical Journal*, vol. 33, no. 5, pp. 573–577, 2016.

[10] B. K. Force, T. P. Vogel, D. M. Nguyen et al., "A A Remarkable Response of Granulomatous Hypophysitis to Infliximab in a Patient With a Background of Crohn's Disease-A Case Report.emarkable response of granulomatous hypophysitis to infliximab in a patient with a background of Crohn's disease - a case report," *Frontiers in Endocrinology*, vol. 11, p. 350, 2020.

[11] C. S. Johns, N. Weare-Regales, C. P. Fernandez, and J. B. Tourtelot, "Unusual Presentation of Central Diabetes Insipidus in a Patient with Crohn's disease. Case reports in classical and unusual causes of hypopituitarism II," *Neuroendocrinology and Pituitary MON-236*, vol. 4, no. 1, JESOCI, 2020.

[12] J S. Malpas, A. J. S. Norton, and A. J. Norton, "Langerhans cell histiocytosis in the adult," *Medical and Pediatric Oncology*, vol. 27, no. 6, pp. 540–546, 1996.

[13] M. Andión Catalán, D. Ruano Domínguez, D. Azorín Cuadrillero, T. de Rojas de Pablos, and L. Madero López, "Histiocitosis de células de Langerhans con afectación gastrointestinal," *Anales de Pediatía*, vol. 83, pp. 279-280, 2015.

[14] N. Grois, U. Pötschger, H. Prosch et al., "Risk factors for diabetes insipidus in langerhans cell histiocytosis," *Pediatric Blood and Cancer*, vol. 46, no. 2, pp. 228–233, 2006.

[15] G. A. Kaltsas, T. B. Powles, J. Evanson et al., "Hypothalamo-pituitary abnormalities in adult patients with langerhans cell histiocytosis: clinical, endocrinological, and radiological features and response to treatment," *The Journal of Cinical Endocrinology and Metabolism*, vol. 85, no. 4, pp. 1370–1376, 2000 Apr.

[16] N. Grois, B. F. Wolfram, A. Heitger, G. H. Mostbeck, J. Hofmann, and H. Gadner, "Diabetes insipidus in Langerhans cell histiocytosis: results from the DAL-HX 83 study." *Medical and Pediatric Oncology*, vol. 24, pp. 248–256, 1995.

[17] M. Minkov, U. Pötschger, N. Thacker, I. Astigarraga, J. Braier, and J. Donadieu, "additive prognostic impact of gastrointestinal involvement in severe multisystem langerhans cell histiocytosis," *Jornal de Pediatria*, vol. 237, pp. 65–70, 2021.

[18] E. Hait, M. Liang, B. Degar, J. Glickman, and V. L. Fox, "Gastrointestinal Tract Involvement in Langerhans Cell Histiocytosis: Case Report and Review of the Literature," *Pediatrics*, vol. 118, no. 5, pp. e1593–e1599, 2006.

[19] A. D. Singhi and E. A. Montgomery, "Gastrointestinal tract Langerhans cell histiocytosis: a clinicopathologic study of 12 patients," *The American Journal of Surgical Pathology*, vol. 35, pp. 305–310, 2011.

[20] I. Baumgartner, A. von Hochstetter, B. Baumert, U. Luetolf, and F. Follath, "Langerhans'-cell histiocytosis in adults," *Medical and Pediatric Oncology*, vol. 28, pp. 9–14, 1997.

19

Heparin-Induced Pituitary Apoplexy Presenting as Isolated Unilateral Oculomotor Nerve Palsy: A Case Report and Literature Review

Bakr Swaid [1] **Frank Kalaba,** [2] **Ghassan Bachuwa** [1] **and Stephen E. Sullivan** [3]

[1] *Department of Internal Medicine, Hurley Medical Center/Michigan State University, Flint, MI, USA*
[2] *Department of Combined Internal Medicine & Pediatrics Residency Program, Hurley Medical Center/Michigan State University, Flint, MI, USA*
[3] *Department of Neurosurgery and the Pituitary and Neuroendocrine Center, University of Michigan, Ann Arbor, MI, USA*

Correspondence should be addressed to Bakr Swaid; bakrswaid@gmail.com

Academic Editor: Carlo Capella

Introduction. Pituitary apoplexy (PA) is a rare and potentially life-threatening clinical syndrome resulting from pituitary gland hemorrhage and/or infarction. Anticoagulation is a risk factor for triggering PA. Isolated oculomotor nerve palsy is an atypical presentation of PA. *Case Presentation.* A 65-year-old African American female with no past medical history of pituitary disease presented to the emergency department (ED) with nonspecific abdominal pain that was thought to be secondary to fecal stasis and subsequently improved with laxatives. She also reported atypical chest pain that was concerning for unstable angina. She was started on aspirin, clopidogrel, and intravenous (IV) heparin. Later, coronary catheterization showed no significant coronary artery disease (CAD). Twelve hours after the procedure, the patient developed acute complete left oculomotor nerve palsy with a severe headache. Magnetic resonance imaging (MRI) of the head showed a large pituitary mass. Pituitary apoplexy was suspected and the patient eventually underwent a successful trans-sphenoidal pituitary resection. *Discussion.* We report a case of PA manifesting as isolated left oculomotor nerve palsy without visual field defects in the setting of using dual antiplatelet therapy (DAPT) and IV heparin for acute coronary syndrome. To the best of our knowledge, this unique combination has not been previously reported.

1. Introduction

Pituitary apoplexy (PA) is a clinical syndrome resulting from pituitary gland hemorrhage and/or infarction usually in the setting of pituitary macroadenoma. When presenting classically, it is characterized by acute onset headache, vomiting, visual changes, ophthalmoplegia, and loss of consciousness [1]. Asymptomatic pituitary hemorrhage and/or infarction, usually detected by imaging, has been described by some as subclinical PA [2]. However, the term PA is usually reserved for classic PA and thus it remains a clinical diagnosis [1]. Catastrophic hemorrhage into the pituitary gland was first reported in 1898 by Pearce Bailey [3]. The first postmortem description of PA was documented by Bleibtreu in 1905 [3]. The term "pituitary apoplexy" was first coined in 1950 by Brougham to describe the full clinical syndrome [3].

PA complicates 2–7% of pituitary adenomas. When it occurs, it is the presenting symptom/sign in 80% of cases [4]. Most PA cases occur in the context of pituitary adenomas, although rare cases of PA resulting from craniopharyngioma [4], primary pituitary carcinoma [5], and pituitary metastasis [6] have been reported. Most cases of PA occur spontaneously. Sibal et al. published a case series of 45 patients with PA and were able to identify at least one precipitating factor in up to 40% of cases [4]. Hypertension is by far the most common precipitating factor (27%). Other reported triggers include major surgery (especially cardiac surgeries), anticoagulants, head trauma, aspirin, pregnancy, coagulopathies, estrogen therapy, radiation therapy, and dynamic pituitary function tests [3].

The most common ocular complication of PA is visual field deficits (71%) resulting from compression on the optic chiasm [1]. PA is also well-known to result in ophthalmoplegia, in 69% of patients according to a case series reported by Randeva et al. in 1999 [1]. The oculomotor nerve III is the most commonly affected nerve (67%), followed by the abducent nerve

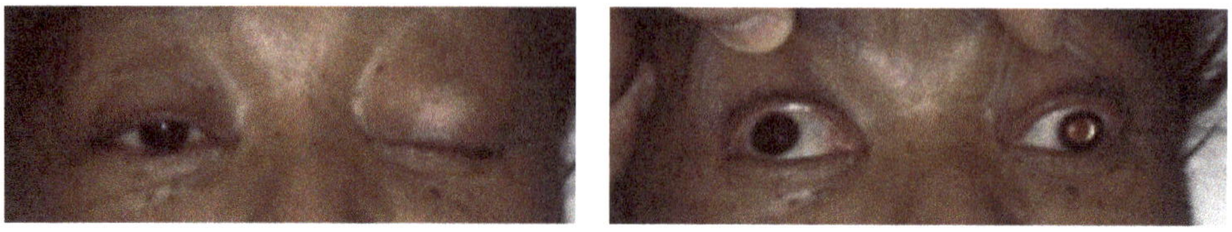

(a) (b)

FIGURE 1: (a) The patient was asked to open both eyes. (b) Both upper eyelids were passively opened. There is a clear anisocoria with down and outward left gaze palsy.

VI (29%). The trochlear nerve IV is the least common to be affected (4%), likely as a result of anatomic advantage [1]. The 3rd, 4th, and 6th cranial nerves (CN) all lie in the cavernous sinus and it is common to have two or more nerves affected simultaneously. In fact, cases of bilateral total ophthalmoplegia (third, fourth, and sixth nerve palsies) caused by PA have been reported [7]. In 2007, Lau et al. reported the first case of spontaneous pituitary apoplexy resulting in isolated bilateral oculomotor nerve palsies [8].

Intracranial hemorrhage is a well-known complication of all antithrombotic pharmacotherapy, including antiplatelets (e.g., aspirin), anticoagulants (e.g., warfarin and heparin), and thrombolytics (e.g., streptokinase). Since PA was recognized as a distinct clinical entity, there have been many case reports of PA attributed to the use of classic antithrombotic therapy. More recently, PA resulting from the use of new oral anticoagulants (NOAs) including dabigatran, apixaban, and rivaroxaban [9], have been reported. In this article, we present a case of PA with atypical presentation of isolated third nerve palsy without visual field deficits likely resulting from the use of IV heparin in the setting of a suspected acute coronary syndrome.

2. Case Presentation

A 65-year-old African American female with past medical history significant for noninsulin-dependent type 2 diabetes mellitus, essential hypertension, dyslipidemia, chronic back pain, morbid obesity (body mass index (BMI) was 41), gastroesophageal reflux disease (GERD), uterine fibroids, generalized anxiety disorder, and former tobacco abuse presented to the emergency department (ED) complaining of generalized abdominal pain of 3 weeks' duration with intermittent diarrhea and constipation. Upon review of systems, she complained of atypical chest pain which was pleuritic and reproducible on palpation. The chest pain was nonexertional but she had exertional dyspnea. Of note, she had no prior history of cardiovascular disease.

Past surgical history was remarkable for cesarean section and hysterectomy. Prior to admission medications included metformin, hydrochlorothiazide, propranolol, ranitidine, and acetaminophen. Family history was remarkable for diabetes. In terms of social history, she was a former tobacco smoker, drank alcohol socially, and denied illicit drug use. She had a history of allergy to hydroxyzine, propoxyphene, and zomepirac.

In the ED, measurement of vital signs showed a temperature of 37.0°C, heart rate of 88 beats per minute, respiratory rate of 18 breaths per minute, blood pressure of 148/82, and pulse oxygen saturation of 99% on room air. Initial physical examination was normal except for obesity, depressed mood, chest wall tenderness, mild abdominal distention with tympanic note to percussion and mild generalized nonspecific tenderness to palpation. Rectal exam showed small nonbleeding external hemorrhoids. Complete blood count and basic metabolic panel were normal except for blood glucose of 240 milligrams/deciliter (mg/dL). Hemoglobin A1c was 9.3%. Troponin I was slightly elevated at 0.07 and it trended down on second measurement. Electrocardiogram showed normal sinus rhythm with new T-wave inversion in the inferolateral leads. Computed tomography angiography (CTA) of the chest, abdomen, and pelvis was only remarkable for fecal stasis in the rectum. Her abdominal pain and constipation was partially relieved after administration of IV morphine and senna-docusate.

She was also given aspirin for the chest pain. After her abdominal symptoms moderately improved, she was placed in the observation unit for cardiology consultation. After evaluation by the cardiologist, she was admitted to a telemetry unit for an inpatient cardiac stress test. She was receiving 81 mg aspirin daily. On day 2 of hospital admission, she underwent myocardial perfusion scan using the standard 0.4 mg regadenoson (LEXISCAN) injection. The stress test showed reversible perfusion defect involving the apex and lateral wall of the left ventricle, suggesting myocardial ischemia. At that time, clopidogrel (Plavix) was added to aspirin and the patient was started on IV heparin per ACS protocol pending cardiac catheterization. On day 4, coronary angiography was performed and it showed no significant occlusive coronary artery disease (CAD). During the catheterization procedure, the patient received IV heparin and IV nitroglycerin in addition to midazolam for sedation and fentanyl for analgesia. The radio contrast used was iohexol (OMNIPAQUE 350). Post-procedure, IV heparin was discontinued while DAPT with aspirin and Plavix were resumed.

After recovery from sedation, the patient complained of a headache which got progressively worse within a few hours. It did not improve with repeated doses of oral hydrocodone and oral/IV acetaminophen. After around 12 hours of cardiac catheterization, the patient developed acute left-sided ptosis, deviated gaze (down and outward palsy), and anisocoria with left pupillary dilation (mydriasis) consistent with acute left 3rd nerve palsy (Figure 1). The patient did not complain of decreased vision and visual field testing by confrontation was normal. She had no other sensory or motor deficits. Her mental status examination did not show evidence of confusion.

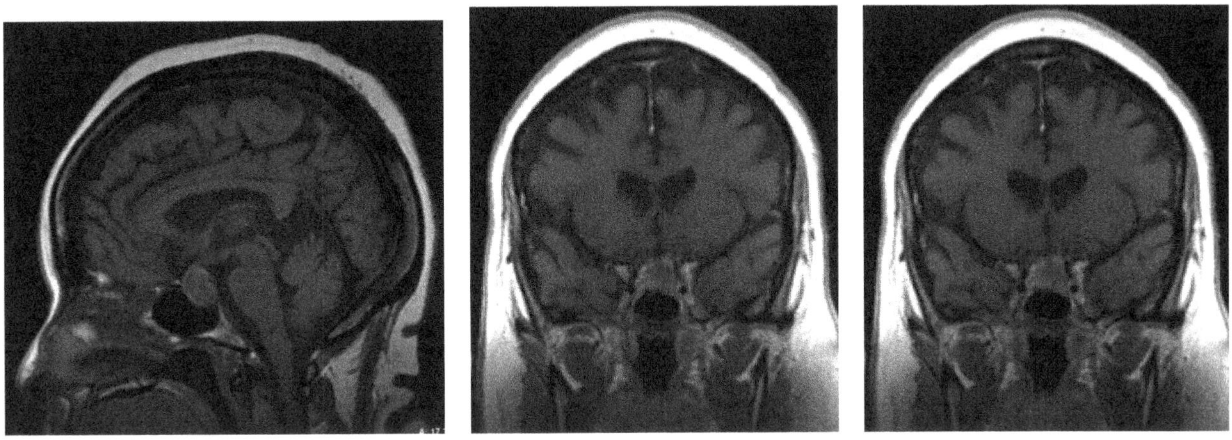

(a) (b) (c)

FIGURE 2: MRI head with contrast T1. (a) Sagittal view showing an enlarged pituitary gland. It measures 1.9 × 2.0 cm in the greatest dimension. The mass is slightly heterogeneous in signal and is slightly impressing on the optic chiasm. (b) and (c) Coronal view with different cuts showing extension on the left cavernous sinus.

TABLE 1: Hormonal workup.

Lab	Result	Reference range
TSH	2.06 μIU/ML	0.3–5.5 micro international unit/milliliter (μIU/ML)
Random plasma cortisol	21 μg/dl	A.M. 4.3–22.4 microgram/deciliter (μg/d) P.M. 3.1–16.7 μg/dL P.M. 3.1–16.7 μg/dL
ACTH	50 pg/mL	≤46 picogram/milliliter (pg/mL)
Prolactin	1.1 ng/mL	1.8–20.3 nanograms per milliliter (ng/mL)
FSH	10.4 mIU/mL	Follicular 2.5–10.2 milli-international units per milliliter (mIU/mL), midcycle 3.4–33.4, luteal 1.5–9.1, pregnant <0.3, postmenopausal 23.0–116.3
LH	2.7 mIU/mL	Follicular 1.9–12.5, midcycle 8.7–76.3, luteal 0.5–16.9, pregnant <1.6, postmenopausal 15.9–54.0, prepubertal <6.1, oral contraceptives 0.7–5.6
Insulin-like growth factor (IGF)	157 ng/mL	41–168 ng/mL
Alpha subunits pituitary glycoprotein	0.2 ng/mL	≤1.2 (females premenopausal) ≤1.8 (female postmenopausal)

Her vital signs were normal. STAT CT head without contrast (per stroke protocol) was read as negative for acute intracranial process. CTA of the head and neck was negative for arterial stenosis or aneurysms. The next day, MRI head and orbit with and without contrast were done using Gadodiamide as the MRI contrast agent. The MRI report, as read in our hospital, indicated a nonenhancing heterogeneous pituitary mass measuring 1.9 × 2.0 cm in the greatest dimension and slightly compressing on the optic chiasm suggestive of pituitary macroadenoma (Figure 2(a)). There was no report of any bleed/infarction by either CT or MRI report.

A multidisciplinary team approach was undertaken with involvement of neurology, endocrinology, ophthalmology, otolaryngology (ENT), and neurosurgery. A full ophthalmological examination was normal except for complete left 3rd nerve palsy and mild cataracts. Visual field testing was normal. Hormonal studies were ordered and the results were as shown in Table 1. Of note, prolactin was lower than normal, while adrenocorticotropic hormone (ACTH) level was above the reference range. Both follicle-stimulating hormone (FSH) and luteinizing hormone (LH) were considered low given the patient's postmenopausal status. The patient had normal random cortisol and free T4 level. She did not receive any IV glucocorticoids. The next day after the third nerve palsy, the patient developed a mild fever at 37.9°C with mild neutrophilic leukocytosis (white blood cell count 14.2 K/UL). The patient was transferred to a neuro step-down unit for close observation. Her vital signs remained mostly normal. Subjectively, she neither had a progression of symptoms nor developed new symptoms. Her headache was controlled with oral hydrocodone/acetaminophen. Her full neurologic examination remained normal except for isolated complete left oculomotor palsy. Leukocytosis gradually normalized over several days.

Pituitary apoplexy was highly suspected as a cause of the third nerve palsy, but the diagnosis was challenged by the fact that our radiologist's interpretation of imaging did not mention bleed or cavernous sinus extension. The diagnosis of diabetic neuropathy of the third nerve from microvascular ischemia was contemplated but it was felt less likely because it is usually pupil-sparing [10]. Neurosurgery requested ENT help for trans-sphenoidal pituitary resection. ENT did not feel comfortable with the plan and recommended transfer to a higher level center. The patient and her family were involved in decision making. They were truthfully told that our medical center is not a high volume center for such pituitary cases and the patient

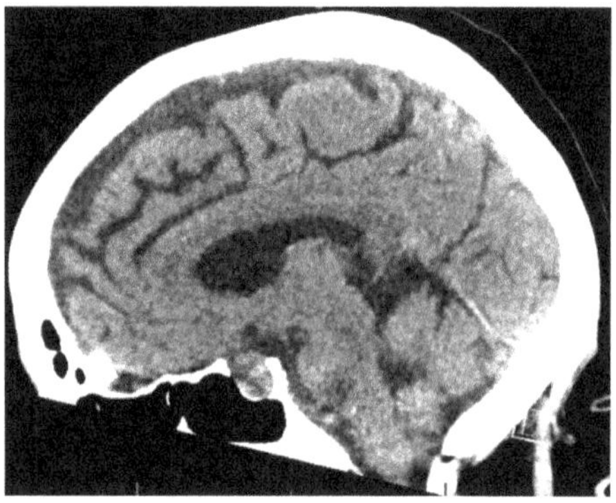

FIGURE 3: CT head without contrast (sagittal view) showing enlarged sella turcica with increased attenuation suggesting a possible hemorrhage within the tumor.

might benefit from a transfer to a more experienced center. They chose to transfer and the patient was transferred by ambulance to an academic center of excellence on day 7 of presentation.

There, neuroradiologists read the images obtained at our hospital differently. The new CT scan report indicated increased attenuation of the sella turcica and in the suprasellar cistern at the site of the patient's pituitary mass, suggestive of possible hemorrhage within the tumor (Figure 3). The new MRI report indicated that there was a sellar/suprasellar mass lesion which appeared to show central intrinsic T1 shortening and hypoenhancement with peripheral right-sided enhancement. There was mass effect on the optic chiasm superiorly. The lesion appeared to extend laterally into the left cavernous sinus with mild mass effect on the cavernous internal carotid artery. The overall hypoenhancing portion measured $2.1 \times 1.9 \times 1.3$ cm (Figures 2(b) and 2(c)).

The physicians in the other hospital decided to proceed with surgical intervention hoping to relieve the pressure on the third nerve. On day 9 of symptoms, the patient underwent successful trans-sphenoidal pituitary resection. Intraoperatively, the neurosurgeon reported a typical contused apoplectic adenoma. A frozen section biopsy report, as well as final pathology report, confirmed necrotic pituitary tumor with evidence of recent hemorrhage. The apoplectic adenoma was removed and the pituitary gland was left intact. Postoperatively, the laboratory assessment indicated central hypothyroidism and secondary adrenal insufficiency. Vital signs were stable. No major sodium abnormalities were noted. The patient was started on oral hydrocortisone and levothyroxine. Otherwise, the immediate postoperative course was uneventful and the patient was discharged home on day 11 of symptoms development. One-month follow-up at the neurosurgeon's office was remarkable for persistence of oculomotor palsy. A six-month follow-up is scheduled.

3. Discussion

In this article, we report a case of a 65-year-old lady with no known history of pituitary disorder prior to admission who suffered from pituitary apoplexy manifesting as severe frontal headache with isolated complete left oculomotor nerve palsy and intact visual fields shortly after coronary angiography, likely resulting from the combination of DAPT and IV heparin given for ACS. To the best of our knowledge, this unique combination has not been previously reported in the literature.

As far as we found, there is no reported case of PA resulting shortly after starting aspirin or other antiplatelets. However, aspirin use was the presumed precipitating factor in 7% of cases of PA according to a case series [4]. The first case of PA resulting from anticoagulant use was reported by Nourizadeh in 1956 [11], six years after Brougham coined the term. It was until 1997, however, when the first case of intravenous (IV) heparin-induced PA was reported by Oo et al. [12]. In 1996, Kelion et al. reported the first case of PA resulting from IV thrombolysis (streptokinase) given for acute MI [13]. In 2007, Tan et al. reported a case of PA triggered by dual antiplatelet therapy (DAPT) along with therapeutic dose of low-molecular weight heparin (LMWH) given for unstable angina in a patient with a known pituitary macroadenoma [14]. The authors raised a concern that treating acute coronary syndrome (ACS) with the combination of DAPT and anticoagulants in the setting of pituitary macroadenoma might be relatively contraindicated.

As mentioned in the previous paragraph, the first case of IV heparin-induced PA was reported in 1997 by Oo et al. [12]. However, that case did not present as CN palsy. Korotinsky et al. reported a similar case to ours in a 68-year-old male with complete right oculomotor palsy following IV heparin and IV nitrates, but their case had an additional clinical presentation with bitemporal superior quadrantanopia which was not present in our case [15]. In 2003, Skljarevski et al. published the first reported case of PA with partial ophthalmoplegia shortly following elective coronary angiography in a patient with atrial septal defect (ASD) in preparation for cardiac surgery [16]. Also in 2003, Nagarajan et al. reported a case of PA with blurry vision, ptosis, and ophthalmoplegia with involvement of the third, fourth, and sixth cranial nerves 36 hours after administering DAPT and therapeutic LMWH for ACS [17]. Moreover, PA stemming from the use of LMWH for thromboprophylaxis in the perioperative period of shoulder arthroplasty was reported by Madhusudhan et al. [18] Again, in that case, the patient had visual deficits and the third nerve palsy was pupil-sparing.

The mechanism of PA is complex and not entirely known [2]. The pituitary gland is a highly vascular organ and pituitary adenomas are known to have increased propensity to bleed when compared to other intracranial tumors [2]. Frequently, pituitary tumors have direct arterial blood supply independent of the hypophyseal portal system that supplies normal pituitary tissue [2]. Also, pituitary adenomas have been shown to have structurally vulnerable blood vessels, decreased angiogenesis, increased sensitivity to glucose deprivation, and high metabolic demand [2]. Hence, PA has been associated with instances of transient hypoperfusion (e.g., major surgeries) or increased metabolic demand (e.g., dynamic hormonal testing and hypoglycemia). The mechanism by which PA results in oculomotor palsy is not entirely known [4]. Suggested mechanisms include direct vascular invasion through the cavernous sinus [8], transmitted pressure from an enlarging sellar mass without extension to the cavernous sinus [4], and interruption of the vasa nervorum supply of the third nerve [19].

In our case, the precipitating factor of PA was likely the use of IV heparin, although many events that happened in our case have been previously reported to trigger PA. These include the use of DAPT [4, 14], iohexol radiocontrast [16], regadenoson [20], IV nitrates use [15], and the coronary angiography procedure itself [16]. A major limitation to our study is the lack of post-operative follow-up and hence the course of pituitary function and third nerve palsy is not known. However, this case has at least three main learning points. First, we should always be cautious when starting IV heparin along with DAPT for ACS, especially if the indication is not very compelling (e.g., atypical chest pain and negative cardiac biomarkers), because of the increased risk of bleeding, including intracranial bleed, and PA. With our patient, unfortunately, IV heparin was commenced 48 hours after ED presentation merely because of a positive stress test despite the patient being free of chest pain at that time. Second, PA can present with a headache followed by isolated unilateral complete third nerve palsy without visual field loss. In contexts similar to our case, a headache could be overlooked because it is a well-recognized side effect of regadenoson and IV nitrates. Therefore, a high index of suspicion is crucial. Third, PA remains a clinical diagnosis supported by radiologic/pathologic evidence. In our case, our radiologist failed to identify bleeding in both the CT and the MRI images. Therefore, when the appropriate clinical context is highly suggestive of PA and the initial radiologist's reading is negative, consultation with a more experienced neuroradiologist is warranted.

References

[1] H. S. Randeva, J. Schoebel, J. Byrne, M. Esiri, C. B. Adams, and J. A. Wass, "Classical pituitary apoplexy: clinical features, management and outcome outcome," *Clinical Endocrinology*, vol. 51, no. 2, pp. 181–188, 1999.

[2] C. Briet, S. Salenave, J.-F. Bonneville, E. R. Laws, and P. Chanson, "Pituitary apoplexy," *Endocrine Reviews*, vol. 36, no. 6, pp. 622–645, 2015.

[3] S. Rajasekaran, M. Vanderpump, S. Baldeweg et al., "UK guidelines for the management of pituitary apoplexy," *Clinical Endocrinology*, vol. 74, no. 1, pp. 9–20, 2011.

[4] L. Sibal, S. G. Ball, V. Connolly et al., "Pituitary apoplexy: a review of clinical presentation, management and outcome in 45 cases," *Pituitary*, vol. 7, no. 3, pp. 157–163, 2004.

[5] R. L. Wright, R. G. Ojemann, and J. H. Drew, "Hemorrhage into pituitary adenomata. report of two cases with spontaneous recovery," *Archives of Neurology*, vol. 12, no. 3, p. 326, 1965.

[6] I. Kruljac, V. Cerina, H. I. Pećina et al., " Pituitary metastasis presenting as ischemic pituitary apoplexy following heparin-induced thrombocytopenia," *Endocrine Pathology*, vol. 23, no. 4, pp. 264–267, 2012.

[7] J. R. Keane, "Acute bilateral ophthalmoplegia," *Neurology*, vol. 36, no. 2, pp. 279–281, 1986.

[8] K. K. Lau, S. M. Joshi, H. Ellamushi, and F. Afshar, "Isolated bilateral oculomotor nerve palsy in pituitary apoplexy: case report and review," *British Journal of Neurosurgery*, vol. 21, no. 4, pp. 399–402, 2007.

[9] S. Ly, A. Naman, B. Chaufour-Higel et al., "Pituitary apoplexy and rivaroxaban," *Pituitary*, vol. 20, no. 6, pp. 709–710, 2017.

[10] C. M. Galtrey, F. Schon, and A. Nitkunan, "Microvascular non-arteritic ocular motor nerve palsies—what we know and how should we treat?," *Neuro-Ophthalmology*, vol. 39, no. 1, pp. 1–11, 2015.

[11] A. R. Nourizadeh and F. W. Pitts, "Hemorrhage into pituitary adenoma during anticoagulant therapy," *JAMA*, vol. 16, no. 193, pp. 623–625, 1965.

[12] M. M. Oo, A. Y. Krishna, G. J. Bonavita, and G. W. Rutecki, "Heparin therapy for myocardial infarction: an unusual trigger for pituitary apoplexy," *The American Journal of the Medical Sciences*, vol. 314, no. 5, pp. 351–353, 1997.

[13] A. D. Kelion, M. Shahi, and J. A. Bell, "An unusual neurological problem in a patient admitted for acute myocardial infarction," *Postgraduate Medical Journal*, vol. 73, no. 864, pp. 669–670, 1997.

[14] T. M. Tan, C. Caputo, A. Mehta, E. C. Hatfield, N. M. Martin, and K. Meeran, "Pituitary macroadenomas: are combination antiplatelet and anticoagulant therapy contraindicated? a case report report," *Journal of Medical Case Reports*, vol. 1, no. 1, article no. 74, 2007.

[15] S. Korotinsky, P. Smadja, S. Goland et al., "Pituitary apoplexy after administration of heparin and isosorbide dinitrate," *Southern Medical Journal*, vol. 95, no. 4, pp. 469–470, 2002.

[16] V. Skljarevski, S. Khoshyomn, and T. J. Fries, "Pituitary apoplexy in the setting of coronary angiography," *Journal of Neuroimaging*, vol. 13, no. 3, pp. 276–279, 2003.

[17] D. V. Nagarajan, D. Bird, and M. Papouchado, "Pituitary apoplexy following anticoagulation for acute coronary syndrome," *Heart*, vol. 89, no. 1, p. 10, 2003.

[18] S. Madhusudhan, T. R. Madhusudhan, R. S. Haslett, and A. Sinha, "Pituitary apoplexy following shoulder arthroplasty: a case report," *Journal of Medical Case Reports*, vol. 5, no. 1, Article ID 284, 2011.

[19] T. Matyskieła, T. Siwek, B. Zwiernik, J. Zwiernik, A. Rakowska, and A. Wińska-Tereszkiewicz, "Case of an isolated oculomotor nerve damage caused by pituitary hemorrhage without cavernous sinus invasion," *Polish Annals of Medicine*, vol. 23, no. 1, pp. 46–48, 2016.

[20] S. Shetty, J. Gnanaraj, S. Jayamani Roshan, and R. El Accaoui, "Pituitary apoplexy after regadenoson myocardial perfusion scan," *Journal of Nuclear Cardiology*, 2018.

20

BYPASS-OMA: Hypoglycemic Hyperinsulinemic Nesidioblastosis after Gastric Bypass Surgery—A Case Report and Review of the Literature

Jessica Cao,[1] **Cindy Kim**,[1] **Thatcher Huynh**,[2] **Amanda Frugoli**,[2] **Heidi Henson**,[2] **Vera Valdez**,[2] **and Tricia Westhoff-Pankratz**[3]

[1]*Western University of Health Sciences, Community Memorial Hospital, Department of Internal Medicine, 147 N Brent St, Ventura, California 93003, USA*
[2]*Community Memorial Hospital, Department of Graduate Medical Education, Department of Internal Medicine, 147 N Brent St, Ventura, California 93003, USA*
[3]*Community Memorial Hospital, Department of Internal Medicine, Department of Endocrinology, 147 N Brent St, California 93003, USA*

Correspondence should be addressed to Amanda Frugoli; afrugoli@cmhshealth.org

Academic Editor: Toshihiro Kita

This rare case vignette describes hypoglycemic, hyperinsulinemic nesidioblastosis in a female patient with prior Roux-en-Y gastric bypass. The patient presented with severe symptomatic hypoglycemia resistant to IV dextrose and diazoxide, requiring surgical resection. Traditional imaging found nonspecific findings, and biochemical analysis was inconsistent with insulinoma. A gallium-68 dotatate PET scan was utilized to successfully localize the tumor in the distal pancreas. She underwent laparoscopic resection of the distal pancreatic lesion with resolution of her symptoms and return to euglycemia. The histological evaluation confirmed the diagnosis of nesidioblastosis. Nesidioblastosis is a rare complication of bariatric surgery that may be more clinically relevant with rising prevalence of obesity. Diagnosis with conventional imaging modalities may be challenging; however, the dotatate PET scan may have high utility in detecting lesions. It is essential for clinicians to consider nesidioblastosis in the differential diagnosis of hyperinsulinemic hypoglycemic conditions and recognize there may be a link with increasing rates of bariatric surgery.

1. Introduction

Hyperinsulinemic hypoglycemia (HH) refers to uncontrolled insulin release from neoplastic beta cells or functionally defective pancreatic beta cells that results in hypoglycemia. This broad term is used to describe a number of disease pathologies with similar mechanisms and clinical presentation. Adult-onset, hyperinsulinemic hypoglycemic syndromes have a wide differential that usually necessitates systematic evaluation. Disease syndromes from endogenous insulin production include insulinoma, nesidioblastosis, and dumping syndrome. The remaining syndromes include surreptitious sulfonylurea or insulin use which needs a biochemical analysis for differentiation.

Although rare, insulinomas are the most common cause of hyperinsulinemic hypoglycemia [1]. Insulinomas represent a type of pancreatic neuroendocrine tumor (pNET) or islet cell tumors. They are usually solitary and benign tumors of the pancreas. They are difficult to distinguish from nesidioblastosis as both disorders result from abnormal pancreatic beta cell function. The ultimate distinction relies on histopathologic evaluation [2]. Without biochemical analysis, insulinoma and factitious hypoglycemia from surreptitious sulfonylurea or insulin use can be indistinguishable. Surreptitious insulin use will show increased insulin with decreased C-peptide levels during the hypoglycemic episode due to the negative feedback imposed by exogenous insulin [3]. The overuse of insulin secretagogue medications such as sulfonylurea may mimic an endogenous insulinoma by stimulating the endogenous release of insulin from pancreatic beta cells and increasing insulin, proinsulin, and C-peptide levels [3]. For this reason, sulfonylurea screens have been developed. Postprandial hypoglycemia or reactive hypoglycemia can be a clinical mimicker for insulinoma or nesidioblastosis but has a distinct pattern with food intake and usually occurs within four hours after eating. Postprandial hypoglycemia can be seen in otherwise healthy patients after eating high-carbohydrate meals. It is most often seen after gastric bypass surgery but can occur after esophagectomy, fundoplication, sleeve, or total gastrectomy. Dumping syndrome was coined to describe the increased amounts of undigested food being rapidly transmitted to the small intestine resulting in a myriad of neuroglycopenia symptoms. This occurs more commonly in patients with gastric bypass surgery due to reduced foregut length [4]. The pathophysiology suggests an increase in neuropeptide release driven by increased incretin secretion stimulating beta cells' insulin production with resulting exaggerated or hyperinsulinemic response [4, 5].

Nesidioblastosis is likely to be an increasing etiology for HH conditions, with rising bariatric rates. Nesidioblastosis was first identified in 1938 by Dr. Laidlaw who described the diffuse proliferation of pancreatic duct epithelium [6]. Over time, the definition has evolved to include a congenital or acquired abnormal function of pancreatic beta cells that results in persistent hypoglycemia that is not explained by insulinoma [7]. In newborns and hyperinsulinemic hypoglycemia of infancy, the underlying pathophysiology is suspected to be sporadic or congenital genetic mutations. These genetic mutations result in either focal or diffuse islet cell changes [8–10]. This pathogenesis is hypothesized to be different for adult onset. The condition is rare for both infants and adults. The prevalence has not been well studied in adults but is the etiology in approximately 0.5–5% of cases of hyperinsulinemia [1].

The acquired form of nesidioblastosis most often occurs following an Roux-en-Y bypass, and pathophysiology remains controversial [8]. Various hypotheses have been proposed, including hindgut theory, foregut theory, presurgical obesity theory, vagus nerve theory, elevated serum bile acid theory, dumping syndrome theory, and other undiscovered pathways. Foregut theory proposes that unidentified anti-incretins released from the foregut are downregulated in bypass surgery. This increases incretin release and stimulates a decrease in blood glucose levels [11]. Hindgut theory proposes that nutrients bypass the foregut, reach the hindgut, and lead to the release of glucagon-like peptide (GLP-1) and peptide YY [11]. After gastric bypass, GLP-1 has been shown to increase postprandially, which is thought to increase the pancreatic β-cell mass [12, 13]. In one study by Service et al., histopathology was compared and nesidioblastosis in obese gastric bypass patients had histological islet cell hypertrophy compared to those in obese patient controls without gastric bypass [14]. The presurgical obesity theory proposes that nesidioblastosis occurs from continued β-cell hypertrophy in response to presurgical obesity [11]. Meire et al. reexamined the six specimens from the study of Service et al. and concluded that patients with post-bypass hypoglycemia did not have an increased β-cell area compared to that of obese controls [14, 15]. During bypass surgery, manipulation of the vagus nerve may suppress ghrelin release, decreasing hunger and increasing insulin secretion [11]. This may exacerbate the propensity for hypoglycemia [14]. Although not fully understood, elevated serum bile acids after surgery have effects similar to bile sequestrants, impacting gluconeogenesis and GLP-1 secretion [11]. It is also possible that there are undiscovered gastrointestinal hormones and pathways, representing a new area of research [11].

It is essential to recognize that hypoglycemia after gastric bypass surgery does not strictly indicate altered pathology but is a side effect of altered anatomy and function. Meier and colleagues examined histopathology from 53 specimens, comparing patients with prior gastric bypass to obese patients and lean controls from autopsies [15]. Not surprisingly, patients with postprandial hypoglycemia after gastric bypass did not have increased beta cells. This is consistent with the most common postprandial hypoglycemia in gastric bypass patients or dumping syndrome. In contrast, cases of insulinoma and nesidioblastosis represent inappropriately increased insulin secretion with associated acquired pathology of an increase in beta cells. These diagnoses are based on biochemical analyses and supporting histopathology.

In this case vignette, we describe a rare hypoglycemic hyperinsulinemic nesidioblastosis in a 37-year-old female patient with prior gastric bypass and review the relevant diagnostic evaluation. As our population continues to have an increased prevalence of obesity, it is also likely that there will be an increase in rates of bariatric surgery and nesidioblastosis [13]. We present this rare case to raise awareness among physicians.

2. Case Presentation

A 37-year-old woman with a history of hypothyroidism, remote amphetamine use, and gastric bypass surgery presented with neuroglycemic episodes. She had gastric bypass surgery with Roux-en-Y 10 years ago and initially lost 120 pounds. In the last four months, she has had recurring bouts of syncope, diaphoresis, and unintentional weight loss of 60 pounds. She reported a history of hypoglycemia and stated she was told a pancreatic mass was found in her previous hospitalization four months earlier. She had no history of diabetes but had self-measured blood glucose levels of less than 50 mg/dL despite using over-the-counter glucose tablets. At the time of her presentation, she had taken up to six glucose tablets daily for low blood sugar. She had severe hypoglycemia of 43 mg/dL, non-anion gap metabolic acidosis, and hypokalemia at 2.8 mmol/L. She required ICU level of care for hourly blood glucose monitoring. A 3-day fast was attempted but her persistent and symptomatic hypoglycemia necessitated dextrose infusion, and her fasting was discontinued before the end of the first day. Diazoxide and continuous intravenous dextrose 5% in water (D5W) were given to attempt to normalize her blood glucose but with poor response to treatment and persistent hypoglycemia.

An endocrinology consult was obtained and a systematic biochemical evaluation was initiated (Table 1). Her blood glucose at the time of the studies was less than 50 mg/dL. Her fasting insulin, C-peptide, and proinsulin were inappropriately normal. Despite her hypoglycemia, the C-peptide and insulin levels were not suppressed as would be expected with normal physiology. Other differentials indicative of sulfonylurea use, autoimmune diabetes, defective cortisol secretion, neuroendocrine tumors, and celiac disease were excluded (Table 2). On hospital day 10, her glucose continued to be low at 47 mg/dL despite diazoxide use. C-peptide and fasting insulin levels at 3.1 ng/mL (reference range: 0.8–3.5 ng/mL) and 3.6 (reference range: 2.0–19.6 ulU/mL) were not suppressed despite severe hypoglycemia (Table 1). Total parenteral nutrition (TPN) was started on her with D20% concentration with amino acids to help manage her hypoglycemia.

She had multiple imaging studies, including abdominal MRI and CT abdomen and pelvis, which had no significant findings except for a contour abnormality near the pancreatic tail identified by MRI imaging (Figure 1). She then underwent endoscopic ultrasound by gastroenterology to assess the pancreas, which was reported as normal. Further testing using a gallium-68 dotatate PET scan demonstrated a focal area of radiotracer concentration in the distal pancreas, possibly consistent with a neuroendocrine tumor (Figure 1).

General surgery was consulted, and she subsequently underwent laparoscopic resection of the distal pancreas and splenectomy. A 0.6 × 0.6 × 0.3 cm pancreatic mass was identified (Figure 2). Pathological analysis staining with chromogranin and synaptophysin highlighted expanded islet cell nests with diffuse expansion of islets of Langerhans and ductal insular complexes consistent with nesidioblastosis (Figures 3–5). There was a focal region of increased density of pancreatic islet cells, which was associated with mild chronic pancreatitis and thought to potentially represent the region identified by increased signal intensity on PET imaging studies (Figure 1). No infiltrative malignant cell population, desmoplastic stromal reaction, or other features suggestive of carcinoma were identified.

The patient had a resolution of symptoms following the distal pancreatectomy and was safely discharged after the appropriate vaccination series for splenectomy.

Table 1: Biochemical evaluation for hypoglycemia.

Lab	Admission	HD#10*	Reference
Glucose (mg/dL)	43	47	70–100
C-peptide (ng/mL)	2.3	3.1	0.8–3.5
Insulin, fasting (ulU/mL)	1.0	3.6	2.0–19.6
Proinsulin (pmol/L)	14.9	N/A	<18

*Patient receiving diazoxide.

Table 2: Serologic exclusion of causes for hypoglycemia.

Lab	Value	Reference
Insulin autoantibody (U/mL)	<0.4	<0.4
Sulfonylurea screen	Negative	N/A
ACTH/cortrosyn stimulation (ug/dL)	1 hour cortisol 19.6	>20 ug/dL
Chromogranin A (ng/mL)	82	25–140
Transglutaminase IgG Abs (U/mL)	0.5	<1
Transglutaminase IgA Abs (U/mL)	0.5	<1
Gliadin peptide Ag IgG (U)	2	<20
Gliadin peptide Ag IgA (U)	3	<20

3. Discussion

Our patient presented with severe symptomatic hypoglycemia resistant to diazoxide, requiring dextrose infusion with TPN. Her resistant hypoglycemia suggested insulinoma, but her biochemical analysis was not consistent with diagnosis. Her C-peptide and insulin levels were inappropriately normal, yet the proinsulin levels were not as elevated as expected. Routine imaging with CT suggested a possible lesion near the pancreas tail but overall was nondiagnostic. Endoscopic Ultrasound was unable to identify any lesion. A gallium-68 dotatate PET scan showed a focal radiotracer concentration in the distal pancreas suggesting a possible neuroendocrine tumor. She underwent laparoscopic resection of the distal pancreas mass, which confirmed nesidioblastosis [16]. In a similar case report, Patti et al. found hypoglycemic patients to have fasting hyperinsulinemia, while in our case, even though our patient presented with blood glucose levels in the 40s, her insulin and C-peptide levels on admission and repeat testing were not elevated from the normal range. More importantly, they were not suppressed, which would be expected with normal physiology [17]. Surreptitious sulfonylurea, insulin use, and malabsorption were excluded. Despite these findings, hyperinsulinemia was still suspected. Our patient was given diazoxide, an oral medication that prevents insulin secretion and is used to treat hyperinsulinism [18]. Despite the use of diazoxide, on hospital day 10, our patient had blood glucose levels in the 40s with nonsuppressed insulin and C-peptide levels, likely indicating increased base-level beta cell function and unregulated insulin secretion.

Diagnosing nesidioblastosis in adults is challenging because traditional imaging techniques lack the sensitivity to differentiate between focal and diffuse hyperinsulinism [7]. Common imaging modalities include computerized tomography, MRI, angiography, and transabdominal ultrasound [19–22]. Endoscopic ultrasound was found to have more than 90% accuracy in detecting lesions smaller than 3 cm, while intraoperative ultrasound was the most sensitive method for detecting tumors smaller than 1 cm [22]. This may not be feasible for patients with a small remnant gastric pouch. If imaging is negative, then an alternative method using arterial calcium stimulation with hepatic venous sampling (ASVS) can be done to localize areas of hyperfunctioning beta cells [17, 22]. If localization is detected, then

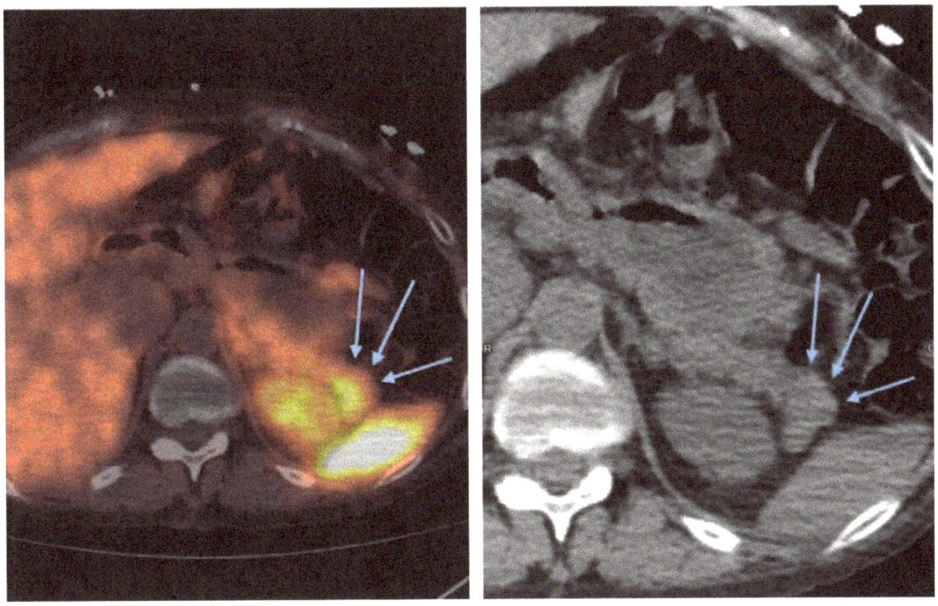

FIGURE 1: Gallium-68 dotatate PET scan and corresponding abdominal CT. Gallium-68 dotatate PET demonstrates a focal area of radiotracer concentration in the distal pancreas consistent with a neuroendocrine tumor in the tail of the pancreas. Compared to CT imaging of the distal pancreas, there is a contour abnormality near the tail, suggesting a possible lesion.

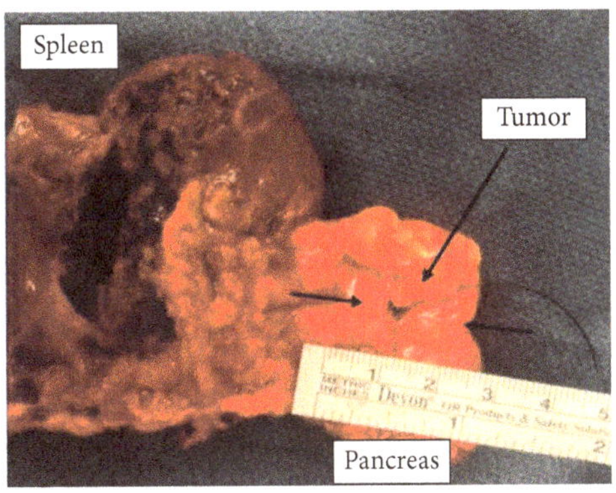

FIGURE 2: Gross pathology demonstrating spleen and pancreas with a 0.6 × 0.6 × 0.3 cm pancreatic mass.

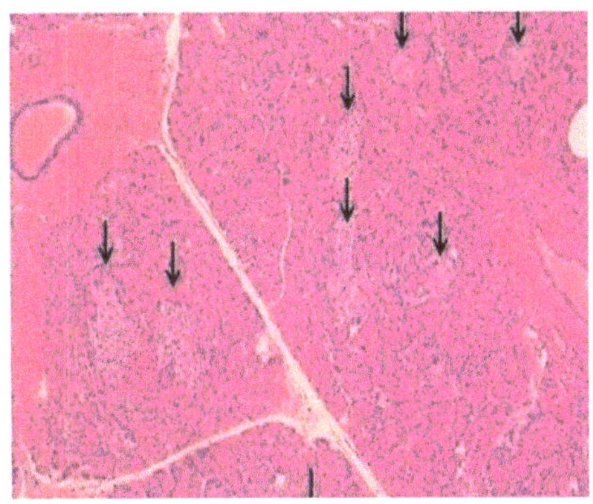

FIGURE 3: Immunohistochemical staining for chromogranin-highlighted expanded islet cell nests with diffuse expansion of islets of Langerhans.

a spleen-preserving distal pancreatectomy is recommended. ASVS can be technically cumbersome, and most cases have been identified via exploratory surgery [14, 17, 20, 23]. Histopathologic evaluation from the resected tissue is required to confirm the diagnosis.

In our literature review, previous cases used selective arterial calcium-stimulation tests to localize and guide partial pancreatectomy [14, 17]. We chose an alternative localization method. There are two other imaging modalities available. Neuroendocrine tumors uniquely express somatostatin receptors, allowing radiolabeled 111In-octreotide to be used in gamma imaging. Unfortunately, 111In-octreotide has a high radiation dose and is taken up physiologically, limiting the detection of smaller lesions [24]. Indium 111 isotope also provides a low image quality [24]. Next, the dotatate PET scan, which uses a radioactive 68-gallium labeled somatostatin analog, has shown to be useful and has a higher sensitivity in locating tumors/hyperplasia than an octreotide scan [25, 26]. The 68-gallium dotatate PET scan was able to localize the lesion in our patient, leading to successful resection and resolution of symptoms (Figure 1). Unfortunately, it is expensive, averaging $8,000 for this case, and the isotope is extremely limited.

Treatment of nesidioblastosis differs for adults and children. Isolate disease in children can present throughout the pancreas and can be cured with partial pancreatectomy of the focal lesion [8, 9]. The diffuse form in children necessitates near-total pancreatectomy [8]. The acquired form of nesidioblastosis most often occurs in adults following a Roux-en-Y bypass. In this setting, the lesions are more likely to be in the pancreatic tail and surgical resction with distal pancreatectomy has been a treatment for some patients [2, 8, 27, 28].

In many cases, surgery can confirm the diagnosis and provide treatment for severe cases [14, 17, 20, 23]. This

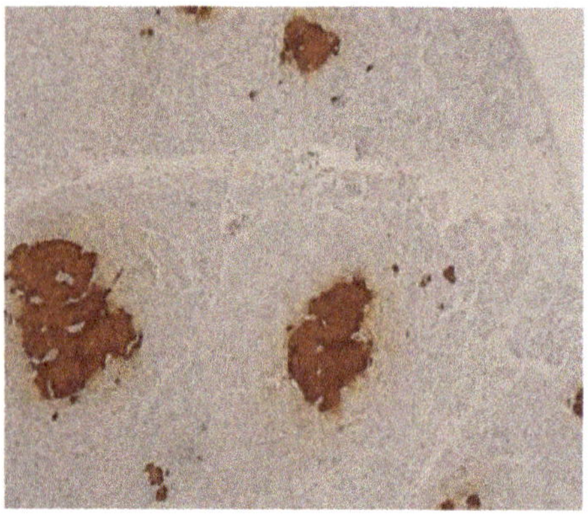

FIGURE 4: Immunohistochemical staining for synaptophysin-highlighted expanded islet cell nests.

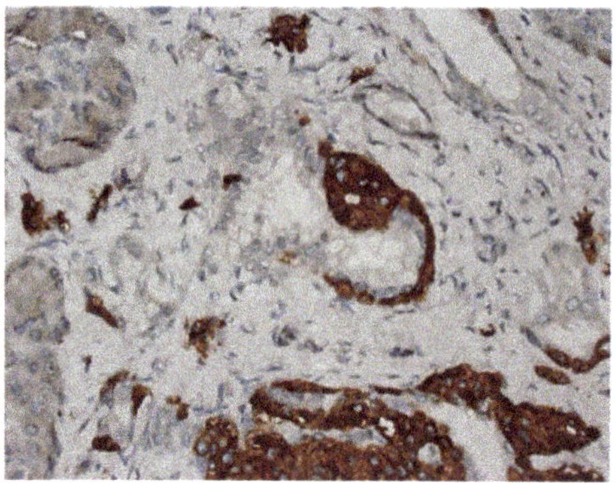

FIGURE 5: Ductuloinsular complexes at 400X with synaptophysin staining.

contrasts with patients without evidence of increased beta islet cell mass. Vanderveen et al. surveyed 48 patients undergoing pancreatic resection for noninsulinoma pancreatogenous hypoglycemia in post-bariatric surgery patients. They found a significant rate of recurrent symptoms; only half of the patients were classified as highly/moderately surgically successful and 25% had no benefit [29]. In our case, distal pancreatectomy provided resolution of our patient's hypoglycemia and post-surgical pathology confirmed the diagnosis of nesidioblastosis.

4. Conclusion

We propose that with increasing rates of obesity and correlating gastric bypass surgeries, more providers will be faced with elucidating the various causes of postprandial and fasting hypoglycemia [13, 30]. We propose that with increased rates of weight loss surgery, hypoglycemic hyperinsulinemic nesidioblastosis will increase in prevalence. Differentiating the etiology can be challenging and requires a stepwise biochemical approach.

References

[1] B. C. H. Van der Wal, R. R. De Krijger, W. W. de Herder et al., "Adult hyperinsulinemic hypoglycemia not caused by an insulinoma: a report of two cases," *Virchows Archiv*, vol. 436, no. 5, pp. 481–486, 2000.

[2] I. Dravecka and I. Lazurova, "Nesidioblastosis in adults," *Neoplasma*, vol. 61, no. 03, pp. 252–256, 2014.

[3] D. H. Awad, S. B. Gokarakonda, and M. Ilahi, *Factitious Hypoglycemia tatPearls [Internet]. Treasure Island (FL)*StatPearls Publishing, Florida, FL, USA, 2022, http://www.ncbi.nlm.nih.gov/books/NBK542310/ S.

[4] P. Berg and R. McCallum, "Dumping syndrome: a review of the current concepts of pathophysiology, diagnosis, and treatment," *Digestive Diseases and Sciences*, vol. 61, no. 1, pp. 11–18, 2016.

[5] J. Tack, J. Arts, P. Caenepeel, D. De Wulf, and R. Bisschops, "Pathophysiology, diagnosis and management of postoperative dumping syndrome," *Nature Reviews Gastroenterology & Hepatology*, vol. 6, no. 10, pp. 583–590, 2009.

[6] G. F. Laidlaw, "Nesidioblastoma, the islet tumor of the pancreas," *American Journal Of Pathology*, vol. 14, no. 2, pp. 125–5, 1938.

[7] A. Raffel, M. Krausch, M. Anlauf et al., "Diffuse nesidioblastosis as a cause of hyperinsulinemic hypoglycemia in adults: a diagnostic and therapeutic challenge," *Surgery*, vol. 141, no. 2, pp. 179–184, 2007.

[8] A. M. Kowalewski, Ł. Szylberg, A. Kasperska, and A. Marszałek, "The diagnosis and management of congenital and adult-onset hyperinsulinism (nesidioblastosis) - literature review," *Polish Journal of Pathology*, vol. 2, no. 2, pp. 97–101, 2017.

[9] C. Crétolle, C. N. Fékété, D. Jan et al., "Partial elective pancreatectomy is curative in focal form of permanent hyperinsulinemic hypoglycaemia in infancy: a report of 45 cases from 1983 to 2000," *Journal of Pediatric Surgery*, vol. 37, no. 2, pp. 155–158, 2002.

[10] A. Reinecke-Lüthge, F. Koschoreck, and G. Klöppel, "The molecular basis of persistent hyperinsulinemic hypoglycemia of infancy and its pathologic substrates," *Virchows Archiv*, vol. 436, no. 1, pp. 1–5, 2000.

[11] H. Ashrafian, T. Athanasiou, J. V. Li et al., "Diabetes resolution and hyperinsulinaemia after metabolic Roux-en-Y gastric bypass," *Obesity Reviews*, vol. 12, no. 5, pp. e257–e272, 2011.

[12] P. Jirapinyo, D. X. Jin, T. Qazi, N. Mishra, and C. C. Thompson, "A meta-analysis of GLP-1 after roux-en-Y gastric bypass: impact of surgical technique and measurement strategy," *Obesity Surgery*, vol. 28, no. 3, pp. 615–626, 2018.

[13] D. E. Cummings, "Gastric bypass and nesidioblastosis - too much of a good thing for islets?" *New England Journal of Medicine*, vol. 353, no. 3, pp. 300–302, 2005 Jul 21.

[14] G. J. Service, G. B. Thompson, F. J. Service, J. C. Andrews, M. L. Collazo-Clavell, and R. V. Lloyd, "Hyperinsulinemic hypoglycemia with nesidioblastosis after gastric-bypass surgery," *New England Journal of Medicine*, vol. 353, no. 3, pp. 249–254, 2005.

[15] J. J. Meier, A. E. Butler, R. Galasso, and P. C. Butler, "Hyperinsulinemic hypoglycemia after gastric bypass surgery is not accompanied by islet hyperplasia or increased β-cell turnover," *Diabetes Care*, vol. 29, no. 7, pp. 1554–1559, 2006.

[16] K. M. Rumilla, L. A. Erickson, F. J. Service et al., "Hyperinsulinemic hypoglycemia with nesidioblastosis: histologic features and growth factor expression," *Modern Pathology*, vol. 22, no. 2, pp. 239–245, 2009.

[17] M. E. Patti, G. McMahon, E. C. Mun et al., "Severe hypoglycaemia post-gastric bypass requiring partial pancreatectomy: evidence for inappropriate insulin secretion and

pancreatic islet hyperplasia," *Diabetologia*, vol. 48, no. 11, pp. 2236–2240, 2005.
[18] A. L. Graber, D. Porte Jr, and R. H. Williams, "Clinical use of diazoxide and mechanism for its hyperglycemic effects," *Diabetes*, vol. 15, no. 3, pp. 143–148, 1966.
[19] E. Christ, D. Wild, K. Antwi et al., "Preoperative localization of adult nesidioblastosis using 68Ga-DOTA-exendin-4-PET/CT," *Endocrine*, vol. 50, no. 3, pp. 821–823, 2015.
[20] R. M. Witteles, F. H. Straus II, S. L. Sugg, M. R. Koka, E. A. Costa, and E. L. Kaplan, "Adult-onset nesidioblastosis causing hypoglycemia," *Archives of Surgery*, vol. 136, no. 6, pp. 656–663, 2001.
[21] S. H. Lee, K. Y. Hyoung, G. S. Seo, B. J. Shin, C. G. Cho, and K. S. Yang, "Diffuse nesidioblastosis of the pancreasin adult with persistent hyperinsulinemic hypoglycemia," *Journal of Korean Endocrine Society*, vol. 11, no. 2, pp. 247–253, 2019.
[22] R. Rinker, "Case report: adult nesidioblastosis A case report and review of the literature," *Digestive Diseases and Sciences*, vol. 43, no. 8, p. 7, 1998.
[23] C. Ferrario, D. Stoll, A. Boubaker, M. Matter, P. Yan, and J. J. Puder, "Diffuse nesidioblastosis with hypoglycemia mimicking an insulinoma: a case report," *Journal of Medical Case Reports*, vol. 6, no. 1, p. 332, 2012.
[24] A. Mojtahedi, S. Thamake, I. Tworowska, D. Ranganathan, and E. S. Delpassand, "The value of (68)Ga-DOTATATE PET/CT in diagnosis and management of neuroendocrine tumors compared to current FDA approved imaging modalities: a review of literature," *American journal of nuclear medicine and molecular imaging*, vol. 4, no. 5, pp. 426–434, 2014.
[25] L. Filippi, P. Pizzichini, O. Bagni, and F. Scopinaro, "Somatostatin receptor analogs (68Ga-dotatoc, 68Ga-dotanoc, 68Ga-dotatate)," in *Radiopharmaceuticals: A Guide to PET/CT and PET/MRI [Internet]*, F. Calabria and O. Schillaci, Eds., Springer International Publishing, Cham, 2020.
[26] S. A. Deppen, E. Liu, J. D. Blume et al., "Safety and efficacy of 68Ga-dotatate PET/CT for diagnosis, staging, and treatment management of neuroendocrine tumors," *Journal of Nuclear Medicine*, vol. 57, no. 5, pp. 708–714, 2016.
[27] G. B. Thompson, F. J. Service, J. C. Andrews et al., "Non-insulinoma pancreatogenous hypoglycemia syndrome: an update in 10 surgically treated patients," *Surgery*, vol. 128, no. 6, pp. 937–945, 2000.
[28] A. A. Lopes, A. C. Miranda, M. S. Maior, R. V. de Mello, and F. A. Bandeira, "Nesidioblastosis associated with pancreatic heterotopia as a differential diagnosis of hypoglycemia: a literature review and case report," *American Journal of Case Reports*, vol. 21, pp. e922778-1–e922778-6, 2020.
[29] K. A. Vanderveen, C. S. Grant, G. B. Thompson et al., "Outcomes and quality of life after partial pancreatectomy for noninsulinoma pancreatogenous hypoglycemia from diffuse islet cell disease," *Surgery*, vol. 148, no. 6, pp. 1237–1246, 2010.
[30] A. Keidar, "Bariatric surgery for type 2 diabetes reversal: the risks," *Diabetes Care*, vol. 34, no. Supplement_2, pp. S361–S266, 2011.
[31] J. M. Neal and W. Han, "Insulin immunoassays in the detection of insulin analogues in factitious hypoglycemia," *Endocrine Practice*, vol. 14, no. 8, pp. 1006–1010, 2008.

21

Pembrolizumab in a Patient with Treatment-Naïve Unresectable BRAF-Mutation Negative Anaplastic Thyroid Cancer

Fadi Nabhan,[1] Elizabeth Kander,[2] Rulong Shen,[3] Amit Agrawal,[4] Vineeth Sukrithan,[2] Ye Zhou,[2] Ashima Goyal,[2] Katie Roll,[1] Manisha Shah,[2] and Bhavana Konda[2]

[1]Division of Endocrinology, Diabetes, and Metabolism, The Ohio State University and Arthur G. James Cancer Center, Columbus, OH 43235, USA
[2]Division of Medical Oncology, Department of Internal Medicine, The Ohio State University Comprehensive Cancer Center, Columbus, OH, USA
[3]Department of Pathology, The Ohio State University Wexner Medical Center, The Ohio State University, Columbus, OH, USA
[4]Department of Otolaryngology—Head and Neck Surgery, The Ohio State University James Cancer Hospital and Solove Research Institute, Columbus, OH, USA

Correspondence should be addressed to Fadi Nabhan; fadi.nabhan@osumc.edu

Academic Editor: Désirée Deandreis

Immune check point inhibitor (ICI) therapy can be a potentially effective salvage treatment for anaplastic thyroid cancer (ATC) with progression despite standard of care therapies. We report a case of unresectable treatment-naïve ATC showing a dramatic and durable response to first-line pembrolizumab therapy. A 69-year-old male presented with a large, right-sided neck mass associated with compressive symptoms. A neck ultrasound showed a large, right-sided, and highly suspicious thyroid nodule. A fine needle aspiration (FNA) biopsy revealed tumor cells consistent with ATC that were positive for PD-L1, with an expression score of >95% and negative for the BRAF V600E mutation. Imaging studies were negative for distant metastases. The disease was declared surgically inoperable, and the patient declined chemotherapy/radiation therapy (XRT), but agreed to ICI therapy with intravenous pembrolizumab 200 mg every three weeks. The patient has received 25 doses of pembrolizumab to date, with rapid resolution of symptoms and a significant reduction in tumor size. He remains alive without disease progression 18 months since initial diagnosis.

1. Introduction

ATC is a rare and aggressive cancer comprising 1.7% of all thyroid cancers [1] that disproportionately accounts for about one-half of thyroid cancer-related deaths [2]. The disease is uniformly lethal, with a median overall survival (OS) of 3-4 months [3]. However, recent reports indicate a trend towards improved survival that is attributed to the development of more effective therapies [4]. Many patients have advanced disease at the time of diagnosis, and 46% of patients had distant metastases at diagnosis in one study [5]. The frequent coexistence of ATA with well-differentiated thyroid cancer (DTC) in tumor specimens, in conjunction with the presence of several shared genomic alterations with DTC suggests that ATC can result from dedifferentiation of DTC. However, the genomic profile of ATC is more complex, and some appear to also arise without evidence of dedifferentiation from DTC [6]. Additionally, ATC has higher mutational burden and genomic disruption than DTC and poorly differentiated thyroid cancer (PDTC) reflecting the significantly higher aggressiveness [7]. Genomic disruption and the acquisition of additional mutations might make ATC an attractive target for immune check point inhibitor therapies de novo. Traditional treatment of ATC depends on the extent of disease at presentation. Stage IVA and resectable stage IVB disease are treated with surgery and external radiation with or without chemotherapy. Chemotherapy and radiation can be considered for unresectable stage IVB and stage IVC patients [2]. The recent FDA approval of dabrafenib (BRAF inhibitor) and trametinib (MEK inhibitor) in advanced BRAF V600E mutated ATC has provided an additional treatment option for this subset of patients [8]. However, progression of disease is frequent which calls for additional therapeutic options. While immunotherapy has been tried as a salvage treatment of patients with ATC [9, 10], there is limited data on its use as a first-line therapy [11]. Here, we report such a case and review-related literature.

2. Case

A 69-year-old male presented with a 2-month history of dysphagia, dysphonia, pain in the right neck and right ear, and a ten-pound weight loss. Thyroid function tests were normal. A physical examination revealed a large, right-sided neck mass. Confirmed by a neck ultrasound, the mass was hypoechoic with macrocalcification and ill-defined borders measuring at least 5.5 cm. A fine needle aspiration (FNA) biopsy at an outside institution revealed malignancy best classified as primary thyroid cancer with high grade and spindle cell origin with suspicion of anaplastic thyroid cancer (ATC). The patient was then referred to our institution for further management. Laryngoscopy revealed right vocal cord paralysis. A CT scan of the neck showed a large, right thyroid lobe mass measuring 7.5 × 4.1 cm, displacing the larynx and trachea to the left and encasing the internal carotid artery by at least 180° (Figures 1 and 2). CT scans of the chest, abdomen, and pelvis and an MRI scan of the brain showed no definitive evidence of distant metastases. Serum thyroglobulin (Tg) level was at 41.5 ng/ml (Beckman Coulter assay with functional sensitivity of 0.1) with undetectable anti-Tg antibodies (Beckman Coulter assay with a functional sensitivity of 0.9). A repeat FNA biopsy of the right thyroid mass revealed discohesive atypical pleomorphic tumor cells consistent with ATC (Figure 3). Immunocytochemistry staining of the both FNA samples were focally positive for TTF 1, variably positive for thyroglobulin and PAX8, and negative for calcitonin, CEA, SOX-10, and p63. PD-L1 22C3 pharmDx—performed on Dako Autostainer Link 48—was positive for high PD-L1 expression with tumor proportion score (TPS) >95% (Figure 4). Molecular testing of the tumor was negative for BRAF (V600/601), KRAS (Exon 2/3/4), and NRAS mutations. Next generation sequencing of the tumor could not be done due to inadequate tissue. Liquid biopsy revealed no reportable genomic alterations. However, this was performed while the patient was on pembrolizumab treatment and not before its initiation. The tumor was deemed unresectable, and the patient declined chemotherapy and radiation therapy. Given the high PD-L1 expression, off-label intravenous pembrolizumab at 200 mg every three weeks was initiated with patient consent and absence of clinical trial accessible to the patient. One week after the first dose, the patient had significant improvement in dysphagia and resolution of pain in the right neck and ear. Restaging scans after four cycles of treatment (one cycle equaling three weeks) revealed a partial response per RECIST v 1.1 (48% decrease in the size of the tumor) (Figures 5 and 6). He

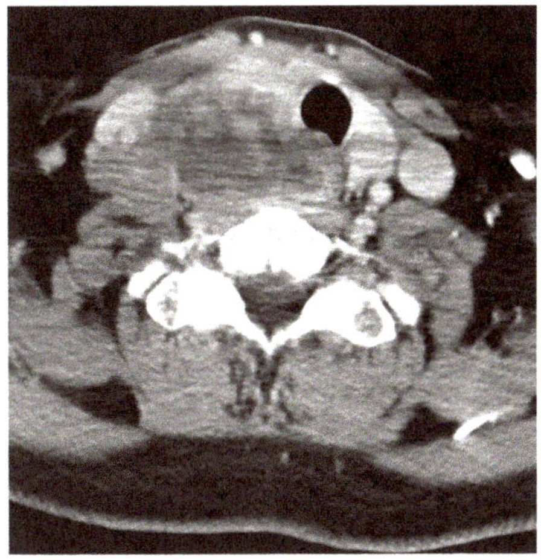

Figure 1: CT scan of the neck at presentation (axial image).

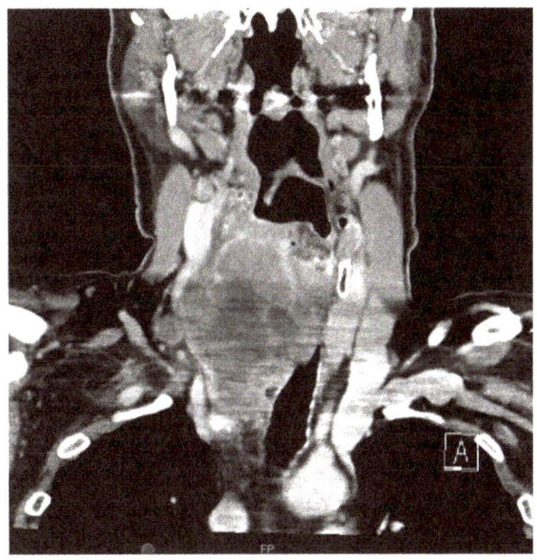

Figure 2: CT scan of the neck at presentation (coronal image).

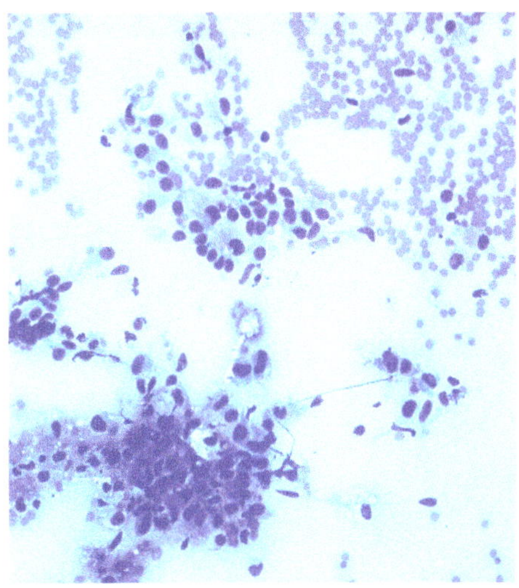

Figure 3: Cytology showing atypical discohesive cells consistent with ATC.

continues to tolerate the treatment well without adverse events, except for the development of immune-mediated thyroiditis. After an initial thyrotoxic phase, the thyroiditis

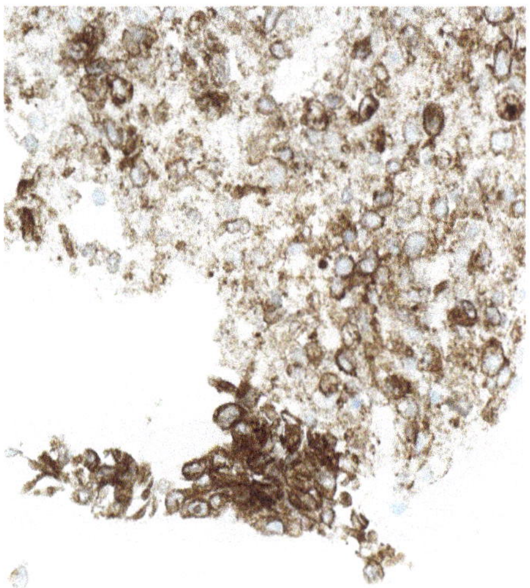

FIGURE 4: Immunocytochemistry staining showing strong positivity for PD-L1.

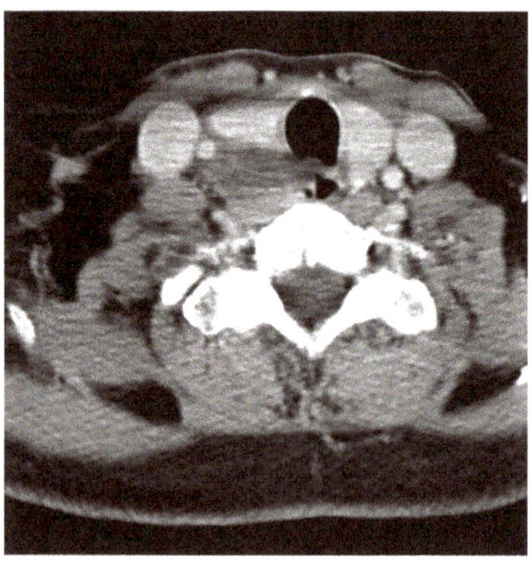

FIGURE 5: First CT scan of the neck after the initiation of pembrolizumab, 4 doses (axial image).

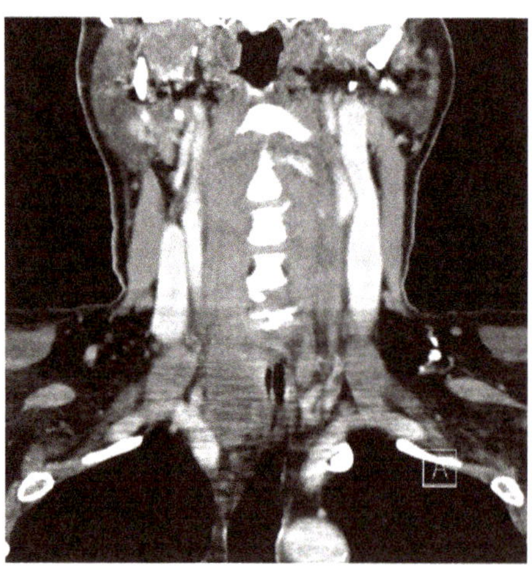

FIGURE 6: First CT scan of the neck after the initiation of pembrolizumab, 4 doses (coronal image).

has progressed toward persistent hypothyroidism and has required thyroid hormone replacement therapy. The patient has received 25 doses of pembrolizumab with continued reduction in size of tumor with most recent scans performed showing approximately 66% reduction in tumor from pretherapy (Figures 7 and 8). The tumor has become resectable but with remaining significant potential high functional morbidity such as possible laryngopharyngectomy and tracheal and esophageal resection given its location. However, the patient continues to decline surgical therapy.

3. Discussion

The evolving understanding of the pathogenesis of ATC at the molecular level has provided insight into its management. ATC differs from well-differentiated thyroid cancer by having a higher mutation burden [7]. However, as stated before, many ATC arise from dedifferentiation of DTC. Genomically, ATC is considered to be composed of three types: one that resembles papillary thyroid cancer (PTC) and has a high prevalence of the *BRAF* V600E mutation; second that resembles follicular thyroid cancer (FTC) and has a high prevalence of the NRAS mutation; and third that has less identifiable genes and appears to resemble hurthle cell thyroid cancer (HCTC) [12]. In ATC patients with the BRAF V600E mutation, which is estimated to be present in 41% of patients [12], the U.S. Food and Drug Administration (FDA) approved the combination of BRAF plus MEK inhibitors (dabrafenib and trametinib, respectively). Subbiah and colleagues [8] reported 16 ATC patients with the BRAF V600E mutation that were treated with dabrafenib and trametinib with an overall response rate of 69% at a median follow-up of 47 weeks.

Immunotherapy has been tried as a treatment for ATC patients who have progressed on other therapies. Iyer and colleagues [9] evaluated 12 patients with ATC on combination therapy of pembrolizumab with tyrosine kinase inhibitors (TKI) where there was a progression of disease on TKI. With combination therapy and a median treatment of 5.6 months, there was a partial response in 42% (5/12) of patients and stable disease in 33% (4/12) of patients [9]. Cabanillas and colleagues [10] reported a case of a patient with ATC where pembrolizumab was used after progression of disease with chemotherapy and dabrafenib/trametinib. The treatment was for approximately ten months, with interruption due to surgery and external radiation, and the patient was alive 12 months after treatment [10]. An ongoing phase 2 study (ATLEP) of the combination of lenvatinib and pembrolizumab showed an interim response rate of 37.5% (6/16; all partial responses) with the rest experiencing stable disease [13]. A phase 2 study of spartalizumab, a PD-1 inhibitor, in ATC reported response rates of 19% (8/42) including three complete responses [14]. Another study of the combination of lenvatinib and pembrolizumab is currently ongoing (NCT04171622).

To the best of our knowledge, there is only one other reported case where ICI therapy was used as a primary treatment for a patient with inoperable and treatment-naïve

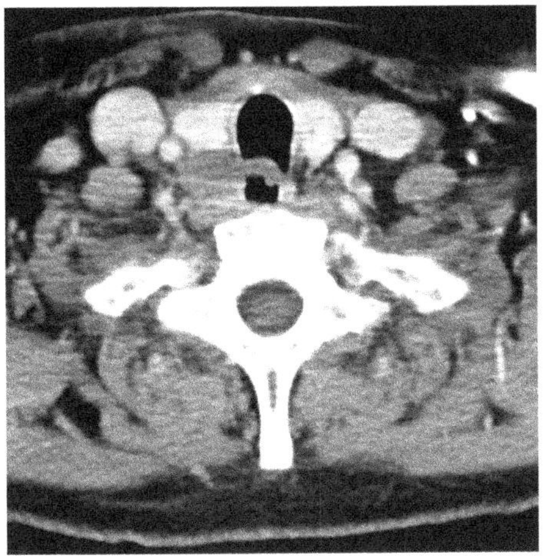

FIGURE 7: CT scan of the neck after 25 doses of pembrolizumab (axial image).

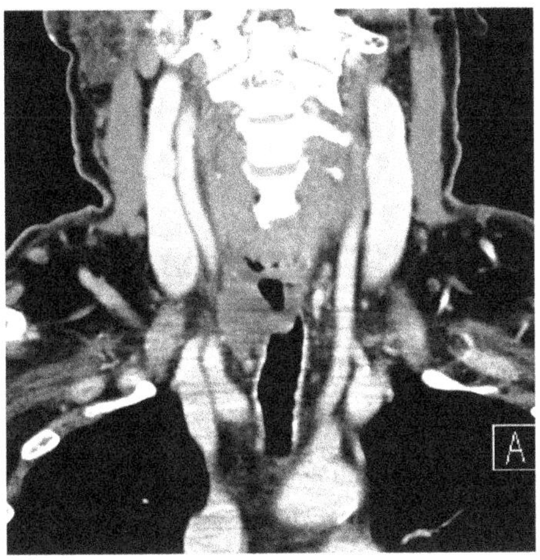

FIGURE 8: CT scan of the neck after 25 doses of pembrolizumab (coronal image).

ATC, with a high PD-L1 expression (60%) in tumor cells [11]. This patient had a near complete response but, however, developed grade 4 colitis after eight cycles of pembrolizumab, which required drug discontinuation, leading to subsequent progression and death 18 months after initial diagnosis [11].

PD-L1 expression has been shown to be as high as 75% in patients with ATC [15]. However, it is important to note that some of the PD-L1 expression may be related to the ensuing immune response to the tumor rather than as an independent process implicated in disease progression. Yet, the association of a worse prognosis with high PD-L1 expression [16] may reflect the latter. Additionally, PD-L1 staining in cytological specimens can be more challenging than in histological ones if the tumor is heterogeneous [17]. When the tumor is homogenous, there is an evidence that the detection and quantification of PD-L1 expression shows a high degree of concordance (>90%) between cytologic and histologic specimens in non-small cell lung cancer [18]. Whether a high PD-L1 expression score is predictive of treatment response in ATC remains unclear. In the present case and another case report [10], the PD-L1 expression was >95%, while the response was irrespective of the degree of PD-L1 expression in a case series by Iyer and colleagues [9].

4. Conclusion

ATC is an aggressive malignancy with a very low survival rate which frequently presents with distant metastases or unresectable disease [19]. This case highlights the possibility of using ICI therapy as a primary treatment modality in treatment-naïve unresectable ATC patients. However, it has yet to be determined whether ICI therapy may be used as a neoadjuvant treatment to allow for surgical intervention or if it may be used as a long-term maintenance therapy when other forms of treatment are refused or when surgery is not feasible. In addition, studies further exploring the use of ICIs as an alternative to chemoradiation are necessary. More studies of immune check point blockade in ATC [20] are in progress, and the results will provide valuable information on the optimal use of these medications in ATC.

Disclosure

This case report was presented as an abstract at the 89th annual meeting of American Thyroid Association under the following title: "Dramatic Response to Pembrolizumab in a Patient with Treatment-Naı¨ve Unresectable Anaplastic Thyroid Cancer."

Acknowledgments

Dr. Manisha Shah reports research funding from Merck and Eli Lilly and Co. Dr. Konda reports research funding from Merck, Eisai, Xencor, Bristol Myers Squibb, and Eli Lilly and Co.

References

[1] R. C. Smallridge and J. A. Copland, "Anaplastic thyroid carcinoma: pathogenesis and emerging therapies," *Clinical Oncology*, vol. 22, no. 6, pp. 486–497, 2010.

[2] R. C. Smallridge, K. B. Ain, S. L. Asa et al., "American thyroid association guidelines for management of patients with anaplastic thyroid cancer," *Thyroid*, vol. 22, no. 11, pp. 1104–1139, 2012.

[3] B. Lin, H. Ma, M Ma et al., "The incidence and survival analysis for anaplastic thyroid cancer: a SEER database analysis," *American Journal of Translational Research*, vol. 11, pp. 5888–5896, 2019.

[4] A. Maniakas, R. Dadu, N. L. Busaidy et al., "Evaluation of overall survival in patients with anaplastic thyroid carcinoma," *JAMA Oncology*, vol. 6, no. 9, pp. 1397–1404, 2020.

[5] B. McIver, I. D. Hay, D. F. Giuffrida et al., "Anaplastic thyroid carcinoma: a 50-year experience at a single institution," *Surgery*, vol. 130, no. 6, pp. 1028–1034, 2001.

[6] J. W. Kunstman, C. C. Juhlin, G. Goh et al., "Characterization of the mutational landscape of anaplastic thyroid cancer via whole-exome sequencing," *Human Molecular Genetics*, vol. 24, no. 8, pp. 2318–2329, 2015.
[7] I. Landa, T. Ibrahimpasic, L. Boucai et al., "Genomic and transcriptomic hallmarks of poorly differentiated and anaplastic thyroid cancers," *Journal of Clinical Investigation*, vol. 126, no. 3, pp. 1052–1066, 2016.
[8] V. Subbiah, R. J. Kreitman, Z. A. Wainberg et al., "Dabrafenib and trametinib treatment in patients with locally advanced or metastatic BRAF V600-mutant anaplastic thyroid cancer," *Journal of Clinical Oncology*, vol. 36, no. 1, pp. 7–13, 2018.
[9] P. C. Iyer, R. Dadu, M. Gule-Monroe et al., "Salvage pembrolizumab added to kinase inhibitor therapy for the treatment of anaplastic thyroid carcinoma," *J Immunother Cancer*, vol. 6, p. 68, 2018.
[10] M. E. Cabanillas, R. Ferrarotto, A. S. Garden et al., "Neoadjuvant BRAF- and immune-directed therapy for anaplastic thyroid carcinoma," *Thyroid*, vol. 28, no. 7, pp. 945–951, 2018.
[11] V. Spalart, B. Legius, K. Segers, J. Coolen, B. Maes, and L. Decoster, "Dramatic response to first line single agent pembrolizumab in anaplastic thyroid carcinoma," *Case Rep Endocrinol*, vol. 2019, Article ID 9095753, 4 pages, 2019.
[12] N. Pozdeyev, L. M. Gay, E. S. Sokol et al., "Genetic analysis of 779 advanced differentiated and anaplastic thyroid cancers," *Clinical Cancer Research*, vol. 24, no. 13, pp. 3059–3068, 2018.
[13] C. Dierks JS, J. Ruf, J. Duyster, O. Thomusch, C. Miething, and A. Zielke, "The lenvatinib/pembrolizumab combination induces long lasting and complete responses in patients with metastatic anaplastic or poorly differentiated thyroid carcinoma: results from a retrospective study and first results from the prospective phase II ATLEP trial," *Annals of Oncology*, vol. 31, p. S1085, 2020.
[14] J. Capdevila, L. J. Wirth, T. Ernst et al., "PD-1 blockade in anaplastic thyroid carcinoma," *Journal of Clinical Oncology*, vol. 38, no. 23, pp. 2620–2627, 2020.
[15] J. J. Bastman, H. S. Serracino, Y. Zhu et al., "Tumor-infiltrating T cells and the PD-1 checkpoint pathway in advanced differentiated and anaplastic thyroid cancer," *The Journal of Clinical Endocrinology & Metabolism*, vol. 101, no. 7, pp. 2863–2873, 2016.
[16] A. V. Chintakuntlawar, K. M. Rumilla, C. Y. Smith et al., "Expression of PD-1 and PD-L1 in anaplastic thyroid cancer patients treated with multimodal therapy: results from a retrospective study," *The Journal of Clinical Endocrinology & Metabolism*, vol. 102, no. 6, pp. 1943–1950, 2017.
[17] D. P. O'Malley, Y. Yang, S Boisot et al., "Immunohistochemical detection of PD-L1 among diverse human neoplasms in a reference laboratory: observations based upon 62,896 cases," *Modern Pathology: An Official Journal of the United States and Canadian Academy of Pathology, Inc*, vol. 32, pp. 929–942, 2019.
[18] J. R. Gosney, A.-M. Boothman, M. Ratcliffe, and K. M. Kerr, "Cytology for PD-L1 testing: a systematic review," *Lung Cancer*, vol. 141, pp. 101–106, 2020.
[19] E. Molinaro, C. Romei, A. Biagini et al., "Anaplastic thyroid carcinoma: from clinicopathology to genetics and advanced therapies," *Nature Reviews Endocrinology*, vol. 13, no. 11, pp. 644–660, 2017.
[20] F. Liotti, N. Prevete, G. Vecchio, and R. M. Melillo, "Recent advances in understanding immune phenotypes of thyroid carcinomas: prognostication and emerging therapies," *F1000 Research*, vol. 8, p. 1, 2019.

22

Prolactin-Secreting Leiomyoma Causing Hyperprolactinaemia Unresponsive to Dopamine Agonist Therapy and Resolution following Myomectomy

Lucinda Barry,[1] **Selvan Pather**,[2] **Ash Gargya**,[1] **and Anthony Marren**[1]

[1]*Royal Prince Alfred Hospital, Sydney, Australia*
[2]*Chris O'Brien Lifehouse, Sydney, Australia*

Correspondence should be addressed to Lucinda Barry; lucinda.barry@health.nsw.gov.au

Academic Editor: Mihail A. Boyanov

Prolactin-secreting leiomyomas are rare, with only eight cases reported in the literature. This case describes a 37-year-old female with hyperprolactinaemia (1846 mIU/L; 85–500 mIU/L) refractory to cabergoline causing infertility and galactorrhea. MRI pituitary was normal. The patient had a known enlarging uterine leiomyoma on serial pelvic ultrasounds (15.2 cm × 9.1 cm × 12.1 cm). The serum prolactin returned to subnormal levels two days postmyomectomy and showed recovery to normal levels in the months following surgery. Immunostaining of the leiomyoma for prolactin was negative. Despite not staining for prolactin, quick resolution of the patient's hyperprolactinaemia after myomectomy supports the diagnosis of a prolactin-secreting fibroid. A prolactin-secreting leiomyoma should be considered in patients with hyperprolactinaemia and normal pituitary MRI which is refractory to dopamine receptor agonist therapy who also have evidence of a uterine fibroid. In patients wishing to seek fertility, myomectomy should be considered to allow for normal ovulation and possibility of future fertility.

1. Introduction

Leiomyomas (uterine fibroids) are common, noncancerous smooth muscle tumours which originate from uterine myometrial cells and are estimated to affect 40–80% of women [1]. Leiomyomas are often asymptomatic and incidentally diagnosed on pelvic ultrasound. However, they can cause abnormal uterine bleeding, pain, mass effect symptoms (urinary or bowel), reduced fertility, and obstetric complications [1]. The cause of leiomyomas is generally unknown; they are, however, known to have oestrogen and progesterone receptors, and their growth is thought to be promoted by these hormones [1]. Leiomyomas typically do not secrete hormones.

Prolactin is a hormone secreted from the anterior pituitary which is regulated by the hypothalamus [2]. It is primarily responsible for stimulating lactation in women postpartum [2].

Prolactin secretion inhibits secretion of gonadotropin-releasing hormone (GnRH) from the hypothalamus which in turn inhibits secretion of follicle-stimulating hormone (FSH) and luteinizing hormone (LH) from the pituitary. FSH and LH are essential in reproduction. In women, a decrease in LH can inhibit ovulation and secretion of oestrogen and progesterone from the ovaries, causing infertility [2].

Prolactin is under tonic inhibition by dopamine that is secreted by the hypothalamus. Pathological hyperprolactinaemia is most commonly caused by a prolactin-secreting pituitary adenoma [2]. Patients with hyperprolactinaemia are often managed with dopamine receptor agonists in order to decrease production of prolactin [2].

We present a case of a patient with leiomyoma who had hyperprolactinaemia unresponsive to medical therapy. The hyperprolactinaemia resolved postresection of her leiomyoma.

2. Case Report

A 37-year-old female underwent investigation for infertility. The patient and her partner were referred to a fertility specialist for review after 14 months of unprotected intercourse without conceiving. Routine fertility investigations of the patient's partner were normal. Her menstrual cycles were irregular (28–75 days). The patient was not taking any regular medications and had no known medical conditions.

Initial routine investigations revealed a mildly elevated prolactin level of 516 mIU/L (85–500 mIU/L), which was not to be significant. TSH was normal. FSH, LH, oestradiol, and progesterone were normal (Table 1). Her antral follicle count was 17 and 19, so she was commenced on letrozole for ovulation induction. The patient did two cycles of letrozole ovulation induction which resulted in ovulation. She developed galactorrhea with a repeat prolactin 990 mIU/L (Figure 1). There was no evidence of interfering macroprolactin on post-PEG (polyethylene glycol) with a recovery of 97%. A post-PEG recovery of greater than 60% excludes the presence of a significant macroprolactin component. MRI pituitary was normal.

A pelvic ultrasound was performed as part of the routine investigations for infertility. This revealed a subserosal leiomyoma measuring 10.3 × 7.2 × 10.5 cm (446 mL). No significant endometrial cavity abnormality was detected.

The patient was commenced on cabergoline; despite increasing the dose of cabergoline to 1 mg/week, the serum prolactin continued to rise to 1856 mIU/L (Figure 1). There was no change to her menstrual cycle with cabergoline.

A repeat pelvic ultrasound was performed a few months later for the suspicion of ectopic prolactin secretion from the leiomyoma given the refractory hyperprolactinaemia. The ultrasound demonstrated significant enlargement of the uterine mass to 15.2 × 9.1 × 12.1 cm (876 mL) with cystic changes and increased vascularity. Sarcomatous change could not be excluded. A subsequent MRI pelvis showed there was no surrounding invasion, so a leiomyosarcoma was thought to be less likely; however, due to the marked increase in size, leiomyosarcoma could not be excluded.

The patient underwent a hysteroscopy, endometrial biopsy, laparoscopy, midline laparotomy, and myomectomy. Saline demonstrated normal ostia bilaterally, normal uterine cavity, and normal endocervical canal. The tubes and ovaries appeared normal bilaterally. There was no evidence of endometriosis. A single port laparoscopy at Palmer's point demonstrated a large pedunculated fundal fibroid. This was converted to a midline laparotomy which revealed a 20 cm vascular pedunculated fibroid, and a myomectomy was performed (Figures 2 and 3).

Histopathology confirmed a benign uterine leiomyoma. There were prominent ischaemic degenerated hydropic and hyaline changes seen as well as degenerative and haemorrhagic areas. Evidence of serosal and subserosal endometriosis with adhesions was also seen on histopathology. Immunostaining of the leiomyoma for prolactin was negative.

Her serum prolactin level two days postoperatively had significantly decreased to subnormal levels (Figure 1).

Table 1: Hormone levels of patient before cabergoline in this case.

	Before cabergoline
FSH (basal RR 1.5–10 IU/L)	5.6 IU/L
LH (basal RR 2.0–12 IU/L)	5.5 IU/L
Oestradiol (follicular RR < 320 pmol/L)	108 pmol/L
Progesterone (follicular RR 0.3–4.0 nmol/L)	0.6 nmol/L

The patient recovered well postoperatively and is planning to commence IVF in the coming months. Her prolactin levels showed recovery towards normal reference range one-month postsurgery.

3. Discussion

This case described a 37-year-old female with hyperprolactinaemia found when investigated for a cause of galactorrhea and infertility. She had a rising prolactin level despite an increasing dose of cabergoline and a normal pituitary MRI. She was found to have an enlarging uterine leiomyoma measuring 15.2 × 9.1 × 12.1 cm. The hyperprolactinaemia rapidly decreased after myomectomy.

There are 8 cases in literature reporting resolution of hyperprolactinaemia after removal of a uterine mass [3–10]. Six of the eight cases revealed leiomyomas on histopathology [3, 5–9]. Of the two other cases, histopathology revealed a low-grade mesenchymal tumour [4] and a uterine tumour resembling ovarian sex cord tumour [10]. Of the six leiomyomas reported, all women were premenopausal (25–47 years). All had no evidence of pituitary adenoma on MRI imaging. The time to diagnosis was 6 months up to 10 years from initial presentation, and the most common presenting complaint was an irregular menstrual cycle. All patients were treated with dopamine agonist therapy, either cabergoline or bromocriptine. The prolactin level continued to rise despite this in all cases (Table 2).

The serum prolactin levels in all 6 patients returned to normal after removal of the leiomyomas, either through hysterectomy or myomectomy, which support the diagnosis of ectopic secretion of prolactin. However, of the 6 leiomyomas reported, only one case reported positive immunostaining for prolactin [3]. Four cases, including this case, did not exhibit immunostaining for prolactin [7–9], and two were not reported [5, 6].

In addition to the anterior pituitary, prolactin has been found to be synthesised and secreted by the uterine myometrium, decidua cells, and leiomyomas [11, 12]. There is evidence that prolactin from decidualised endometrial stroma has an important role in maintaining healthy pregnancies, while myometrial prolactin likely plays a role in maintaining regular menstrual cycles [13]. Two studies found that prolactin acts as an autocrine or paracrine growth factor for leiomyomas and myometrial cells, promoting their proliferation [14, 15]. However, each leiomyoma has been found to have different sensitivities to prolactin [16]. Another study found that prolactin secretion from leiomyoma is greater than myometrial prolactin secretion in the same patient [17]. In addition, prolactin secretion from a leiomyoma increases with time, whereas myometrial prolactin

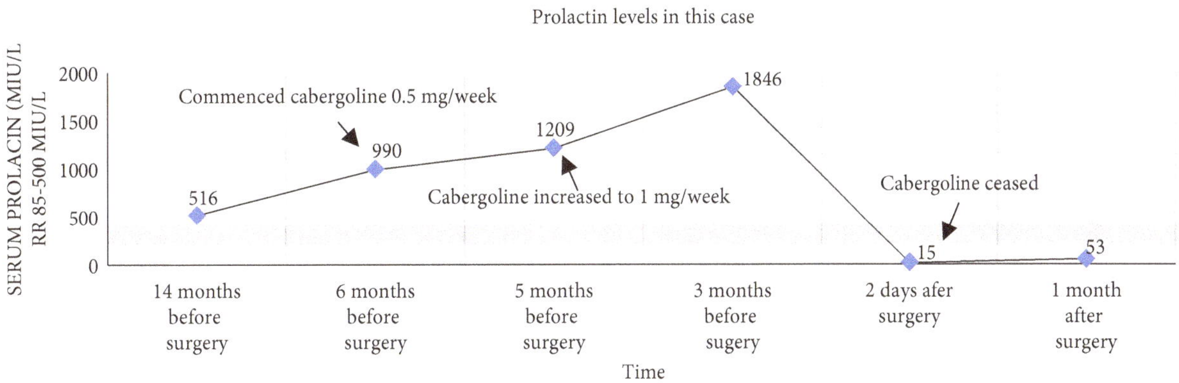

FIGURE 1: Prolactin levels before and after surgery in this case.

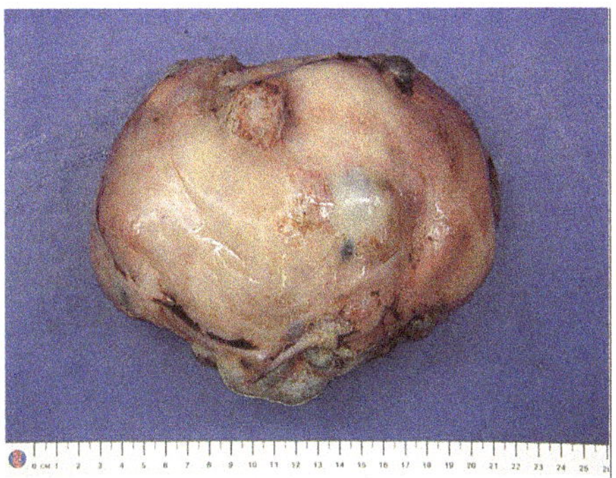

FIGURE 2: Macroscopic image of leiomyoma.

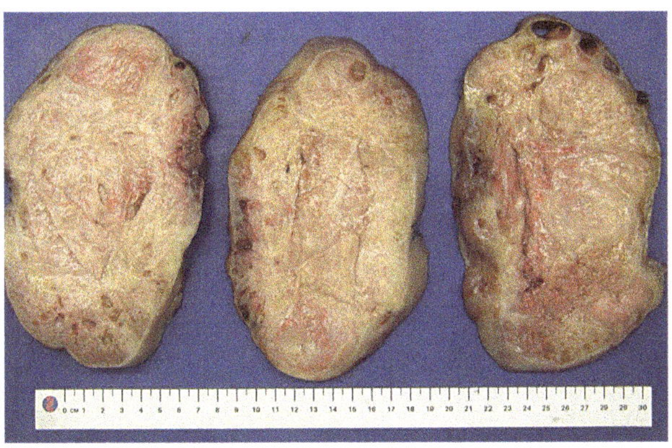

FIGURE 3: Macroscopic image of leiomyoma—cross-section.

did not. The study also found that as prolactin secretion from a leiomyoma increased, the prolactin receptors on the leiomyoma also increased [17], which likely contributed to growth.

Dopamine receptors have also been found on leiomyomas, with overexpression of dopamine receptors correlating to proliferation of leiomyomas [18]. A study of patients with leiomyomas but no evidence of serum hyperprolactinaemia showed statistically significant shrinkage of the tumour with 0.5 mg of cabergoline once weekly for 6 weeks [19], confirming the presence of dopamine receptors. Another study found significant improvement in symptoms related to leiomyoma like per vaginal bleeding and pain, as well as a decrease in the size of the leiomyoma with cabergoline 0.5 mg per week for 3 months. All patients's serum prolactin was tested prior to the study and found to be normal [16]. The leiomyoma in this case did not respond to either cabergoline. The leiomyomas in the other case reports also did not respond to dopamine agonist therapy. Letrozole (aromatase inhibitor) has also been reported to shrink the size of leiomyomas [18]. Letrozole in this case was only used for five days for ovulation induction, so it was not expected to affect the leiomyoma in this case.

Some leiomyomas appear to be more sensitive to prolactin as a growth factor causing unregulated growth and clinically significant hyperprolactinaemia. Complete resistance or paradoxical rise on dopamine agonists may act as a red flag for ectopic prolactin secretion. As discussed, leiomyomas with increased prolactin secretion also had increased prolactin receptors. Dopamine receptors have been found on leiomyomas, and shrinkage of some has been seen with dopamine agonist therapy in patients without hyperprolactinaemia. The leiomyoma in this case was sensitive to prolactin and hence continued to proliferate until hyperprolactinaemia was evident. As discussed, high levels of prolactin caused an increase in prolactin receptors on leiomyomas. It is plausible that while this leiomyoma may have had dopamine receptors, the unregulated proliferation of prolactin and significantly increased expression of prolactin receptors meant that it did not respond to dopamine agonist therapy. Further research is required to further determine the underlying cause of this phenomenon and diagnostic indicators.

With regards to pituitary prolactinomas, serum prolactin is generally directly proportionate to the size of the tumour, with a tumour >4 cm correlating to a serum prolactin level of ≥5276 mIU/L [20]. Each of the six cases including this case reported large leiomyomas >8 cm [3, 9], but all with moderately raised prolactin levels (≤5900 mIU/L). This suggests the leiomyomas are likely poorly differentiated with only small focal areas secreting prolactin. This is confirmed by the case which was positive when immunostaining for prolactin as it reported "focal but intense" positive areas of prolactin-secreting cells [3]. It is possible that the cases where immunostaining was negative also had small focal areas of prolactin-secreting cells which were not seen in the

Table 2: Published case reports of ectopic secretion of prolactin from uterine leiomyomas.

Article reference	Age of patient	First clinical manifestations	Peak prolactin reported (mIU/L)	Dopamine agonist therapy	Dose cabergoline	Prolactin response	Histopathology	Size of leiomyoma	Time to diagnosis	Immunostaining for prolactin
[3]	47	Galactorrhoea	4765	Cabergoline	2 mg/week	Refractory	Leiomyoma	13.9 × 10.4 × 11.8 cm	10 months	Positive
[5]	44	Amenorrhoea	4638	Bromocriptine	30 mg/day	Refractory	Leiomyoma	8 × 7 cm	10 years	Not reported
[6]	36	Irregular menstrual cycle, galactorrhea, and headaches	2127	Bromocriptine	15 mg/day	Refractory	Leiomyoma	5.5 cm	6 months	Not reported
[7]	25	Irregular menstrual cycle and galactorrhoea	3191	Cabergoline bromocriptine	Dose not specified	Refractory	Leiomyoma	6 × 7.2 × 8 cm	3 years	Negative
[8]	45	Not reported	Not reported	Bromocriptine	Not reported	Refractory	Leiomyoma	9 cm	6 months	Negative
[9]	41	Amenorrhea and galactorrhea	5900	Dopamine agonist—not specified	Not reported	Refractory	Leiomyoma	Not reported	6 years	Negative
This case	37	Irregular menstrual cycle and galactorrhea	1846	Cabergoline	1 mg/week	Refractory	Leiomyoma	15.2 cm × 9.1 cm × 12.1 cm	14 months	Negative

samples. This may have been complicated by the areas of haemorrhage and ischaemic changes which were seen on histopathology in this case.

The serum prolactin levels of each case were not directly proportionate to the size of the leiomyoma and could not be correlated to immunostaining positivity (Table 2).

This case is significant, in that it supports the current few reports of ectopic secreting prolactin from a leiomyoma. Despite not staining for prolactin, the patient's prolactin level decreased to subnormal levels within two days post-operatively. This was due to suppression of anterior pituitary lactotroph cells from ectopic hyperprolactinaemia. The prolactin then normalised. Quick resolution of the patient's hyperprolactinaemia after myomectomy supports the diagnosis of a prolactin-secreting fibroid.

A prolactin-secreting leiomyoma should be considered in patients with hyperprolactinaemia and normal pituitary MRI which is refractory to dopamine receptor agonist therapy who also have evidence of a uterine fibroid. In patients wishing to seek fertility, myomectomy should be considered to allow for normal ovulation and possibility of future fertility.

Consent

The consent is obtained.

References

[1] H. Kaganov and A. Ades, "Uterine fibroids: investigation and current management trends," *Australian Family Physician*, vol. 45, no. 10, pp. 722–725, 2016.

[2] M. Al-Chalabi, A. N. Bass, and I. Alsalman, *Physiology, Prolactin*, StatPearls, Treasure Land, FL, USA, 2020.

[3] S. Sachdev, M. C. Reyes, and P. J. Snyder, "Ectopic prolactin secretion from a uterine leiomyoma," *Journal of the Endocrine Society*, vol. 16, no. 4, Article ID bvaa035, 2020.

[4] I. Y. Simsir, G. U. Kocabas, S. B. Sahin et al., "A case of an ectopic prolactinoma," *Gynecological Endocrinology*, vol. 28, no. 2, pp. 148-149, 2012.

[5] V. Cordiano, "Complete remission of hyperprolactinemia and erythrocytosis after hysterectomy for a uterine fibroid in a woman with a previous diagnosis of prolactin-secreting pituitary microadenoma," *Annals of Hematology*, vol. 84, no. 3, pp. 200–202, 2005.

[6] A. G. Herzog, "Migraine with ectopic hyperprolactinemia from uterine fibroids," *Neurology*, vol. 55, no. 1, pp. 148-149, 2000.

[7] S. N. Sendur, F. Aktoz, A. Usubutun, Z. S. Tuncer, and T. Erbas, "Hyperprolactinaemia associated with giant uterine myoma, description of a case and review of literature," *Journal of Obstetrics and Gynaecology*, vol. 39, no. 7, pp. 1034–1036, 2019.

[8] H. Sato, Y. Asami, R. Shiro et al., "Resolution of dopamine agonist-resistant hyperprolactinemia by hysterectomy: a case report," *Gynecological Endocrinology*, vol. 34, no. 3, pp. 199–201, 2018.

[9] R. Upreti, M. Dray, and M. S. Elston, "Uterine fibroid causing hyperprolactinemia and paradoxical prolactin rise with dopamine agonist: case report and systematic review," *SN Comprehensive Clinical Medicine*, vol. 2, no. 4, pp. 464–467, 2020.

[10] G. K. Dimitriadis, D. S. Wajman, J. Bidmead et al., "Ectopic hyperprolactinaemia due to a malignant uterine tumor resembling ovarian sex cord tumors (UTROCST)," *Pituitary*, vol. 23, no. 6, pp. 641–647, 2020.

[11] R. S. Auriemma, G. Del Vecchio, R. Scairati et al., "The interplay between prolactin and reproductive system: focus on uterine pathophysiology," *Frontiers in Endocrinology*, vol. 11, Article ID 594370, 2020.

[12] R. J. Marano and N. Ben-Jonathan, "Minireview: extrapituitary prolactin: an update on the distribution, regulation, and functions," *Molecular Endocrinology*, vol. 28, no. 5, pp. 622–633, 2014.

[13] Y. Hiraoka, K. Tatsumi, M. Shiozawa et al., "A placenta-specific 5' non-coding exon of human prolactin," *Molecular and Cellular Endocrinology*, vol. 75, pp. 71–80, 1991.

[14] R. A. Nowak, S. Mora, T. Diehl, A. R. Rhoades, and E. A. Stewart, "Prolactin is an autocrine or paracrine growth factor for human myometrial and leiomyoma cells," *Gynecologic and Obstetric Investigation*, vol. 48, no. 2, pp. 127–132, 1999.

[15] A. R. DiMauro, A. Dahal, I. Okeke et al., "SAT-003 prolactin is expressed in uterine leiomyomas and may promote their growth," *Journal of the Endocrine Society*, vol. 4, no. Suppl 1, 2020.

[16] M. Vahdat, M. Kashanian, N. Ghaziani, and N. Sheikhansari, "Evaluation of the effects of cabergoline (dostinex) on women with symptomatic myomatous uterus: a randomized trial," *European Journal of Obstetrics & Gynecology and Reproductive Biology*, vol. 206, pp. 74–78, 2016.

[17] R. Baban, S. Al-Suheiri, and Y. Farid, "Prolactin receptors in uterine leiomyoma," *Saudi Medical Journal*, vol. 29, no. 11, pp. 1593–1596, 2008.

[18] B. Gurates, C. Parmaksiz, G. Kilic, H. Celik, S. Kumru, and M. Simsek, "Treatment of symptomatic uterine leiomyoma with letrozole," *Reproductive BioMedicine Online*, vol. 17, no. 4, pp. 569–574, 2008.

[19] A. Elbareg, M. Elmahasi, and F. Essadi, "Effectiveness of dopamine agonist, cabergoline (dostinex) treatment on uterine myoma regression in comparison to the effect of gonadotropin-releasing hormone analog (GnRHa) goserelin (zoladex)," *Fertility and Sterility*, vol. 100, no. 3, p. S33, 2013.

[20] W. T. Burke, D. L. Penn, J. P. Castlen et al., "Prolactinomas and nonfunctioning adenomas: preoperative diagnosis of tumor type using serum prolactin and tumor size," *Journal of Neurosurgery*, vol. 14, pp. 1–8, 2019.

23

Lack of Catch-Up Growth with Growth Hormone Treatment in a Child Born Small for Gestational Age Leading to a Diagnosis of Noonan Syndrome with a Pathogenic *PTPN11* Variant

Daniel J. Olivieri,[1] Lauren J. Massingham,[2] Jennifer L. Schwab,[2] and Jose Bernardo Quintos[3]

[1]*The Warren Alpert Medical School of Brown University, Providence, RI, USA*
[2]*Division of Genetics, Hasbro Children's Hospital/Warren Alpert Medical School of Brown University, 593 Eddy Street, Providence, RI 02903, USA*
[3]*Division of Pediatric Endocrinology and Diabetes, Hasbro Children's Hospital/Warren Alpert Medical School of Brown University, 593 Eddy Street, Providence, RI 02903, USA*

Correspondence should be addressed to Jose Bernardo Quintos; jbquintos@brown.edu

Academic Editor: J. Paul Frindik

Background. Growth hormone (GH) treatment increases the adult height of short children born small for gestational age (SGA). Catch-up growth is associated with a younger age, shorter height, and prepubertal status at the onset of GH treatment. We report a 12 11/12-year-old girl born SGA who received GH for 5 years without catch-up growth and was diagnosed with Noonan Syndrome (NS). *Results.* A 5-year-and-9-month-old 46, XX girl born SGA was started on GH treatment at a dose of 0.32 mg/kg/week. Her midparental target height is 158.6 cm. Endocrine work up showed an IGF-1 level 69 ng/ml (Normal (N): 55–238 ng/ml), IGFBP3 2.6 mg/L (N: 1.9–5.2 mg/L), TSH 3.2 mIU/L (N: 0.35–5.5 mIU/L), and a normal skeletal survey. Height was 96 cm (0.1%; Ht SDS −2.9), weight 14 kgs (1%; Wt SDS −2.3), and Tanner 1 breast and pubic hair were observed. Due to the poor catch-up growth on GH treatment, she was referred to Genetics to elucidate genetic or syndromic causes of short stature. She was noted to have posteriorly rotated ears and slight down slanting of the palpebral fissures. Genetic findings showed a heterozygous pathogenic variant in *PTPN11* (c.922A > G (p.Asn308Asp)) diagnostic for NS. This finding is de novo given negative parental testing. She was noted to have a heterozygous missense variant of unknown significance (VUS) in *FGFR3*: c.746C > A (p.Ser249Tyr). *FGFR3* is associated with multiple skeletal dysplasias including thanatophoric dysplasia, achondroplasia, and Crouzon syndrome and hypochondroplasia. Clinical correlation is poor for these syndromes. *Conclusion.* Diminished catch-up growth and response to GH treatment in a child born SGA led to the diagnosis of NS. The concomitant diagnosis of SGA and NS may have affected the responsiveness of this child to the growth promoting effect of GH treatment.

1. Introduction

Small for gestational age (SGA) has a global incidence of 3–10% and results in a higher risk for metabolic dysregulation and reduced fetal growth [1, 2]. While over 85% of infants will "catch-up" to their peers by two years of age, nearly 10% of SGA infants will continue to fall below the 3rd percentile of height until adulthood [3]. Failure to "catch-up" to peers—children two standard deviations below the mean for age and sex at two years of age per Food and Drug Administration criteria or four years of age per European Medicines Agency criteria—can warrant Growth Hormone (GH) pharmacologic treatment [4, 5]. Nonresponders to GH treatment warrant complete metabolic and genetic workup to determine the etiology [6–9]. We present a patient born SGA who was refractory to GH treatment and later found to have an *FGFR3* variant of unknown significance (VUS) and a PTPN11 pathogenic variant of Noonan Syndrome (NS).

Initial clinical presentation, serial measurements, workup, and case management are discussed.

2. Case Presentation

The patient initially presented to the pediatric endocrinologist at Hasbro Children's Hospital (Providence, RI, USA) as a five years and two months old female for growth evaluation.

She was born to a 32-year-old G1P0 ⟶ 2 mother at 37 weeks, 2 days gestation, via cesarean section and her twin brother (discordant) during an uncomplicated pregnancy. Her birth was notable for intrauterine growth restriction (IUGR) with weight and length more than two standard deviations below the mean (1.75 kg and 38.1 cm length). The perinatal course included a 1-week hospital stay for catch-up growth but no NICU stay. Her twin brother was born at 5 pounds, 1 ounce, and 18 inches length. Maternal medications included levothyroxine, and the mother's past medical history was notable for papillary thyroid cancer. No drugs, alcohol, or cigarettes were reported nor documented in pregnancy. She required early intervention at 6 months for a motor delay (inability to sit up). Her predicted midparental target height is 157 cm ± 10 cm (62 inches ± 4 inches) with a lower limit of 147 cm (58 inches).

A concern for failure to catch up in growth by age four years led to a referral to the pediatric endocrine clinic at five years and two months of age. Her parents denied polyuria, polydipsia, headache, fatigue, fever, weight loss, cold intolerance, sleep disturbance, abdominal pain, and constipation.

The initial laboratory investigation was normal (Table 1). The physical examination findings included a height of 96.1 cm (0.2%; SDS of −2.9), a weight of 14.0 kg (1%; SDS of −2.3), and a BMI of 15.1 kg/m^2 (50.3%). She had Tanner 1 breast and pubic hair and otherwise unremarkable physical examination. Given the height of 2.9 standard deviations below the mean at age 4 years, GH treatment was warranted [10]. She began recombinant growth hormone at a dose of 0.6 mg administered subcutaneously every night at a starting dose of 0.32 mg/kg/week.

A six-month follow-up visit was notable for an excellent annualized growth rate of 10.4 cm/year. GH dose was increased from 0.6 mg SQ to 0.65 mg SQ every night to maintain a dosage of 0.32 mg/kg/week. She denied side effects of GH injections including symptoms of pseudotumor cerebri, such as headaches, blurry vision, or vomiting. The subsequent annual growth velocities and height standard deviations (Ht SDS) are presented in Table 2. Additionally, there was a 9-month treatment lapse from years two, three due to financial cost (i.e., high health insurance deductible), resulting in diminished growth (Figures 1 and 2). GH therapy treatment was reinitiated at an age of 8 years.

Due to the continued diminished growth, she was referred to the Division of Genetics at 10 years and 9 months of age to elucidate genetic or syndromic causes of short stature. She was noted to have posteriorly rotated ears and slightly downward slanting of the palpebral fissures. A comprehensive Short Stature Syndrome Panel Plus (sequencing and deletion/duplication) from Blueprint Genetics analyzed 374 genes including IGF-1, IGF-1 receptor, IGF-ALS (insulin-like growth factor-binding protein, acid-labile subunit), GH, GH receptor, GH releasing hormone receptor, and STAT5b demonstrated a heterozygous pathogenic variant in *PTPN11* (c.922A > G (p.Asn308Asp)) diagnostic for NS. This finding is de novo as parental testing for the *PTPN11* variant was negative. She was noted to have a heterozygous missense variant of unknown significance (VUS) in *FGFR3*: c.746C > A (p.Ser249Tyr). *FGFR3* is associated with multiple skeletal dysplasias including thanatophoric dysplasia, achondroplasia, Crouzon syndrome, and hypochondroplasia. Clinical correlation is poor as our patient's findings are not as severe as typically described for these syndromes. The patient then received comprehensive screening for NS, including a renal ultrasound, EKG, skeletal survey, ophthalmic evaluation, and thyroid panel.

Table 1: Initial laboratory values.

Description	Value	Reference range
Genetic		
Karyotype	46, XX	—
Thyroid markers		
TSH, high sensitivity	2.977 uIU/mL	0.350–5.5 uIU/mL
Thyroglobulin Ab	<15.0 U/mL	0.0–60.0 U/mL
Thyroid peroxidase Abs	<28.0 IU/mL	1.0–60.0 IU/mL
Endocrine		
IGF-1 binding protein 3	2.6 mg/L	1.1–5.2 mg/L
IGF-1	69 ng/mL	55–238 ng/mL
Renal		
Ultrasound	Normal findings	—
Inflammatory markers		
Celiac disease	Negative	—

At the last endocrine visit at 12 years and 11 months of age, the patient's height was 138 cm (0.4%; SDS = −2.6) and weight was 32.4 kg (2.3%; SDS = −2.0) on 2.2 mg/day subcutaneous GH treatment injections (0.5 mg/kg/week). Additionally, she was noted to have Tanner 3 breast development and Tanner 4 pubic hair. Other notable physical examination findings included frontal bossing and triangular facies. Her most recent annualized growth was 5.2 cm/year (69%; SDS = 0.52). Her most recent bone age was 11 years–11 years and 6 months, with a predicted adult height of148.5 cm–150 cm vs. the midparental target height is 157 cm ± 10 cm (62 inches ± 4 inches) with a lower limit of 147 cm (58 inches). The plan is to discontinue GH treatment once the bone age is 14-15 years and growth rate is <2.5 cm/year.

3. Discussion

We report a 12 11/12-year-old girl born SGA who received GH for 5 years without catch-up growth and was diagnosed with NS with a *PTPN11* pathogenic variant. The concomitant diagnosis of SGA and NS may have affected the responsiveness of this child to the growth-promoting effect of GH treatment.

TABLE 2: Annual growth parameters.

Year	Height standard deviations[a] below mean for age and sex	Growth rate (cm/year)
0	−2.9	—
1	−2.5	7.5
2	−2.2	6.7
3	−2.2	4.5
4	−2.2	5.1
5	−2.5	5.1

[a]Height standard deviations refers to the number of standard deviations below the mean height for age and sex.

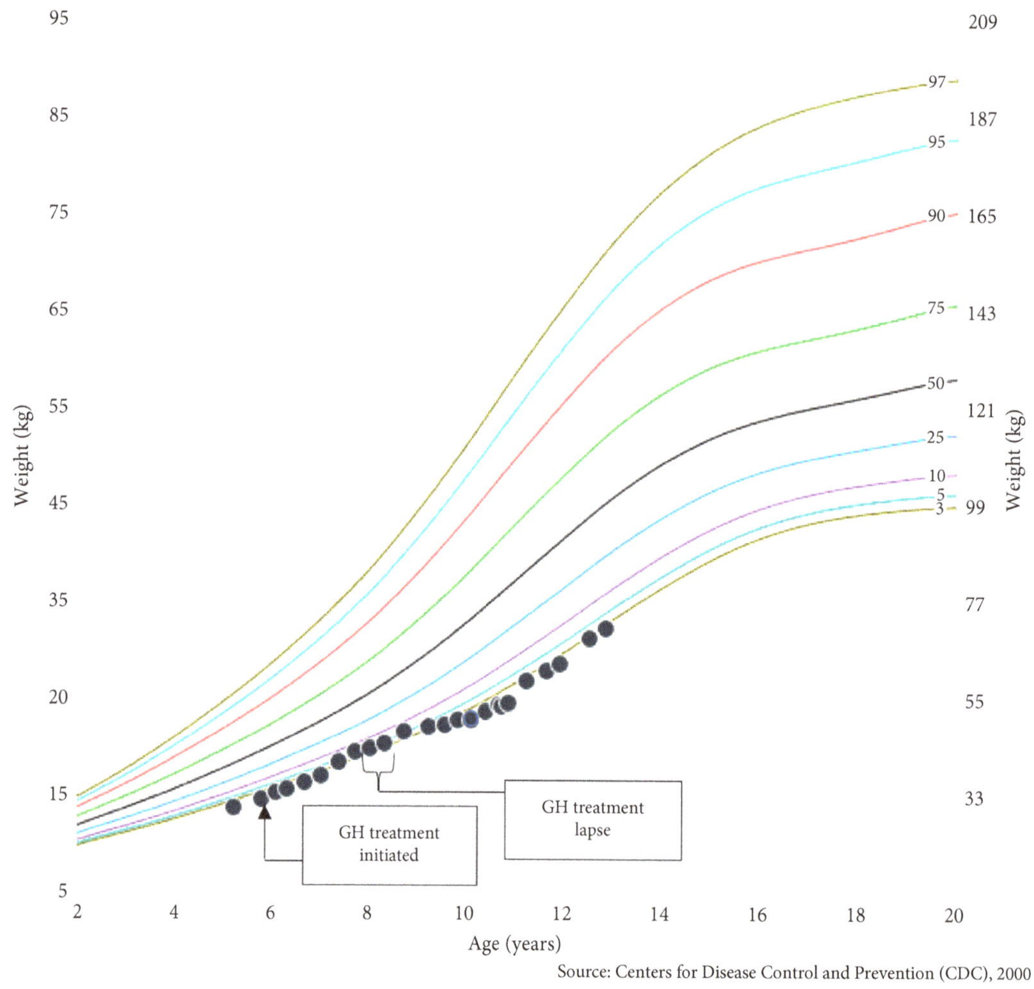

FIGURE 1: Plotted weight-for-age percentiles for Jane Doe. Centers for Disease Control and Prevention (CDC) weight-for-age percentiles, girls 2 to 20 years old.

Children born SGA require careful follow-up and monitoring to evaluate for developmental and growth-related complications [10]; children born SGA on average weigh less and are shorter than their non-SGA counterparts [1, 11]. While the majority of SGA infants experience "catch-up" growth, nearly 15% of SGA infants will not "catch-up" by two years of life [12]. Children who remain two or greater standard deviations below the mean for their age and sex warrant consideration for GH treatment [13]. The efficacy of GH treatment in children born SGA has been correlated to earlier treatment initiation, shorter starting height, and decreased starting weight [14]. Important considerations for GH treatment include financial cost, treatment compliance, and the psychological effects of short stature [15–17]. Despite the strong efficacy of GH treatment associated with children who fit FDA or EMA criteria, some children will remain two standard deviations below their midparental target height refractory to GH therapy [18]. Potential causes of children refractory to GH include mutations in the GH receptor, IGF-1 gene, and GH signaling pathway [19]. Specifically, in regard to children born SGA, variability in response to GH treatment has been reported and may be explained through genetic mutations in the GH/GH receptor transduction signaling pathway [19, 20]. More recent studies

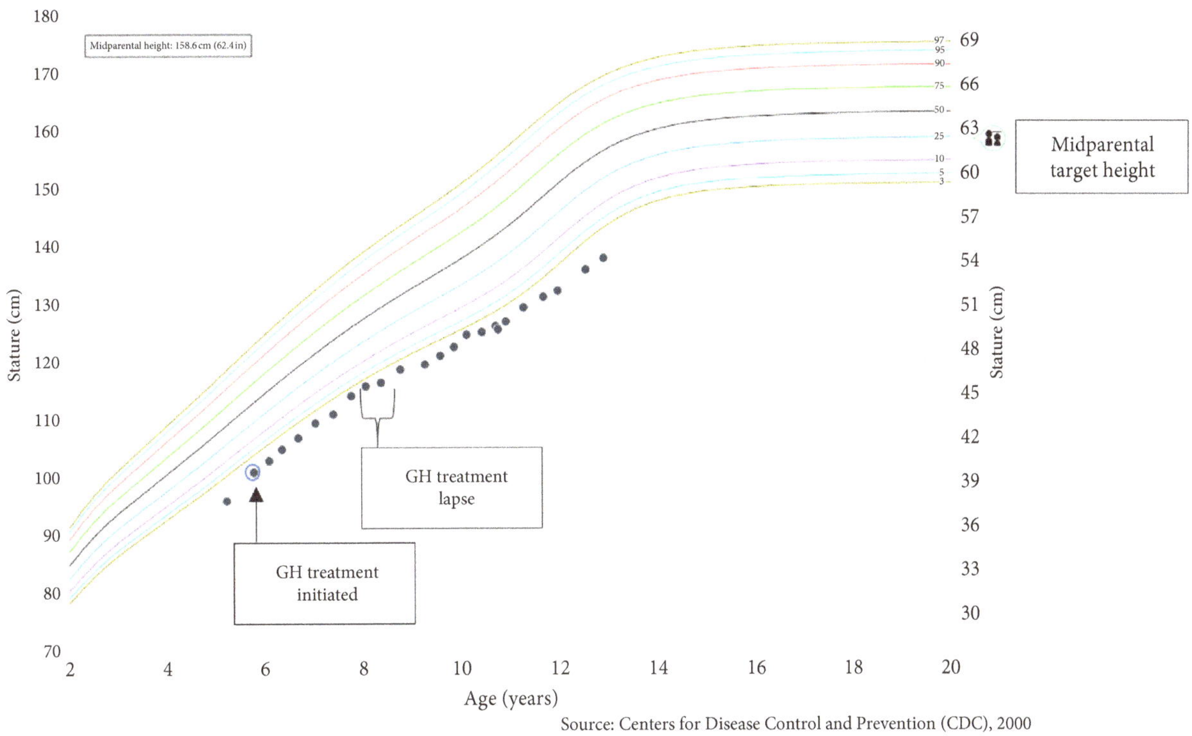

Figure 2: Plotted stature-for-age percentiles for Jane Doe. Centers for Disease Control and Prevention (CDC) stature-for-age percentiles, girls 2 to 20 years old.

analyze the role of growth-plate-related genes including COL2A1, COL11A1, ACAN, and FLNB [21, 22]. GnRH agonists may be indicated in children born SGA who are in puberty with predicted adult height 2.5 standard deviations below the mean for their corresponding age and sex [23]. Some children born SGA who are short at the start of puberty may benefit from the combined use of GH and GnRH agonist treatment [23–25].

NS is a genetic condition associated with short stature and is inherited in either an autosomal dominant or de novo (sporadic variant) manner [26]. The incidence of NS is approximately 1 in 1,000–2,500 births. Besides short stature, it is also commonly associated with cardiac abnormalities, characteristic facies, lymphatic dysplasias, and coagulation defects [26–28]. Studies have shown that, in children with NS, prepubertal GH treatment has resulted in increased growth at a rate equivalent to girls with Turner syndrome, although not to the level of children with idiopathic GH deficiency [27, 28]. The thought is there is a possibly impairment of the GH IGF1 axis. Therefore, GH treatment is an FDA-approved indication for children diagnosed with NS, with nearly 60% of children with NS obtaining an adult height within one standard deviation of their midparental target height [29]. Without GH treatment, nearly 70% of children with NS will have short stature throughout adulthood [29, 30]. Side effects from GH treatment in children with NS are infrequently reported. Most notable in regard to NS, GH treatment does not influence cardiac morphogenesis [29, 31]. One potential mechanism for the GH resistance in NS relates to the *PTPN11* variant. *PTPN11* encodes SHP2, a protein tyrosine phosphatase involved in GH signaling [20, 32]. Therefore, postreceptor GH signaling mutations in SHP2 might explain the mild resistance to GH treatment sometimes seen in NS patients [32]. Additionally, the downstream signaling mutation in SHP2 might also explain the compensatory elevated GH secretion occasionally seen in NS patients [32]. Finally, although recombinant IGF-1 therapy may be a potential treatment in children with NS, to the best of our knowledge, there have been no reports showing the efficacy of IGF-1 in children with NS [33].

Our patient born SGA was also diagnosed with *PTPN11*-related NS after extensive genetic testing. Additionally, genetic testing was not diagnostic for other conditions that could explain her short stature, including GH receptor, IGF-1 gene, or GH signaling pathway abnormalities. While children born SGA and children with NS can have significant increases in growth with GH treatment [34], our patient had poor response to GH treatment. Therefore, we hypothesize that the concomitant diagnosis of SGA and *PTPN11*-related NS may have affected the responsiveness of our patient to the growth-promoting effect of GH therapy. Additionally, it is important to note that genetic workup also elucidated a nondiagnostic VUS in the FGFR3 gene (c.746C > A (p.Ser249Tyr)). While pathogenic variants in this gene can be associated with several genetic syndromes including thanatophoric dysplasia, achondroplasia, Crouzon syndrome, and hypochondroplasia, our patient's phenotype did not fit these diagnoses, and at this time, the significance of this molecular finding is still unclear.

4. Conclusions

We present a case of a 12 11/12-year-old girl born SGA who received GH for 5 years without catch-up growth and was later diagnosed with NS. In turn, the concomitant diagnosis of SGA and NS may have altered the child's ability to respond to GH treatment.

References

[1] G. T. Mandy, L. E. Weisman, and M. S. Kim, "Infants with fetal (intrauterine) growth restriction," 2021, https://www.uptodate.com.
[2] W. K. Cho, B.-K. Suh, and B.-K. Suh, "Catch-up growth and catch-up fat in children born small for gestational age," *Korean Journal of Pediatrics*, vol. 59, no. 1, pp. 1–7, 2016.
[3] J. Argente, O. Mehls, and V. Barrios, "Growth and body composition in very young SGA children," *Pediatric Nephrology*, vol. 25, no. 4, pp. 679–685, 2010.
[4] A. D. Rogol, "Growth hormone treatment for children born small for gestational age," 2021, https://www.uptodate.com/contents/growth-hormone-treatment-for-children-born-small-for-gestational-age.
[5] A. Deodati and S. Cianfarani, "The rationale for growth hormone therapy in children with short stature," *Journal of Clinical Research in Pediatric Endocrinology*, vol. 9, no. S2, pp. 23–32, 2017.
[6] G. Johannsson, M. Bidlingmaier, B. M. K. Biller et al., "Growth hormone research society perspective on biomarkers of GH action in children and adults," *Endocrine Connections*, vol. 7, no. 3, pp. R126–R134, 2018.
[7] N. Møller and J. O. L. Jørgensen, "Effects of growth hormone on glucose, lipid, and protein metabolism in human subjects," *Endocrine Reviews*, vol. 30, no. 2, pp. 152–177, 2009.
[8] G. H. Seo and H.-W. Yoo, "Growth hormone therapy in patients with noonan syndrome," *Annals of Pediatric Endocrinology & Metabolism*, vol. 23, no. 4, pp. 176–181, 2018.
[9] C. C. J. Smeets, S. R. Judith, M. v. d. Steen, and A. C. S. Hokken-Koelega, "Metabolic health and long-term safety of growth hormone treatment in silver-russell syndrome," *The Journal of Clinical Endocrinology & Metabolism*, vol. 102, no. 3, pp. 983–991, 2017.
[10] P. E. Clayton, S. Cianfarani, P. Czernichow, G. Johannsson, R. Rapaport, and A. Rogol, "Management of the child born small for gestational age through to adulthood: a consensus statement of the international societies of pediatric endocrinology and the growth hormone research society," *The Journal of Clinical Endocrinology & Metabolism*, vol. 92, no. 3, pp. 804–810, 2007.
[11] J. Karlberg and K. Albertsson-Wikland, "Growth in full- term small-for-gestational-age infants: from birth to final height," *Pediatric Research*, vol. 38, no. 5, pp. 733–739, 1995.
[12] A. C. Hokken-Koelega, M. A. D. Ridder, R. J. Lemmen, H. D. Hartog, S. M. D. M. Keizer-Schrama, and S. L. Drop, "Children born small for gestational age: do they catch up?" *Pediatric Research*, vol. 38, no. 2, pp. 267–271, 1995.
[13] P. A. Lee, S. D. Chernausek, A. C. S. Hokken-Koelega, and C. Paul, "International small for gestational age advisory board consensus development conference statement: management of short children born small for gestational age," *Pediatrics*, vol. 111, no. 6, pp. 1253–1261, 2003.
[14] J. Dahlgren and K. A. Wikland, "Final height in short children born small for gestational age treated with growth hormone," *Pediatric Research*, vol. 57, no. 2, pp. 216–222, 2005.
[15] D. E. Sandberg and L. D. Voss, "The psychosocial consequences of short stature: a review of the evidence," *Best Practice & Research Clinical Endocrinology & Metabolism*, vol. 16, no. 3, pp. 449–463, 2002.
[16] C. J. Kelnar, "Which children should receive growth hormone treatment. cost-benefit analysis is the key," *Archives of Disease in Childhood*, vol. 83, no. 2, pp. 176–178, 2000.
[17] J. M. Lee, M. M. Davis, S. J. Clark, T. P. Hofer, and A. R. Kemper, "Estimated cost-effectiveness of growth hormone therapy for idiopathic short stature," *Archives of Pediatrics & Adolescent Medicine*, vol. 160, no. 3, pp. 263–269, 2006.
[18] A. Grimberg, S. A. DiVall, C. Polychronakos et al., "Guidelines for growth hormone and insulin-like growth factor-I treatment in children and adolescents: growth hormone deficiency, idiopathic short stature, and primary insulin-like growth factor-I deficiency," *Hormone Research in Paediatrics*, vol. 86, no. 6, pp. 361–397, 2016.
[19] R. G. Rosenfeld, "IGF-I therapy in growth disorders," *European Journal of Endocrinology*, vol. 157, no. s1, pp. S57–S60, 2007.
[20] S. Loche, L. Carta, A. Ibba, and C. Guzzetti, "Growth hormone treatment in non-growth hormone-deficient children," *Annals of Pediatric Endocrinology & Metabolism*, vol. 19, no. 1, pp. 1–7, 2014.
[21] L. Plachy, V. Strakova, L. Elblova et al., "High prevalence of growth plate gene variants in children with familial short stature treated with GH," *The Journal of Clinical Endocrinology & Metabolism*, vol. 104, no. 10, pp. 4273–4281, 2019.
[22] J. B. Quintos, M. H. Guo, and A. Dauber, "Idiopathic short stature due to novel heterozygous mutation of the aggrecan gene," *Journal of Pediatric Endocrinology & Metabolism: JPEM*, vol. 28, no. 7-8, pp. 927–932, 2015.
[23] M. J. J. Finken, M. van der Steen, C. C. J. Smeets et al., "Children born small for gestational age: differential diagnosis, molecular genetic evaluation, and implications," *Endocrine Reviews*, vol. 39, no. 6, pp. 851–894, 2018.
[24] M. van der Steen, A. J. Lem, D. C. M. v. d. van der Kaay, and A. C. S. Hokken-Koèelega, "Puberty and pubertal growth in GH-treated SGA children: effects of 2 years of GnRHa versus no GnRHa," *The Journal of Clinical Endocrinology & Metabolism*, vol. 101, no. 5, pp. 2005–2012, 2016.
[25] A. J. Lem and D. C. M. v. d. van der Kaay, M. A. J. d. Ridder et al., "Adult height in short children born SGA treated with growth hormone and gonadotropin releasing hormone analog: results of a randomized, dose-response GH trial," *The Journal of Clinical Endocrinology & Metabolism*, vol. 97, no. 11, pp. 4096–4105, 2012.
[26] A. A. Romano, J. E. Allanson, J. Dahlgren et al., "Noonan syndrome: clinical features, diagnosis, and management guidelines," *Pediatrics*, vol. 126, no. 4, pp. 746–759, 2010.
[27] P. A. Lee, J. L. Ross, B.T. Pedersen, P. Kotnik, J. A. Germak, and H. T. Christesen, "Noonan syndrome and turner syndrome patients respond similarly to 4 years' growth-hormone therapy: longitudinal analysis of growth-hormone-naïve patients enrolled in the NordiNet® international outcome study and the ANSWER program," *International Journal of Pediatric Endocrinology*, vol. 2015, no. 1, pp. 1–9, 2015.
[28] N. Zavras, C. Meazza, A. Pilotta et al., "Five-year response to

growth hormone in children with noonan syndrome and growth hormone deficiency," *Italian Journal of Pediatrics*, vol. 41, no. 1, pp. 71–76, 2015.

[29] J. A. Noonan, A.-M. Kappelgaard, and A.-M. Kappelgaard, "The efficacy and safety of growth hormone therapy in children with noonan syndrome: a review of the evidence," *Hormone Research in Paediatrics*, vol. 83, no. 3, pp. 157–166, 2015.

[30] J. A. Noonan, R. Raaijmakers, and B. Hall, "Adult height in noonan syndrome," *American Journal of Medical Genetics Part A*, vol. 123, no. no. 1, pp. 68–71, 2003.

[31] A. M. Cotterill, W. J. McKenna, A. F. Brady et al., "The short-term effects of growth hormone therapy on height velocity and cardiac ventricular wall thickness in children with noonan's syndrome," *The Journal of Clinical Endocrinology & Metabolism*, vol. 81, no. 6, pp. 2291–2297, 1996.

[32] G. Binder, K. Neuer, M. B. Ranke, and N. E. Wittekindt, "PTPN11 mutations are associated with mild growth hormone resistance in individuals with noonan syndrome," *The Journal of Clinical Endocrinology & Metabolism*, vol. 90, no. 9, pp. 5377–5381, 2005.

[33] P. F. Collett-Solberg and M. Misra, "The role of recombinant human insulin-like growth factor-I in treating children with short stature," *The Journal of Clinical Endocrinology & Metabolism*, vol. 93, no. 1, pp. 10–18, 2008.

[34] A.-M. Kappelgaard and T. Laursen, "The benefits of growth hormone therapy in patients with turner syndrome, noonan syndrome and children born small for gestational age," *Growth Hormone & IGF Research*, vol. 21, no. 6, pp. 305–313, 2011.

24

Central Hyperthyroidism due to Thyroid-Stimulating Hormone-Secreting Pituitary Microadenoma in an Adolescent Boy: Case Report and Review of the Literature

Le Hoang Bao,[1] Nguyen Minh Duc,[2,3,4] Phan Cong Chien,[5] Thieu-Thi Tra My,[2] Tran Viet Thang,[1] and Tran Quang Nam[1]

[1]*Department of Endocrinology, University Medical Center, Ho Chi Minh City, Vietnam*
[2]*Department of Radiology, Hanoi Medical University, Ha Noi, Vietnam*
[3]*Department of Radiology, Pham Ngoc Thach University of Medicine, Ho Chi Minh City, Vietnam*
[4]*Department of Radiology, Children's Hospital 2, Ho Chi Minh City, Vietnam*
[5]*Department of Radiology, University Medical Center, Ho Chi Minh City, Vietnam*

Correspondence should be addressed to Nguyen Minh Duc; bsnguyenminhduc@pnt.edu.vn

Academic Editor: J. Paul Frindik

Thyroid-stimulating hormone- (TSH-) secreting pituitary adenoma (TSH-oma) is a rare cause of secondary hyperthyroidism and can be misdiagnosed as primary hyperthyroidism. We report a case of a 15-year-old male patient who was one of two monozygotic twins and exhibited hyperthyroidism syndrome. The laboratory results showed secondary hyperthyroidism, with increased levels of free T3 (FT3) and free T4 (FT4) and no TSH inhibition. Magnetic resonance imaging (MRI) and histopathological examination of the pituitary gland confirmed pituitary microadenoma. The patient was treated with methimazole, propranolol, and somatostatin analogs to restore euthyroidism before undergoing an endoscopic transsphenoidal resection of the pituitary tumor. After surgery, the hyperthyroidism symptoms improved, thyroid hormones normalized, and MRI of the pituitary gland showed the complete removal of the tumor with no recurrence after 2 years of follow-up.

1. Introduction

Thyroid-stimulating hormone- (TSH-) secreting pituitary adenoma (TSH-oma) is a rare cause of hyperthyroidism [1], accounting for 0.5% to 3% of all functioning pituitary tumors and fewer than 1% of all hyperthyroidism cases [2]. The prevalence of TSH-oma in the general population is estimated to be 1-2 cases per million population [3]. TSH-omas are characterized by autonomous TSH secretion that is unresponsive to the negative feedback exerted by thyroid hormones [3]. This continuous TSH overstimulation leads to T4 and T3 hypersecretion, which is classified as either central hyperthyroidism or secondary hyperthyroidism [4]. Although Graves' disease and other common causes of hyperthyroidism typically occur more frequently in women than in men, TSH-omas occur with equal frequency in men and women, and the mean age at presentation ranges from 41 to 45 years [5, 6].

In the past, TSH-omas were diagnosed when they reached the invasive macroadenoma stage. Currently, unsuppressed TSH secretion in hyperthyroid patients is more readily detected by ultrasensitive immunometric assays for TSH and the measurement of circulating free thyroid hormones (FT4 and FT3) [3]. The current screening strategies that measure FT4 only when abnormal TSH levels are detected fail to recognize both central hypothyroidism and hyperthyroidism, leading to the misdiagnosis of TSH-oma [3]. In Vietnam, TSH-oma is a rare cause of hyperthyroidism and receives less attention than primary hyperthyroidism, and case reports remain limited.

2. Case Presentation

A 15-year-old male patient presented to the clinic reporting exertion palpitations and feeling hot, with no other complaints. The patient had no growth chart until he came to our hospital. The patient did not gain weight as well as his monozygotic twin brother (Figure 1).

A physical examination revealed the following: pulse, 120 beats per minute; blood pressure, 140/80 mmHg; weight, 50 kg; height, 173 cm; body mass index (BMI) 16.7 kg/m^2; and BMI percentile according to age, 6.1. No abnormalities in the heart, lung, abdomen, or nerve were detected. However, he presented signs of hand tremor at rest, and an enlarged thyroid gland was detected with a firm density. No eye abnormalities due to hyperthyroidism and no signs of acromegaly, gynecomastia, or galactorrhea were detected. He had normal secondary sexual characteristics, with his genitalia and pubic hair (Tanner stage 3). The patient had no history of prior thyroid disease. The monozygotic twin brother presented no clinical symptoms of hyperthyroidism, with a normal thyroid function test.

2.1. Investigation. The test results revealed secondary hyperthyroidism, with elevated FT3 levels at 23.08 pmol/L, FT4 levels of 86.32 pmol/L, and TSH levels of 8.25 mUI/L. Investigations of other hormones, including cortisol, adrenocorticotropic hormone (ACTH), testosterone, luteinizing hormone (LH), insulin-like growth factor-1 (IGF-1), and prolactin, showed normal results (Table 1).

Thyroid ultrasound revealed that the thyroid gland was heterogeneous, without increased vascularity. Magnetic resonance imaging (MRI) of the pituitary showed a pituitary lesion with mild hyperintensity on the T2-weighted image (Figure 2(a)), which was less enhancing than the surrounding pituitary parenchyma (Figure 2(b)) and measured 5 × 6 × 7 mm in size. This lesion was suspected to be a pituitary microadenoma.

2.2. Treatment. The patient could not afford the cost of somatostatin analog; therefore, thyroid hormone levels were normalized by methimazole (20 mg per day) and propranolol (10 mg three times per day) before performing an endoscopic transsphenoidal resection of the pituitary tumor. When the patient was admitted to the hospital for surgery, he received a short-term treatment with sandostatin (0.1 mg three times a day), propylthiouracil (PTU), and propranolol. Because the patient was treated with oral methimazole 20 mg per day for 5 months and still had high serum FT4 before surgery, we switched to PTU to prevent thyroid storm during surgery. Postoperative pathology results revealed an adenoma of the pituitary gland (Figure 3).

After surgery, the doses of PTU and propranolol were gradually reduced. Two weeks following the operation, the patient was stabilized, PTU and propranolol were discontinued, and he was discharged from the hospital. Serum TSH and FT4 levels were evaluated and showed a decreasing tendency after treatment (Figure 4).

2.3. Outcome and Follow-Up. After discharge, the patient presented no clinical symptoms of hyperthyroidism. His weight was 50 kg before surgery and, 2 years later, it was 60 kg (gain 10 kg in 2 years); his height was 173 cm before surgery and later, his height was 175 cm. Hormonal testing after discharge was performed after 2 months, 6 months, and 18 months, and serum TSH, FT4, ACTH, and cortisol levels were detected in the normal range. MRI of the pituitary gland after 1 (Figure 2(c)) and 2 years (Figure 2(d)) showed the complete removal of the tumor, with no recurrence.

3. Discussion

We reported a case of a TSH-secreting pituitary adenoma that occurred in one of two monozygotic twins, who presented with exertion palpitations, feeling hot, trembling, lack of weight gain, tachycardia, and a diffuse, enlarged thyroid. With normal prolactin, IGF-1, cortisol, ACTH, testosterone, and LH levels, our patient was diagnosed with solitary TSH-oma, with no associated pituitary insufficiency. In 70% of cases, TSH-omas secrete TSH alone, and the remaining 30% are mixed adenomas that may cosecrete TSH and other anterior pituitary hormones (growth hormone, PRL, and LH/FSH; Table 2). The presence of these mixed adenomas can be explained by the expression of common transcription factors, such as Prop-1 and Pit-1, by thyrotrope, somatotrope, and lactotrophic cells [7].

Most patients have the typical symptoms and signs of hyperthyroidism (e.g., palpitations, tremors, and heat intolerance), but a few patients have mild or even no hyperthyroid symptoms [8]. In addition, patients may have symptoms related to the expanding tumor mass, such as the compression of the normal pituitary gland or the optic chiasm, or the secretion of growth hormone or prolactin [9]. The characteristic signs of Graves' ophthalmopathy (proptosis and periorbital edema) are absent without the coexistence of Graves' disease [10, 11].

The size of our patient's pituitary tumor on MRI was quite small, only 5 × 6 × 7 mm. In the past, MRI of the pituitary gland was more likely to detect a macroadenoma than a microadenoma [8], with an average tumor diameter of 3.1 cm [12]. In the last decade, microadenomas (diameter ≤1 cm) have been increasingly recorded (up to 30%–35%) due to the introduction of more sensitive and specific assays for the evaluation of thyroid function and increased awareness among endocrinologists and general practitioners [13].

Pediatric functioning pituitary adenoma is very rarely encountered in clinical practice; therefore, few pediatric cases of TSH-oma have been published in the literature (Table 3).

The diagnosis of TSH-secreting pituitary adenoma is critical to the success of treatment. According to Beck-

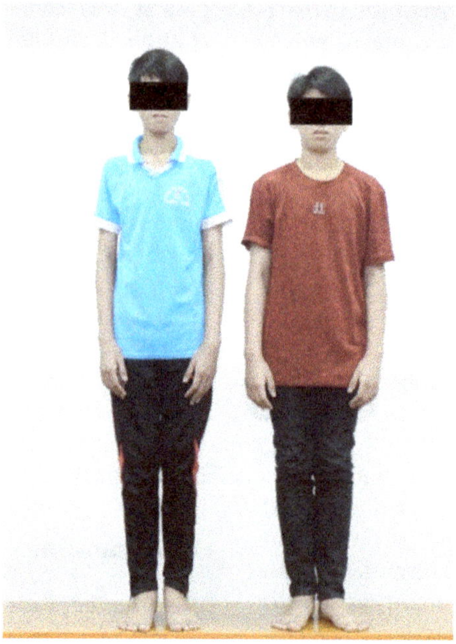

FIGURE 1: The patient (left) did not gain weight as well as his monozygotic twin brother (right).

TABLE 1: Hormonal results.

Investigations	Level	Reference range
FT4 (pmol/L)	**86.32**	12–22
FT3 (pmol/L)	**23.08**	3.1–6.8
TSH (mUI/L)	**8.25**	0.27–4.2
Cortisol (nmol/L)	261.3	118.6–618
ACTH (pmol/L)	9.2	1.6–13.9
Testosterone (nmol/L)	12.94	12–29
LH (mUI/mL)	2.55	1.24–8.62
IGF-1 (ng/mL)	291	100–1000
Prolactin (ng/mL)	16.64	4.04–15.2

FT4: free T4; FT3: free T3; TSH: thyroid-stimulating hormone; ACTH: adrenocorticotropic hormone; LH: luteinizing hormone; IGF-1: insulin-like growth factor-1. Bold levels are out of the normal range.

Peccoz, approximately one-third of patients with TSH-oma underwent an inappropriate thyroidectomy or received radioiodine treatment due to an incorrect diagnosis of primary hyperthyroidism (i.e., Graves' disease or toxic multinodular goiter) [3].

The most appropriate definitive therapy for patients with TSH-omas is initial medical therapy to restore euthyroidism prior to a transsphenoidal resection of the tumor [2]. The preferred medical therapy is somatostatin analogs, which can reduce the size of the tumor and normalize serum thyroid hormone levels prior to surgery [3]. In a review of 43 TSH-secreting pituitary adenoma cases, 26 patients received somatostatin analogs as initial therapy, a reduction in TSH levels of greater than 50% occurred in 88% of cases, and the normalization of free T4 was reported in 85% of patients [8]. Somatostatin analogs are very expensive, and side effects include nausea, abdominal discomfort, bloating, diarrhea, glucose intolerance, and cholelithiasis. If somatostatin analogs are not well tolerated, dopamine agonists (such as bromocriptine and cabergoline) may be effective in select cases, particularly in patients whose tumors also secrete prolactin [8].

Antithyroid drugs (such as methimazole or PTU) can be combined with somatostatin analogs and propranolol to restore euthyroidism before surgery, according to the recommendations of the European Thyroid Association [2]. However, because our patient could not afford to pay for a somatostatin analog, we choose to use antithyroid drugs combined with propranolol to restore euthyroidism before the endoscopic transsphenoidal resection of the pituitary tumor [20].

The transsphenoidal resection of the pituitary adenoma is the definitive therapy of choice for patients with TSH-secreting adenomas. Adenoma resection cures the majority of patients with microadenomas and approximately 50%–60% of patients with macroadenoma [2, 8, 21]. Patients who do not recover

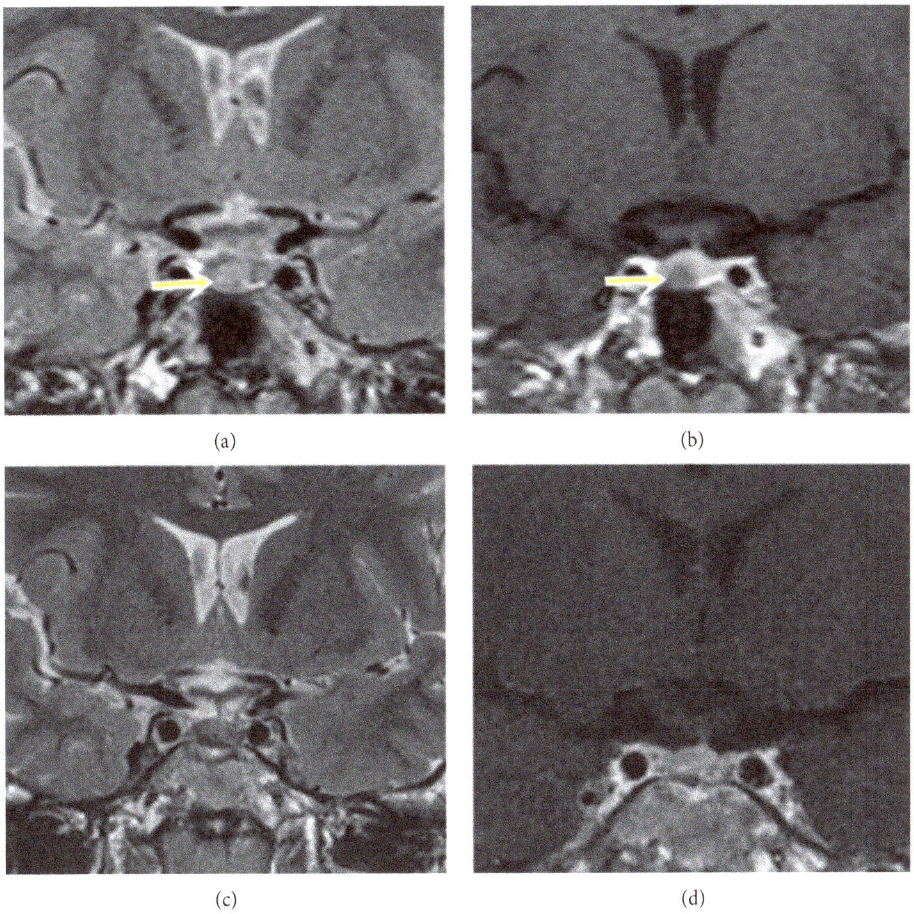

FIGURE 2: Preoperative (a, b) and postoperative (c, d) pituitary MRI results. Coronal T2-weighted image (a) and T1-weighted image with contrast enhancement (b) showed a pituitary lesion that was hyperintense on T2-weighted image and hypoenhancing compared with the surrounding pituitary parenchyma on T1-weighted image (arrows). The postoperative pituitary MRI showed no evidence of recurrence (c, d).

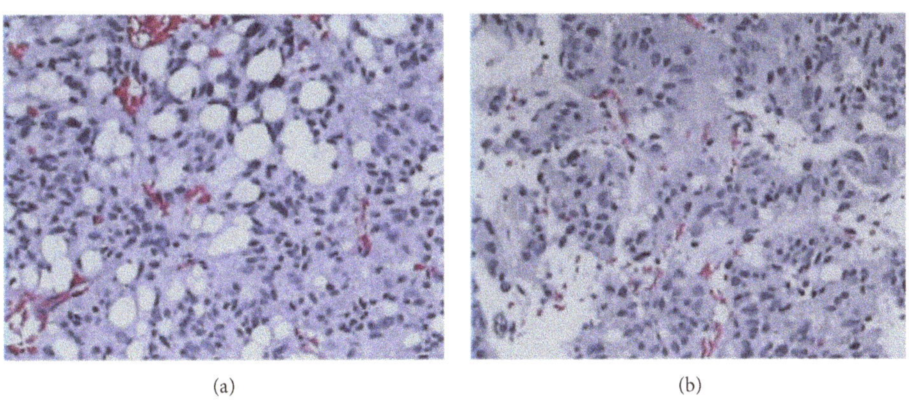

FIGURE 3: Hematoxylin and eosin staining of the patient's pituitary adenoma (a, b, × 200). Tumor tissue was composed of cytoplasmic-rich glandular cells arranged in clusters and featuring rounded nuclei. Cells arranged around the blood vessels and formed papillary structures with little mitosis.

following surgery can continue treatment with either radiotherapy or long-term somatostatin analogs [8].

The recommendations established by the European Thyroid Association in 2013 [2] confirmed the inability to clearly define cure criteria for TSH-oma patients after surgery or radiation therapy. The recommendations also outlined additional factors that could be considered when determining whether a cure has been achieved, including clinical improvements in hyperthyroidism and neurological symptoms and the absence of hormone and imaging

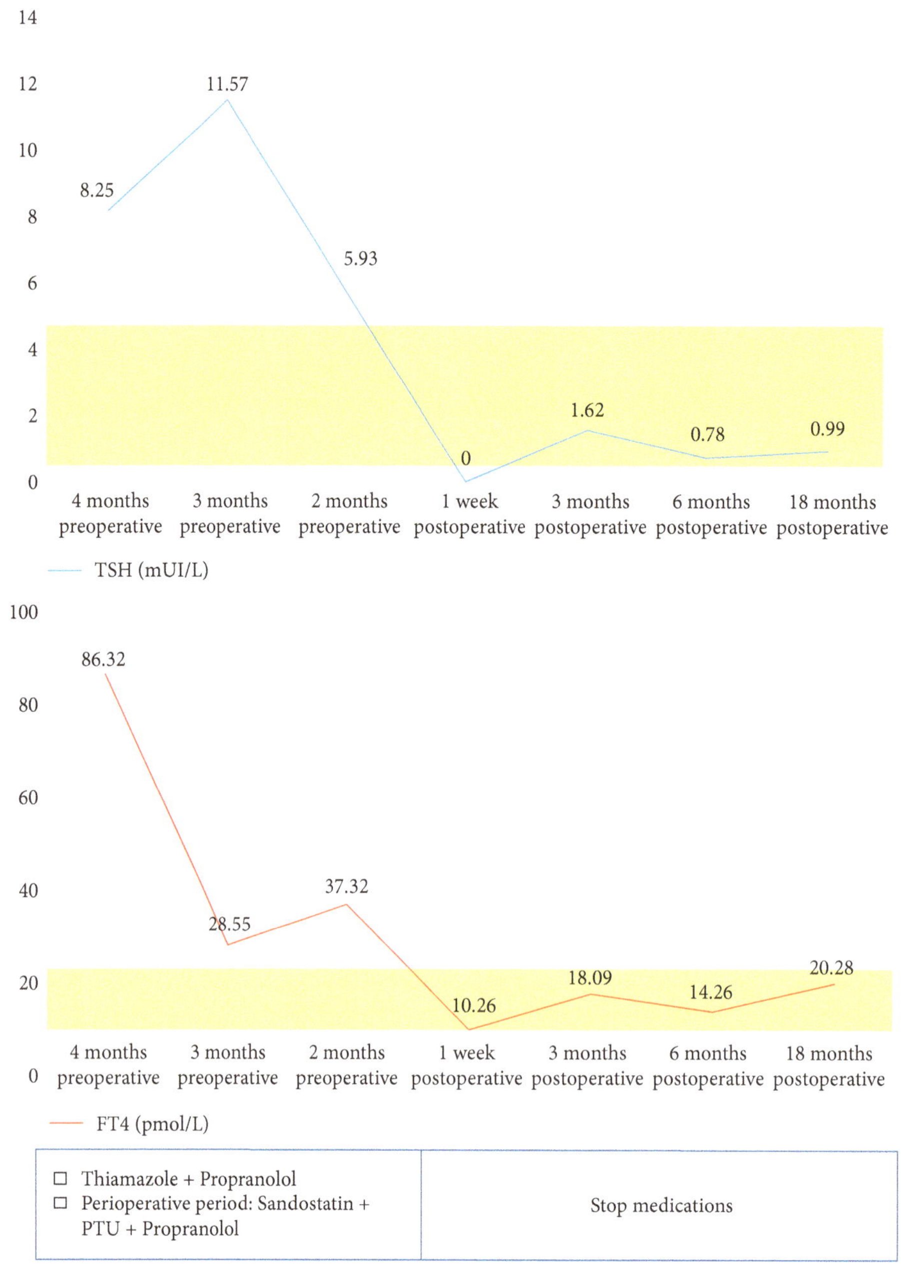

Figure 4: TSH and FT4 assay results showed decreasing trends after treatment.

Table 2: Different types of TSH-secreting pituitary adenomas [3].

	No.	% of total
TSH-omas	461	100
Solitary TSH-oma	324	70.3
Mixed TSH-oma	137	29.7
TSH/GH-omas	84	18.3
TSH/prolactin-omas	45	9.7
TSH/gonadotropin-omas	8	1.7

TSH: thyroid secreting hormone; GH: growth hormone.

abnormalities. Thus, our patient meets the posttreatment cure criteria, including no longer presenting symptoms of hyperthyroidism, the normalization of thyroid hormones, and the absence of a residual tumor on MRI.

Although no published protocols exist for TSH-omas, patients should be assessed clinically and biochemically 2 to 3 times during the first postoperative year and once per year thereafter. The evaluation should include the levels of TSH,

TABLE 3: Summary of the 7 cases reported in the literature of pediatric TSH-secreting pituitary adenomas and the present case.

Presentation	Tumor size	Function	Complications	Remission through surgery	Reference
15-year-old boy with hyperthyroidism	30 × 30 × 30 mm	TSH/GH/FSH/LH-omas	Inferior and superior extension	No	[14]
11-year-old girl after adenomectomy	48 × 62 × 58 mm	TSH/FSH-omas	Suprasellar, right temporal lobe extension	No	[15]
13-year-old boy with hyperthyroidism	20 × 15 mm	Solitary TSH-oma	Suprasellar extension Intratumor hemorrhage Diabetes insipidus Hypopituitarism Postoperative bacterial meningitis	No	[16]
16-year-old boy with goiter and hypertension	17 × 15 mm	TSH/FSH-omas	Suprasellar extension	No	[17]
13-year-old girl asymptomatic	28 × 25 × 29 mm	Solitary TSH-oma	Intrasellar and suprasellar extension	Successful treatment with somatostatin analogs	[18]
8-year-old boy with hyperthyroidism	Macroadenoma	Solitary TSH-oma	Suprasellar and sphenoidal extension	Yes	[19]
13-year-old boy with hyperthyroidism	40 × 45 mm	TSH/GH-omas	Compressing the surrounding structures Secondary adrenal insufficiency	No	[7]
15-year-old boy with hyperthyroidism	5 × 6 × 7 mm	Solitary TSH-oma	No	Yes	Present case

FT3, FT4, and other pituitary hormones, as necessary. An MRI of the pituitary gland should be repeated every 2-3 years and should be performed if an increase in TSH and thyroid hormones is detected or clinical symptoms appear that suggest the potential for relapse [2].

Our patient was followed for 2 years after surgery and showed good results, with a normal thyroid function test and no evidence of recurrent tumor on pituitary gland MRI. In a series of 43 cases, which were followed for a mean of 8 years, two patients died (ages 75 and 86 years); 19 patients were cured after pituitary surgery alone; 17 patients displayed symptom of residual disease after surgery, which was controlled with somatostatin analogs, pituitary radiation, or both; and seven were controlled by somatostatin analogs alone [8].

4. Conclusion

TSH-oma is an uncommon cause of secondary hyperthyroidism, which can be easily misdiagnosed as primary hyperthyroidism. Other pituitary hormones should be evaluated to determine the presence of cosecretory tumors or pituitary insufficiency due to tumor compression. The principal treatment is initial medical therapy to normalize thyroid hormone levels prior to an endoscopic transsphenoidal resection of the pituitary tumor. This patient was cured due to an accurate preoperative diagnosis and multimodal therapy.

Consent

Appropriate informed consent for patient information to be published in this article was obtained.

Disclosure

Le HB and Nguyen MD are considered as co-first authors.

Authors' Contributions

Le HB and Nguyen MD contributed equally to this article.

References

[1] L. Önnestam, K. Berinder, P. Burman et al., "National incidence and prevalence of TSH-secreting pituitary adenomas in Sweden," *The Journal of Clinical Endocrinology & Metabolism*, vol. 98, no. 2, pp. 626–635, 2013.

[2] P. Beck-Peccoz, A. Lania, A. Beckers, K. Chatterjee, and J.-L. Wemeau, "2013 European thyroid association guidelines for the diagnosis and treatment of thyrotropin-secreting pituitary tumors," *European Thyroid Journal*, vol. 2, no. 2, pp. 76–82, 2013.

[3] P. Beck-Peccoz, C. Giavoli, and A. Lania, "A 2019 update on TSH-secreting pituitary adenomas," *Journal of Endocrinological Investigation*, vol. 42, no. 12, pp. 1401–1406, 2019.

[4] P. Beck-Peccoz, A. Lania, and L. Persani, "Chapter 24. TSH-producing adenomas," *Endocrinology*pp. 266--274, W.B. Saunders Ltd, Philadelphia, PA, USA, 7th edition, 2015.

[5] P. Beck-Peccoz, F. Brucker-Davis, L. Persani, R. C. Smallridge, and B. D. Weintraub, "Thyrotropin-secreting pituitary tumors ∗," *Endocrine Reviews*, vol. 17, no. 6, pp. 610–638, 1996.

[6] G. Cossu, R. T. Daniel, K. Pierzchala et al., "Thyrotropin-secreting pituitary adenomas: a systematic review and meta-analysis of postoperative outcomes and management," *Pituitary*, vol. 22, no. 1, pp. 79–88, 2019.

[7] B. D. Pereira, L. Raimundo, O. Mete, A. Oliveira, J. Portugal, and S. L. Asa, "Monomorphous plurihormonal pituitary adenoma of pit-1 lineage in a giant adolescent with central hyperthyroidism," *Endocrine Pathology*, vol. 27, no. 1, pp. 25–33, 2016.

[8] H. Socin, P. Chanson, B. Delemer et al., "The changing spectrum of TSH-secreting pituitary adenomas: diagnosis and management in 43 patients," *European Journal of Endocrinology*, vol. 148, no. 4, pp. 433–442, 2003.

[9] P. Beck-Peccoz, L. Persani, D. Mannavola, and I. Campi, "TSH-secreting adenomas," *Best Practice & Research Clinical Endocrinology & Metabolism*, vol. 23, no. 5, pp. 597–606, 2009.

[10] Y. Ogawa and T. Tominaga, "Thyroid-stimulating hormone-secreting pituitary adenoma presenting with recurrent hyperthyroidism in post-treated Graves' disease: a case report," *Journal of Medical Case Reports*, vol. 21, pp. 7–27, 2013.

[11] M. Kamoun, M. D'Herbomez, C. Lemaire et al., "Coexistence of thyroid-stimulating hormone-secreting pituitary adenoma and Graves' hyperthyroidism," *European Thyroid Journal*, vol. 3, no. 1, pp. 60–64, 2014.

[12] M. J. Clarke, D. Erickson, M. R. Castro, and J. L. D. Atkinson, "Thyroid-stimulating hormone pituitary adenomas," *Journal of Neurosurgery*, vol. 109, no. 1, pp. 17–22, 2008.

[13] E. Malchiodi, E. Profka, E. Ferrante et al., "Thyrotropin-secreting pituitary adenomas: outcome of pituitary surgery and irradiation," *The Journal of Clinical Endocrinology & Metabolism*, vol. 99, no. 6, pp. 2069–2076, 2014.

[14] J. M. Stanley and S. S. Najjar, "Hyperthyroidism secondary to a TSH-secreting pituitary adenoma in a 15-year-old male," *Clinical Pediatrics*, vol. 30, no. 2, pp. 109–111, 1991.

[15] A. Avramides, A. Karapiperis, E. Triantafyllidou, S. Vayas, A. Moshidou, and A. Vyzantiadis, "TSH-secreting pituitary macroadenoma in an 11-year-old girl," *Acta Paediatrica*, vol. 81, no. 12, pp. 1058–1060, 1992.

[16] M. Phillip, E. Hershkovitz, P. Kornmehl, A. Cohen, and E. Leiberman, "Thyrotropin secreting pituitary adenoma associated with hypopituitarism and diabetes insipidus in an adolescent boy," *Journal of Pediatric Endocrinology and Metabolism*, vol. 8, no. 1, pp. 47–50, 1995.

[17] M. Kessler, R. David, M. Pawelczak, A. Hanono, and B. Shah, "Thyrotropin-secreting pituitary adenoma in an adolescent boy: challenges in management," *Pediatrics*, vol. 126, no. 2, pp. e474–e478, 2010.

[18] S. Rabbiosi, E. Peroni, G. M. Tronconi, G. Chiumello, M. Losa, and G. Weber, "Asymptomatic thyrotropin-secreting pituitary macroadenoma in a 13-year-old girl: successful first-line treatment with somatostatin analogs," *Thyroid*, vol. 22, no. 10, pp. 1076–1079, 2012.

[19] Y. Nakayama, S. Jinguji, S.-I. Kumakura et al., "Thyroid-stimulating hormone (thyrotropin)-secretion pituitary adenoma in an 8-year-old boy: case report," *Pituitary*, vol. 15, no. 1, pp. 110–115, 2012.

[20] M. W. Dyer, A. Gnagey, B. T. Jones et al., "Perianesthetic management of patients with thyroid-stimulating hormone-secreting pituitary adenomas," *Journal of Neurosurgical Anesthesiology*, vol. 29, no. 3, pp. 341–346, 2017.

[21] F. Brucker-Davis, E. H. Oldfield, M. C. Skarulis, J. L. Doppman, and B. D. Weintraub, "Thyrotropin-secreting pituitary tumors: diagnostic criteria, thyroid hormone sensitivity, and treatment outcome in 25 patients followed at the National Institutes of Health," *The Journal of Clinical Endocrinology & Metabolism*, vol. 84, no. 2, pp. 476–486, 1999.

Gonadoblastoma with Dysgerminoma Presenting as Virilizing Disorder in a Young Child with 46, XX Karyotype: A Case Report and Review of the Literature

Prathamesh Chandrapattan,[1] Amitabh Jena,[1] Rashmi Patnayak,[2] Swayamsidha Mangaraj,[3] Sujata Naik,[2] and Saroj Panda[4]

[1]*Department of Surgical Oncology, IMS & SUM Medical College and Hospital, Bhubaneswar, Odisha, India*
[2]*Department of Pathology, IMS and SUM Medical College and Hospital, Bhubaneswar, Odisha, India*
[3]*Department of Endocrinology, IMS & SUM Medical College and Hospital, Bhubaneswar, Odisha, India*
[4]*Department of Medical Oncology, IMS & SUM Medical College and Hospital, Bhubaneswar, Odisha, India*

Correspondence should be addressed to Swayamsidha Mangaraj; drsmangaraj@gmail.com

Academic Editor: Osamu Isozaki

Gonadoblastoma is a neoplasm containing an intimate mixture of germ cells and elements resembling immature granulosa or Sertoli cells. It has been considered as in situ germ cell malignancy that can be associated with malignant components. The tumor has been reported to almost exclusively develop in various types of gonadal gene mutation syndromes, such as in pure or mixed gonadal dysgenesis and among females carrying Y chromosome material. However, it can be rarely present in normal women with 46, XX karyotype. Ovarian gonadoblastoma presenting with signs of contrasexual puberty in a young female child with normal 46, XX karyotype is an extremely rare clinical entity and seldom reported in the literature. We report a case of a nine-year-old girl child who presented with signs of virilization and contrasexual pubertal development. A detailed clinical evaluation along with supportive biochemical and radiological findings pointed to the presence of a virilizing ovarian tumor. The patient underwent right salpingo-oophorectomy, pelvic node dissection, and infracolic omentectomy. The excised tumor was confirmed to be gonadoblastoma which was overgrown by dysgerminoma on histopathological evaluation. The presence of associated malignant tumors (like dysgerminoma) should always be ruled out in cases of gonadoblastoma.

1. Introduction

Various inherited and acquired causes can lead to hyper-androgenism and its resultant manifestations in a female child. In young children, androgen-producing ovarian and adrenal tumors can lead to features of virilization in a relatively short span of time. Gonadoblastoma is a relatively rare ovarian tumor comprised of sex cord and primitive germ cell components. Though being benign themselves, they are frequently associated with invasive germ cell malignant tumors [1]. These tumors are frequently seen among individuals with 46, XY gonadal dysgenesis. However, they have been rarely described in individuals with normal 46, XX karyotype [1–6]. This presentation is even rarer in children less than ten years, and only one such case has been previously reported [5]. We present an interesting case of a young girl who presented with features of contrasexual pubertal development which was subsequently attributed to right ovarian gonadoblastoma with dysgerminoma. We describe her clinical presentation and management outcome along with a review of the literature describing cases of gonadoblastoma arising in individuals with normal 46, XX karyotype.

2. Case Report

A nine-year-old girl presented for evaluation of progressively increased hair growth over androgen-dependent areas, deepening of voice, and abdominal distension. The patient had first episode of bleeding per vaginum at the age of 7 years and 6 months. Following it, she had an irregular menstrual bleeding pattern for the next five months. Subsequently, the bleeding episodes had ceased on its own without any drug intake, and she was amenorrhoeic for the last one year. However, no medical consultation or evaluation was done at that point of time for this precocious pubertal event. The parents had also noticed a significant height gain in comparison with her peers in the preceding one and half years. There was no history of any chronic drug intake or prior surgery. There was no history of a similar disorder in any family member. She was born out of a nonconsanguineous marriage and delivered at term by normal vaginal delivery. The perinatal period was uneventful. On clinical examination, the girl was thin built with muscular appearance. Her anthropometric parameters were as follows: height of 145 cm (>97th percentile) and weight of 41 kg (90th–97th percentile). She had evidence of virilization characterized by a significant degree of hirsutism (Ferriman–Gallaway score of 16/36), clitoromegaly (clitoral length 16 mm and clitoral index 56 mm^2), and lack of breast development. No Turner syndrome stigmata were noted. Her vitals were within a normal range. On abdominal palpation, a mobile abdominal mass (around 10 cm × 10 cm) was noted in the right lower abdomen with the presence of shifting dullness and bulging flanks. Ultrasonography of the abdomen and pelvis revealed a large lobulated adnexal mass (around 11 cm × 6 cm × 9 cm) arising from the right ovary along with ascites. The left ovary was morphologically normal. A pubertal uterus (dimension of around 7.5 cm × 5 cm × 3.6 cm) with a normal endometrial echogenicity of 3 mm was also noted. Her bone age was advanced by two years in contrast to her chronological age. Contrast enhanced computed tomography revealed a large lobulated solid mass of size 11.9 cm × 6.5 cm × 9.4 cm arising from the right ovary, morphologically normal looking left ovary, and presence of gross ascites (Figure 1). The right ovarian mass was characterized by heterogeneous post-contrast enhancement and punctuate internal calcification along with multiple intratumor tortuous vascular channels (Figure 1). Serum lactate dehydrogenase (LDH) (361 U/L, normal: 140-280 U/L), serum beta human chorionic gonadotropin (hCG) (447.2 m·IU/ml, normal: <5.0 m·IU/ml), and CA-125 (56.93 U/ml, normal: <35 U/ml)) levels were elevated. Serum alpha-fetoprotein (AFP) level (4.2 ng/ml, normal: <5.8 ng/ml) was normal. Hormonal evaluation revealed significantly elevated levels of serum testosterone (12.51 ng/ml, normal: 0.06–0.52 ng/ml), low luteinizing hormone level (0.26 m·IU/ml, normal: >0.6 m·IU/ml for pubertal response), and slightly elevated estradiol level (30 pg/ml, normal: <20 pg/ml). Serum dehydroepiandrostenedione sulphate (DHEAS) levels were within a normal range. Karyotype analysis from peripheral blood sample revealed a normal female 46, XX pattern. Fluorescence in situ hybridization (FISH) from peripheral blood did not reveal any Y chromosome material. Based on the above clinical, biochemical, and supportive radiological findings, a diagnosis of virilizing ovarian tumor leading to contrasexual puberty was considered. Intraoperative findings revealed a 15 cm × 10 cm firm and lobulated mass arising from the right ovary whereas the left ovary appeared morphologically normal. The patient underwent right salpingo-oophorectomy, pelvic lymph node dissection, and infracolic omentectomy along with left ovarian biopsy (Figure 2). Around three liters of straw-coloured ascitic fluid was drained. The patient had an uneventful recovery in the postoperative period. Ascitic fluid cytology was negative for malignant cells. Histopathologic examination of excised tumor revealed greyish yellow tumor with focal areas of myxoid changes and haemorrhage with an intact capsule. The tumor cells were present in sheets and nests separated by fibrous septa with lymphoid infiltration. Occasional primordial follicles were also seen in between. The tumoral cells were large with prominent nucleoli and mitotic activity. At places, bizarre tumor cells with areas of calcification (suggestive of burned out gonadoblastoma) were seen. Regional lymph node assessment revealed reactive hyperplasia. Based on the above characteristic findings, a diagnosis of dysgerminoma associated with burned out gonadoblastoma was made (Figure 3). The left ovary biopsy sample revealed normal ovarian histology. Pathological staging was pT1aN0Mx. However, a cytogenetic study for assessing Y chromosome material from affected ovarian tumor tissue was not performed. The patient was started on chemotherapy comprising of bleomycin, etoposide, and cisplatin combination for four cycles. The virilization features decreased over the course of next three months with significant improvement in hirsutism, voice change, and other physical characteristics. The patient is on regular follow-up for the past one year with no evidence of tumor recurrence till now and menstrual cycles have not resumed. The hormonal evaluation revealed normalization of testosterone levels (0.2 ng/ml) and normal early pubertal gonadotropin levels.

3. Discussion

The diagnosis of virilization in a young girl can be clinically challenging at times. The causes include various inherited and acquired conditions such as disorders of sex development (DSD), virilizing ovarian tumors, adrenal tumors, and exogenous androgen exposure. DSD such as various forms of congenital adrenal hyperplasia (CAH), ovotesticular DSD, and aromatase deficiency can present with features of hyperandrogenism in females. They can be distinguished from other tumoral causes of virilization by the presence of genital ambiguity since birth, presence of associated findings (maternal virilization during pregnancy in case of aromatase deficiency, history of salt wasting in certain forms of CAH), usually slower rate of androgenization in contrast to virilizing tumors and characteristic hormonal profile. Similarly, ovarian and adrenal tumors are usually characterized by rapid progression and more severe virilization in affected individuals. The presence of cushingoid features in addition to signs of virilization may point towards the presence of underlying adrenocortical carcinoma. Elevated androgen levels (serum testosterone level of more than 2 ng/ml and serum dehydroepiandrostenedione sulphate level of more than 8 μg/mL) are characteristic of virilizing ovarian and

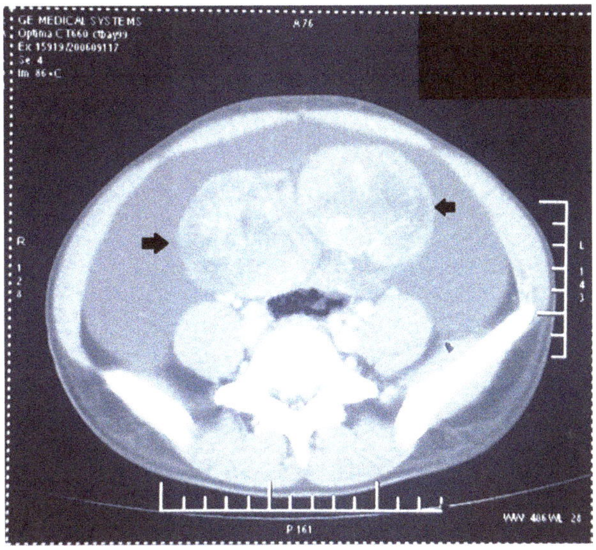

FIGURE 1: A large lobulated solid heterogeneously enhancing mass (solid black arrows) arising from the right ovary of size 11.9 cm × 6.5 cm × 9.4 cm with punctuate internal calcification and ascites.

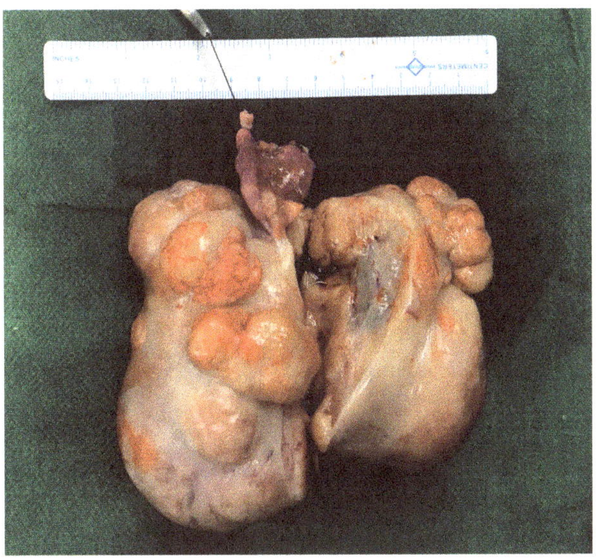

FIGURE 2: Resected specimen showing cut opened the right ovary with an attached fallopian tube. The right ovary measures around 15 cm × 10 cm with a bosselated outer surface. The ovary is entirely replaced by a solid mass which greyish-yellow with focal areas of myxoid changes and haemorrhage with an intact capsule. The fallopian tube appears normal.

adrenal tumors, and these tumors may be identified by necessary dedicated imaging studies. The common age of presentation of gonadoblastomas is in the second and third decade [7]. The common clinical manifestations of these ovarian tumors include hirsutism, virilization, menstrual abnormalities, and abdominal pain/distension [7]. The characteristic features of virilization seen in gonadoblastomas are due to excessive production of testosterone by

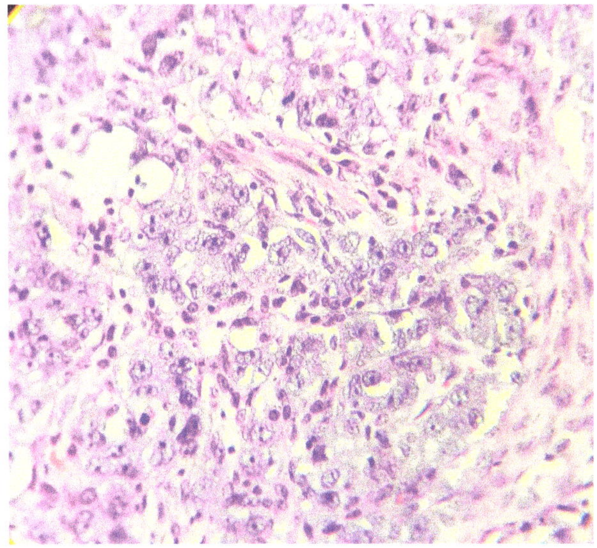

FIGURE 3: Histological findings showing nests of germ cells separated by fibrous septa infiltrated by lymphoid cells. Tumor cells are large, high N : C ratio with prominent nucleoli. (hematoxylin and eosin (H&E), 200x).

these tumors [1, 8]. On the other hand, ovarian dysgerminomas are usually hormonally inert. Rarely ovarian dysgerminoma can be associated with elevated estradiol levels due to the presence of syncytiotrophoblastic giant cells or due to malignant transformation [9]. Pure gonadoblastomas are usually small in size but may acquire large size due to invasive component overgrowth [8]. Around 40% or more cases of gonadoblastoma are bilateral [7, 10, 11]. The pathological hallmark of these tumors is the presence of sex cord and primitive germ cell components. The presence of calcification serves as an important diagnostic clue [2, 7, 8, 10].

It is customary to rule out the presence of invasive malignancy in every case of gonadoblastoma. This is due to the fact that malignant germ cell tumors are associated with 50–60% of gonadoblastomas. The most common malignancy is pure dysgerminoma, whereas other variants include immature teratoma, embryonal carcinoma, yolk sac tumor, and choriocarcinoma [3, 4, 7, 12]. Gonadoblastomas are found among 25–30% of patients with XY gonadal dysgenesis and among 15–20% of patients with 45, X/46, XY karyotype [2]. This finding underscores the importance of karyotype analysis. Normal 46, XX karyotype is observed in rare cases [1–6]. Hence, cytogenetic assessment of Y chromosome in blood/affected tissue is advocated. In our case, although we had conducted FISH analysis from peripheral blood, we could not do cytogenetic assessment of Y chromosome from affected tissue. Pure gonadoblastomas are benign in nature, and it has been reported that cases with dysgerminomas also have a favorable prognosis [3]. However, association of other tumor types such as the yolk sac tumor may have unfavorable prognosis [3, 13]. We have summarized relevant cases of patients having 46, XX karyotype and gonadoblastoma described in the literature in Table 1 [1, 3–6, 8, 10, 11, 14–17]. Our case is unique as

Table 1: Summary of similar cases published in the literature with gonadoblastoma and normal 46, XX karyotype.

Author	Year	Clinical presentation	Age in years	Precocity	Karyotyping	Laterality	Management	Additional findings in histopathology (in addition to gonadoblastoma)	Adjuvant therapy
Erhan et al. [14]	1992	Abdominal mass	26	No	46, XX	Right	TAH + BSO	Dysgerminoma	Combination chemotherapy
Obata et al. [15]	1995	Abdominal pain	10	No	46, XX	Bilateral	B/L oophorectomy	Left with dysgerminoma, right with yolk sac tumour	Combination chemotherapy
Zhao et al. [16]	2000	Abdominal mass	27	No	46, XX	Unilateral	USO + chemotherapy + later TAH + USO + LND + omentectomy	Choriocarcinoma, embryonal carcinoma, yolk sac tumor, immature teratoma, and dysgerminoma	Chemotherapy
Erdemoglu & Ozen [17]	2007	Abdominal mass	19	No	46, XX	Unilateral	Unilateral oophorectomy	Endodermal sinus tumor	—
Gorosito et al. [10]	2010	Pregnancy with ovarian mass	17	No	46, XX	Left	Left oophorectomy	Dysgerminoma	Chemotherapy
Yilmaz et al. [11]	2010	Abdominal distention with mass	20	No	46, XX	Bilateral	BSO	Dysgerminoma	Chemotherapy (bleomycin, etoposide, and cisplatin) and radiation
Esin et al. [3]	2011	Irregular vaginal bleeding Pelvic pain	15	No	46, XX	Left	Left oophorectomy with right ovary wedge biopsy	Dysgerminoma	—
Kanagal et al. [8]	2013	Abdominal distention and mass	14	No	46, XX	Left	USO + cytoreductive surgery + right ovarian wedge biopsy	Mixed germ cells and sex cord cell derivatives	Combination chemotherapy
Kulkarni et al. [4]	2016	Abdominal pain	20	No	46, XX	Left	USO + omental biopsy	Dysgerminoma	—
McCuaig et al. [6]	2017	Oligomenorrhea and menorrhagia	20	No	46, XX	Left	USO	Dysgerminoma with syncytiotrophoblastic differentiation	Observation
Roth et al. [5]	2019	Abdominal pain and mass	9	No	46, XX	Right	USO	Malignant mixed germ cell tumour	Cisplatin based combination chemotherapy
Rafeey et al. [1]	2020	Abdominal pain and mass	10	No	46, XX	Bilateral	USO with cytoreduction with right ovarian biopsy, para-aortic LN sampling with Partial Omentectomy	Dysgerminoma	Chemotherapy (Bleomycin, Etoposide and Cisplatin)

BSO: bilateral salpingo-oophorectomy, LND: lymph node dissection, USO: unilateral salpingo-oophorectomy, and TAH: total abdominal hysterectomy.

similar presentation is extremely rarer in children less than ten years and only one such case has been reported earlier [5]. Cases of dysgerminoma presenting with precocious puberty in children have also been described rarely in children [9, 18]. The presentation of 46, XY complete gonadal dysgenesis as pubertal virilizing disorder in adolescent due to underlying virilizing ovarian tumor (presence of concomitant gonadoblastoma and dysgerminoma) has been well described in the literature [19].

Surgery remains the main modality of treatment. The extent of surgery includes oophorectomy accompanied by salpingectomy, hysterectomy, omentectomy, and lymph node dissection depending on the disease status [3, 8, 11]. Germ line and tumoral Y chromosome analysis are helpful in deciding regarding contralateral oophorectomy in young patients keeping in mind fertility issues. The coexistence of invasive malignancy in gonadoblastoma requires adjuvant chemotherapy [2, 9, 11].

4. Conclusion

The presence of virilizing features in a young girl should be thoroughly evaluated. Gonadoblastoma is a rare virilizing ovarian tumor that usually arises in dysgenetic gonads. Although frequently associated with presence of Y chromosome, these tumors can rarely be seen in individuals with normal 46, XX karyotype. The presence of concomitant malignancy associated with gonadoblastoma should be always ruled out due to important therapeutic and prognostic implications.

Consent

Written informed consent was obtained from the patient for publication of this case report and any accompanying images.

Disclosure

All authors have no financial relationship related to this article to disclose.

References

[1] R. M. Abdur, M. Abdulwaasey, S. Samia Fatima, Z. Uddin, and M. U. Tariq, "Bilateral gonadoblastoma with dysgerminoma in a phenotypically normal female with 46XX karyotype: report of a rare case and literature review," *Cureus*, vol. 7, 2020.

[2] M. Jung, H. Jeong Ahn, J. Young Kim, and K. R. Kim, "Gonadoblastoma overgrown by dysgerminoma in women with 46, XX karyotype: a report of two cases," *Korean Journal of Pathology*, vol. 1, pp. 66–70, 2003.

[3] S. Esin, E. Baser, T. Kucukozkan, and H. A. Magden, "Ovarian gonadoblastoma with dysgerminoma in a 15-year-old girl with 46, XX karyotype: case report and review of the literature," *Archives of Gynecology and Obstetrics*, vol. 285, pp. 447–451, 2012.

[4] M. M. Kulkarni, S. G. Sinai Khandeparkar, A. Joshi, and P. V. Bhayekar, "Unilateral gonadoblastoma with dysgerminoma in normal fertile woman having a child: extremely rare occurrence with characteristic immunohistomorphology," *Indian Journal of Pathology and Microbiology*, vol. 59, p. 527, 2016.

[5] L. M. Roth, M. M. Davis, and B. Czernobilsky, ""Classic and "Dissecting" Gonadoblastoma in a Phenotypic Girl With a 46, XX Peripheral Karyotype and No Evidence of a Disorder of Sex Development," *International Journal of Gynecological Pathology*, vol. 38, pp. 581–587, 2019.

[6] J. M. McCuaig, A. Noor, B. Rosen et al., "Case report: use of tumor and germline Y chromosomal analysis to guide surgical management in a 46, XX female presenting with gonadoblastoma with dysgerminoma," *International Journal of Gynecological Pathology*, vol. 36, pp. 466–470, 2017.

[7] J. Prat, D. Cao, S. G. Carinelli, F. F. Nogales, R. Vang, and C. J. Zaloudek, "Germ cell-sex cord-stromal tumors," *WHO Classification of Tumours of Female Reproductive System*, pp. 67-68, International Agency For Research On Cancer Press, Lyon, France, 4th edition, 2014.

[8] D. V. Kanagal, K. Prasad, A. Rajesh et al., "Ovarian gonadoblastoma with dysgerminoma in a young girl with 46, XX karyotype: a case report," *Journal of Clinical and Diagnostic Research*, vol. 7, pp. 2021-2022, 2013.

[9] E.-S. Song, J.-P. Lee, J.-H. Han et al., "Dysgerminoma of the ovary with precocious puberty: a case report," *Gynecological Endocrinology*, vol. 23, pp. 34–37, 2007.

[10] M. Gorosito, B. Pancera, S. Sarancone, and A. L. Nocito, "Gonadoblastoma: an unusual ovarian tumor," *Annals of Diagnostic Pathology*, vol. 14, pp. 247–250, 2010.

[11] B. Yilmaz, T. Gungor, H. Bayramoglu, S. Soysal, and L. Mollamahmutoglu, "Bilateral ovarian gonadoblastoma with coexisting dysgerminoma in a girl with 46, XX karyotype," *Journal of Obstetrics and Gynaecology Research*, vol. 36, pp. 697–700, 2010.

[12] I. Gelincik, S. Ozen, and I. Bayram, "Left ovarian gonadoblastoma with yolk sac tumor in a young woman," *Indian Journal of Pathology and Microbiology*, vol. 53, p. 345, 2010.

[13] Y.-C. Changchien, I. Haltrich, T. Micsik et al., "Gonadoblastoma: case report of two young patients with isochromosome 12p found in the dysgerminoma overgrowth component in one case," *Pathology, Research & Practice*, vol. 208, pp. 628–632, 2012.

[14] Y. Erhan, A. S. Toprak, N. Ozdemir, and B. Tiras, "Gonadoblastoma and fertility," *Journal of Clinical Pathology*, vol. 45, pp. 828-829, 1992.

[15] N. H. Obata, N. Nakashima, M. Kawai, F. Kikkawa, S. Mamba, and Y. Tomoda, "Gonadoblastoma with dysgerminoma in one ovary and gonadoblastoma with dysgerminoma and yolk sac tumor in the contralateral ovary in a girl with 46XX karyotype," *Gynecologic Oncology*, vol. 58, pp. 124–128, 1995.

[16] S. Zhao, N. Kato, Y. Endoh, Z. Jin, Y. Ajioka, and T. Motoyama, "Ovarian gonadoblastoma with mixed germ cell tumor in a woman with 46, XX karyotype and successful pregnancies," *Pathology International*, vol. 50, pp. 332–335, 2000.

[17] E. Erdemoglu and S. Ozen, "Ovarian gonodoblastoma with yolk sac tumor in a young 46, XX female: case report," *European Journal of Gynaecological Oncology*, vol. 28, pp. 516–518, 2007.
[18] N. M. Kamal, U. Khan, S. Mirza, K. Mazoun, F. M. Mirza, and M. Jundi, "Ovarian dysgerminoma with normal serum tumour markers presenting in a child with precocious puberty," *Journal of Cancer Research and Therapeutics*, vol. 11, p. 661, 2015.
[19] S. Alam, H. Boro, A. Goyal, and R. Khadgawat, ""46, XY complete gonadal dysgenesis with pubertal virilisation due to dysgerminoma/gonadoblastoma," *BMJ Case Reports*, vol. 13, Article ID e235501, 2020.

26

The Highs and Lows of an Unknown Pheochromocytoma in an Elderly Patient

Christina N. DiMaria, Lorena I. Rasquin, and Wikien A. Hung Pinto

Department of Internal Medicine, Einstein Medical Center, Philadelphia, PA, 19141, USA

Correspondence should be addressed to Christina N. DiMaria; dimariac@einstein.edu

Academic Editor: Takeshi Usui

Pheochromocytomas are rare catecholamine producing neuroendocrine tumors. The incidence of these tumors is estimated to affect 0.8 per 100,000 person-years and is most common in the fourth to fifth decade of life with equal prevalence in men and women. We describe a case of an 84-year-old male who presented with cycling episodes of severe hypertension and hypotension after an elective cardiac catheterization. Workup of the labile blood pressure revealed a large suprarenal mass and free serum metanephrines (MN) 104 nmol/L (reference range 0.0-0.49 nmol/L) and normetanephrines (NMN) of 24 nmol/L (reference range 0.0-0.89 nmol/L), confirming the diagnosis of a pheochromocytoma. The patient's labile blood pressure was a challenge to manage medically and improved only after aggressive hydration and an alpha-adrenergic antagonist. Of note, this is the second eldest patient known to be published to date with a pheochromocytoma.

1. Introduction

Pheochromocytomas are rare catecholamine producing neuroendocrine tumors. The incidence of these tumors is estimated to affect 0.8 per 100,000 person-years and are most common in the fourth to fifth decade of life with equal prevalence in men and women [1, 2]. Most of these tumors (85%) arise from the adrenal medulla. Those arising from the extra-adrenal neural ganglia are called paragangliomas.

Due to a large production of catecholamines, such as epinephrine, norepinephrine, and dopamine, patients can present with the classic triad of symptoms of sweating, headaches, and tachycardia [3]. Other patients can present during a pheochromocytoma induced "spell," with sudden onset of paroxysmal hypertension that is self-limited [4]. However, it is important to note most patients do not present with the classic triad or during a pheochromocytoma spell [5, 6]. The diagnosis of pheochromocytoma is made by biochemical testing in urine and serum for metanephrine (MN) and normetanephrine (NMN) end products of catecholamine metabolism, followed by imaging studies such as a computerized tomography (CT) scan.

In this report, we describe a case of an 84-year-old male diagnosed with a pheochromocytoma and cycling episodes of hypertension and hypotension. Of note, this is the second eldest patient known to be published to date with a pheochromocytoma.

2. Case Presentation

We present the case of an 84-year-old male with past medical history of hypertension, benign prostatic hyperplasia, former alcohol and cocaine abuse, chronic kidney disease stage 3A, severe malnutrition, and frequent falls who presented from a nursing home for elective left heart catheterization. The patient had an NSTEMI two months earlier but had refused catheterization at the time with new left ventricular systolic dysfunction and an ejection fraction of 45%.

During the catheterization, the patient developed hypertensive emergency with flash pulmonary edema and the procedure had to be aborted. He was admitted to the Cardiac Critical Care Unit for hypertensive emergency and was started on antihypertensive drips. Urine drug screen was negative. He was weaned off the drips after 36 hours. After which he developed labile blood pressures, fluctuating in minutes, and ranging from 68/31 mmHg to 323/115 mmHg with his heart rate ranging from 90 bpm to 140 bpm. These blood pressure readings were measured in four extremities with a manual manometer and confirmed with an arterial line. During the rapid shifts in blood pressure the patient would develop blank staring episodes and nonresponsiveness that would last approximately 30 seconds to 1 minute. An immediate head CT showed no acute ischemic changes, hemorrhagic stroke, or cerebral edema. Electroencephalogram showed generalized slowing consistent with moderate metabolic encephalopathy. In addition, the patient developed acute kidney injury with maximum creatinine of 2.6 mg/dl from a baseline of 1.3 mg/dl.

Workup of the labile blood pressure, including an abdominal CT scan without contrast because of the patient's kidney injury revealed a large 9.4 x 8.7 x 8.1 cm round, slightly lobulated left suprarenal mass with mixed cystic and solid components and no calcifications with Hounsfield units ranging from 15 to 45. Free serum metanephrines (MN) were 104 nmol/L (reference range 0.0-0.49 nmol/L) and normetanephrines (NMN) were 24 nmol/L (reference range 0.0-0.89 nmol/L), with a ratio of MN to NMN of 4:1, which were drawn at the peak of a hypertensive cycle. Because of the labile blood pressures, the patient was on no antihypertensive medications, including alpha or beta blockers or calcium channel antagonists, at the time when then the serum and urine metanephrines were drawn. His UDS was negative for cocaine and the patient was not on tricyclic antidepressant or other drugs that can cause false positive elevations of plasma and urinary catecholamines or metanephrines [7]. The findings confirmed the diagnosis of pheochromocytoma.

The patient was started on prazosin and, however, developed worsening hypotension again, even while receiving aggressive fluid resuscitation. After the patient was euvolemic, the prazosin was able to be titrated up to goal with stabilization of his blood pressure. Due to his advanced age, severe malnutrition, no family support, worsening mental status, and comorbidities he was deemed not an appropriate surgical candidate. Patient was discharged under hospice care.

3. Discussion

In this case report we present the second eldest patient to date, based on literature review, to be diagnosed with a pheochromocytoma at age 84 years old. The eldest patient to date was an 87-year-old male from Buffet et al.'s study on germline mutations in a metastatic paragangliomas [8]. Previously, Chenguan et al. presented a case of a giant malignant pheochromocytoma in an 81-year-old male that measured 13.5x10.6x9.8 cm [9]. Our patient's pheochromocytoma was comparable in size and there was suspect it had been partially controlled and disguising as primary hypertension, as the patient was on prazosin for benign prostatic hyperplasia and on multiple antihypertensive medications.

In our patient's case, he did not receive perioperative blockade as his pheochromocytoma was unknown at the time of the procedure, his prazosin was held, and the stress of the cardiac catheterization precipitated a pheochromocytoma spell, causing a hypertensive emergency. He was initially started on intravenous nitroglycerin that was changed to nicardipine for better blood pressure control. Per the Endocrine Clinical Practice Guidelines, patients with functional pheochromocytomas and paragangliomas should receive perioperative blockade in addition to a high-sodium diet and fluid intake prior to the surgery [10]. Perioperative blockade consists of alpha-adrenergic receptor blockers as the first-choice drug class to minimize perioperative complications and calcium channel blockers are the most often used add on drug to control blood pressure. Beta-adrenergic receptor blockers are indicated to control tachycardia, but only after alpha-adrenergic receptor blockade has been achieved.

By day two the patient's blood pressure began to wildly fluctuate. The intravenous nicardipine was discontinued. From the standpoint of the medical team, this labile blood pressure was extremely challenging to manage. Each time the team tried to intervene on the elevated blood pressure his blood pressure suddenly plummeted and vice versa. There was concern which extreme was more harmful to the patient and was there a balance in treatment.

There are multiple cases describing such cyclic episodes of hypotension and hypertension with pheochromocytomas [11–13]. A review by Kobal et al. of seven cases found an association of labile blood pressures with tumors that predominantly secrete epinephrine [14]. This corresponds with our case's findings, showing serum catecholamine markers as primarily metanephrine, a metabolite of epinephrine.

There are a few proposed mechanisms for this cyclic blood pressure; however the exact mechanism is uncertain. One proposed mechanism is based on autoregulation by baroreceptors. A surge in catecholamines, primarily epinephrine, would cause vasoconstriction and decreased blood volume leading to decreased cardiac output triggering further release of catecholamines. The baroreceptors would then sense the vasoconstriction causing negative feedback of the sympathetic and parasympathetic nervous system resulting in hypotension [15]. Another proposed mechanism is that posture affects tumor secretions. Oishi et al. proposed that an increase in intra-abdominal pressure leads to a surge in catecholamines release and noted that when patients lay supine that their blood pressure would fluctuate [10]. While other theories suggest intravascular volume depletion and ischemic response of the central nervous system as cause of the varying blood pressures [16], our patient's blood pressure remained labile after starting prazosin and only stabilized after aggressive fluid resuscitating, supporting the latter mechanism.

There was discussion which alpha-blockade to initiate. The patient was on prazosin, a short acting alpha-1-adrenergic blocker, for BPH with blood pressure control prior to admission. Phenoxybenzamine, an irreversible, long acting, and nonselective alpha receptor antagonist, is the preferred drug for preoperative preparation to control blood pressure. Doxazosin, a selective alpha-1-adrenergic blocker, was another option [10]. However, with the labile pressures and concern for hypotension, there was concern for using a long acting antagonist and prazosin was initiated because of its ability to be up titrated. In the end, the patient's blood pressure was able to be managed with fluid resuscitation and prazosin without the need for a second antihypertensive agent.

The only curative modality for pheochromocytoma is tumor excision, with a laparoscopic approach being the procedure of choice for patients with a solitary intra-adrenal pheochromocytomas without malignant radiologic features [10]. As noted, the patient's advanced age, severe malnutrition, worsening mental status, being with no family made him a poor surgical candidate. These factors also contributed to the decision to not proceed with genetic evaluation, as the Endocrine Clinical Practice Guidelines recommend all patients be engaged in shared decision-making for genetic testing [10].

4. Conclusion

In conclusion, pheochromocytoma can be seen in elderly patients. It is important to note that alpha-adrenergic antagonist medications may mask an insidious pheochromocytoma unless provoked by a stressor, like a surgery. The composition of the tumor secretions, epinephrine versus norepinephrine versus dopamine, can lead to varying presentations of patients that should trigger pheochromocytoma workup. Lastly, patients with pheochromocytomas that present with rapid cyclic fluctuations of hypertension and hypotension may benefit from fluid repletion in addition to an alpha-adrenergic antagonist.

References

[1] C. M. Beard, S. G. Sheps, L. T. Kurland, J. A. Carney, and J. T. Lie, "Occurrence of pheochromocytoma in Rochester, Minnesota, 1950 through 1979," *Mayo Clinic Proceedings*, vol. 58, no. 12, pp. 802–804, 1983.

[2] M. A. Guerrero, J. M. J. Schreinemakers, M. R. Vriens, I. Suh, J. Hwang, and W. T. Shen, "Clinical spectrum of pheochromocytoma," *Journal of the American College of Surgeons*, vol. 209, no. 6, pp. 727–732, 2009.

[3] P. P. Stein and H. R. Black, "A simplified diagnostic approach to pheochromocytoma: a review of the literature and report of one institution's experience," *Medicine*, vol. 70, no. 1, pp. 46–66, 1991.

[4] W. F. Young and D. E. Maddox, "Spells: in search of a cause," *Mayo Clinic Proceedings*, vol. 70, no. 8, pp. 757–765, 1995.

[5] Y. C. Kudva, W. F. Young, G. B. Thompson et al., "Adrenal incidentaloma: an important component of the clinical presentation spectrum of benign sporadic adrenal pheochromocytoma," *The Endocrinologist*, vol. 9, no. 2, pp. 77–80, 1999.

[6] J. Baguet, L. Hammer, T. Mazzuco et al., "Circumstances of discovery of phaeochromocytoma: a retrospective study of 41 consecutive patients," *European Journal of Endocrinology*, vol. 150, no. 5, pp. 681–686, 2004.

[7] K. R. Feingold, B. Anawalt, A. Boyce, G. Chrousos, K. Dungan, A. Grossman et al., *Endotext [Internet]*, Endotext. MDText.com, Inc., 2000, http://www.ncbi.nlm.nih.gov/pubmed/25905160.

[8] A. Buffet, A. Morin, L. Castro-Vega et al., "Germline mutations in the mitochondrial 2-oxoglutarate/malate carrier (SLC25A11) gene confer predisposition to metastatic paragangliomas," *Endocrine Abstracts*, 2018.

[9] E. Sun and B. Lu, "Giant malignant pheochromocytoma in an elderly patient," *Medicine*, vol. 97, no. 19, Article ID e0614, 2018.

[10] J. W. M. Lenders, Q.-Y. Duh, and G. Eisenhofer, "Pheochromocytoma and paraganglioma : an endocrine society clinical practice guideline," *The Journal of Clinical Endocrinology & Metabolism*, vol. 99, no. 6, pp. 1915–1942, 2014.

[11] E. L. Bravo, "Evolving concepts in the pathophysiology, diagnosis, and treatment of pheochromocytoma," *Endocrine Reviews*, vol. 15, no. 3, pp. 356–368, 1994.

[12] M. A. Baxter, P. Hunter, G. R. Thompson, and D. R. London, "Phaeochromocytomas as a cause of hypotension," *Clinical Endocrinology*, vol. 37, no. 3, pp. 304–306, 1992.

[13] S. Oishi, M. Sasaki, M. Ohno, T. Umeda, and T. Sato, "Periodic fluctuation of blood pressure and its management in a patient with pheochromocytoma: case report and review of the literature," *Japanese Heart Journal*, vol. 29, no. 3, pp. 389–399, 1988.

[14] S. L. Kobal, E. Paran, A. Jamali, S. Mizrahi, R. J. Siegel, and J. Leor, "Pheochromocytoma: cyclic attacks of hypertension alternating with hypotension," *Nature Clinical Practice Cardiovascular Medicine*, vol. 5, no. 1, pp. 53–57, 2008.

[15] C. N. Ionescu, O. V. Sakharova, M. D. Harwood, E. A. Caracciolo, M. H. Schoenfeld, and T. J. Donohue, "Cyclic rapid fluctuation of hypertension and hypotension in pheochromocytoma," *The Journal of Clinical Hypertension*, vol. 10, no. 12, pp. 936–940, 2008.

[16] A. Ganguly, C. E. Grim, M. H. Weinberger, and D. P. Henry, "Rapid cyclic fluctuations of blood pressure associated with an adrenal pheochromocytoma," *Hypertension*, vol. 6, no. 2, Pt 1, pp. 281–284, 1984.

27

Atypical Presentation of Testicular Adrenal Rest Tumor (TART) Leading to Bilateral Partial Orchiectomy in a 31-Year-Old Adult Revealing Primary Adrenal Insufficiency with *CYP11A1* Deficiency

Cyril Garcia,[1] Marie Dusaud,[2] Paul Chiron,[2] Mathilde Sollier,[1] Sika Nassouri,[1] Lionel Groussin,[3] Mathilde Sibony,[4] Claire Goursaud,[5] Florence Roucher-Boulez,[5] and Lyse Bordier[1]

[1]*Hôpital d'Instruction des Armées BEGIN, Service d'endocrinologie, 69 avenue de Paris, Saint-Mande 94160, France*
[2]*Hôpital d'Instruction des Armées BEGIN, Service d'urologie, 69 avenue de Paris, Saint-Mande 94160, France*
[3]*Hôpital COCHIN, Service d'endocrinologie, 27 rue du Faubourg Saint Jacques, Paris 75014, France*
[4]*Hôpital COCHIN, Service d'anatomopathologie, 27 rue du Faubourg Saint Jacques, Paris 75014, France*
[5]*Hospices Civils de Lyon-Bron, Laboratoire de Biochimie et Biologie Moléculaire Grand Est, Lyon 69000, France*

Correspondence should be addressed to Cyril Garcia; garcia.cyril@free.fr

Academic Editor: Mihail A. Boyanov

Adrenogenital syndrome is commonly associated with a deficiency in 21-hydroxylase but can be present in other rare enzymatic blocks. We report here the case of a 31-year-old man who presented with bilateral painful testicle lesions leading to bilateral partial orchiectomy as they were suspected for malignancy. These lesions were finally identified as benign testicle adrenal rest tumors (TARTs), and the patient was actually belatedly diagnosed with primary adrenal insufficiency due to 2 mutations of the *CYP11A1* gene encoding the cholesterol side-chain cleavage enzyme (P450scc); the mutations were 940G > A (p.Glu314Lys) and c.1393C > T (p.Arg465Trp). The same mutations were found in his 29-year-old sister, who was then also diagnosed for primary adrenal insufficiency. Deficiency in P450scc is an extremely rare genetic autosomal recessive disorder with around 40 described families in the literature and 30 different mutations. As the diagnosis of delayed onset of P450Scc mutation is difficult, this case illustrates the need for a systematic endocrinological assessment in any case of bilateral testicle lesions, thus avoiding unnecessary surgery.

1. Introduction

Adrenogenital syndrome is commonly associated with an enzymatic block and congenital adrenal hyperplasia (CAH), in which gonadal lesions develop from adrenal-like cells. In these cases, increased levels of ACTH are associated with hyperplasia of ACTH-sensitive tissues, mainly the adrenals, but also within other sites like the testis or ovaries [1]. These testicle lesions are benign and so-called TTAGS (testicular tumor of adrenogenital syndrome) or better known as TARTs (testicular adrenal rest tumors) [1, 2].

TARTs were mainly described in defects in 21-hydroxylase, which are the most frequent enzymatic blocks representing 90 to 94% of CAH [1, 3]. TARTs can be present in other blocks, such as in 17alpha hydroxylase, P450Scc, 3 beta-hydroxysteroid dehydrogenase, and 11 beta-hydroxylase deficiencies [4]. TARTs can never occur in adrenal insufficiency of autoimmune origin, despite high rates of ACTH [4].

We report here the cases of a young man and his sister, who were belatedly diagnosed with primary adrenal insufficiency due to mutations of the *CYP11A1* encoding the cholesterol side-chain cleavage enzyme (P450scc), the first rate-limiting step of steroidogenesis.

2. Case Report

A 31-year-old man was referred to the urologist for painful bilateral testicular lesions. No other genital lesions were observed, and in particular, no hypospadias. The patient did not report any decrease in libido or erectile dysfunction and had normal ejaculations. The blood pressure was 106/63 mmHg, the heart rate was 67 beats per minute, the height was 174 cm, the weight was 66 kg, and the BMI was 21.8 kg/m^2. In his family, his sister's height was 1.58 m, her weight was 52 kg, and her BMI was 20.8 kg/m^2. As his mother's height was 155 cm and his father's height was 158 cm, the target height was estimated at 163 cm ((mother + father)/2). The patient was classified as Tanner stage V because the penis was of adult size. Only facial hair was limited requiring only one shave per week. Electrolyte values were as follows: urea 1.9 mmol/L, creatinine 61 µmol/L, sodium 141 mmol/L, and potassium 4.2 mmol/L. Despite the fact that testosterone measurement was not performed, hypogonadism was suggested by bone densitometry, which showed osteopenia; the lumbar T score was -1.8 SD and the femoral T score was -1.2 SD.

Ultrasonography revealed bilateral, heterogeneous, and vascularized lesions, localized on the top of both testicles, within the testicle hilus. Testicles were found to be hypotrophic as measured at 6 to 7 ml (normal range, 15–30 ml). The ultrasound report did not point to a benign tumor (notably, it did not formally rule out a testicular germ cell tumor). The extemporaneous analysis of the tumor suspected a Leydig cell tumor. Therefore, bilateral inguinal testicular exploration with partial orchiectomy was performed in the first instance, according to the Cancerology Committee of the French Association of Urology (CCFAU) recommendations and the European Association of Urology (EAU) recommendations. Bilateral partial orchiectomy was performed to preserve fertility (Figure 1). No preoperative hormonal analysis was made as no endocrine aetiology was evoked at that time.

The lesions were first considered as benign Leydig cell hyperplasia at anatomopathology. The tumors were measured macroscopically at 2 and 2.5 cm for the right and left lesions, respectively. They were found to be brown to orange and multimicronodular. Microscopically, the tumors were made of eosinophilic cells with regular round nuclei. In some cells, brown pigments of lipofuscin were observed. Calcification and adipose metaplasia were also observed. As the surgeon first considered these lesions as potentially malignant, classical immunohistochemistry was performed in this setting; however, these cells were first difficult to differentiate from normal Leydig cells, as immunochemistry was not specific. Lastly, because of bilateral lesions, testicular adrenal rest tumors (TARTs) were suspected, although no Reinke crystals were seen [1, 5–7].

The patient was then referred to the endocrinologist for testosterone replacement and hormonal evaluation. Presentation was marked by diffuse melanodermia and important asthenia, since adolescence.

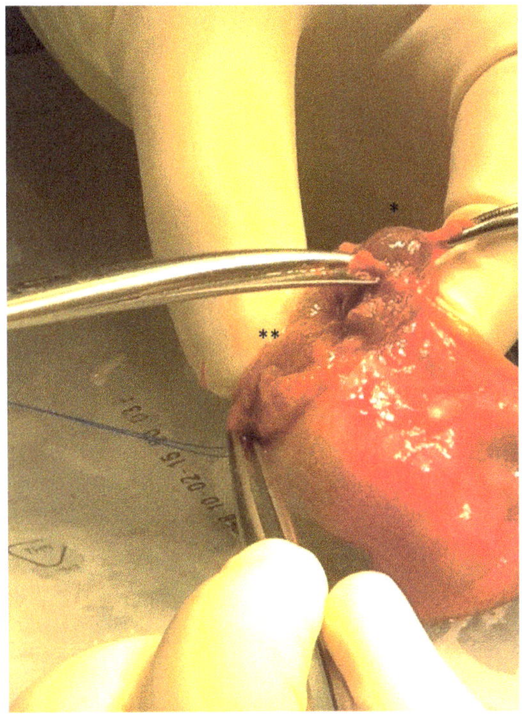

Figure 1: Perioperative view: partial right orchiectomy. Open testicular albuginea, tumor enucleation, and adjacent healthy parenchyma. *Testicular adrenal rest tumor. ** Healthy testicular pulp.

Patient's hormone profile is presented in Table 1. Results were consistent with postoperative hypergonadotropic hypogonadism (low testosterone and elevated gonadotrophins, FSH, and LH), but primary adrenal insufficiency was also revealed (low cortisol with elevated ACTH). Antibodies against 21-hydroxylase were <0.2 mUI/L. Adrenal androgens and most of the steroids of the adrenal cortex were low (Table 1). Atrophic adrenal glands were observed on computed tomography. As the patient was then explained that a genetic aetiology was suspected, he asked for his 29-year-old sister to also be screened for adrenal insufficiency as she has suffered from unexplored asthenia since childhood. This young woman also presented melanodermia. The first menstruation occurred at 9.5 years old. The same hormone profile was observed with primary adrenal insufficiency (Table 2, because of oral contraceptive medication, only a few hormones were dosed).

This hormone profile was not consistent with the diagnostic of the most common enzymatic blocks, as no elevation of any single steroid was observed. However, this was suggesting an enzymatic deficiency at a very early step in steroid biosynthesis. As the patient's adrenals did not appear enlarged on computed tomography, STAR deficiency was highly improbable. The hypothesis of P450Scc deficiency was conducted by *CYP11A1* gene analysis by next-generation sequencing (NM_000781 [8]). Both patients were then found to be compound heterozygous for the mutations 940G > A (p.Glu314Lys) and c.1393C > T (p.Arg465Trp), and haplotype segregation was confirmed by parental genetic analysis. The past medical history of the father was marked by surgery

Table 1: Hormone profiles of the 31-year-old male patient harboring compound heterozygous mutations in the *CYP11A1* gene.

Hormone	Unit	Result	Normal range
Cortisol	nmol/L	72	110.7–609.2
ACTH	pg/ml	>1250	10–60
Total testosterone	nmol/L	7.9	6–27
Free testosterone	pmolL	14.2	28.8–139
Estradiol	pmol/L	92	33–228
SHBG	nmol/L	48.83	14.5–48.4
FSH	UI/L	74	1.3–9.2
LH	UI/L	31.9	1.2–8.6
Delta 4 androstenedione	ng/ml	0.24	0.5–3.5
Dehydroepiandrosterone sulfate	ng/ml	497	1600–4490
Progesterone	nmol/L	0.8	<0.64
17-Hydroxyprogesterone	nmol/L	0.79	1.81–6.6
Pregnenolone	nmol/L	0.32	0.6–1.9
17-Hydroxypregnenolone	nmol/L	0.6	1.8–10.2
11-Deoxycortisol	nmol/L	0.29	0.6–3.2
11-Deoxycorticosterone	pmol/L	191	121–514
Corticosterone	nmol/L	5.8	5.7–23
Aldosterone	pmo/L	180	117–580
Active renin	mUI/L	18.54	<36

Table 2: Hormone profile of the 29-year-old female patient harboring compound heterozygous mutations in the *CYP11A1* gene.

Hormone	Unit	Result	Normal range
Cortisol	nmol/L	226	186.1–664.8
ACTH	pmol/L	>440	1.1–13.2
Testosterone	nmol/L	0.14	<3.3
Delta 4 androstenedione	nmol/L	0.7	1.4–9.78
Dehydroepiandrosterone sulfate	nmol/L	1437	2680–9230
Aldosterone	pmol/L	294	117–580
Active renin	mUI/L	12.8	<36

for hypospadias. In addition, to testosterone replacement for the male patient, treatment consisted in glucocorticoid substitution without the need for mineralocorticoids, as blood pressure, natremia, and kaliemia were normal in both patients.

3. Discussion

TART frequency in enzymatic blocks is estimated between 14 and 86% according to a publication gathering 33 studies in this field, with underestimation probably due to undone screenings [7]. These lesions should be actually clinically palpable if the size is more than 20 mm and are bilateral in almost 80% of cases [7]. Studies show that TARTs can be present from childhood, with a higher prevalence during puberty [3]. Their prevalence could be correlated with ACTH levels in patients treated with hydrocortisone, as suggested in a cohort study of 25 patients where the increasing dose of hydrocortisone led to a size reduction of lesions in 35.7% of cases and a remission in 42.9% at 6 month follow-up [9]. These lesions are thus reversible. In summary, TARTs were reported mainly in CAHs with bad hormone control, but it is to know that TARTs can also develop in well-controlled patients, and conversely, bad-controlled patients can be free from TART occurrence [7].

The TART origin could be due to the development of embryonic primordial adrenogenital cells or from urogenital cell ridges [10]. These tumors could be made of fœtal Leydig cells or precursors of Leydig cells [10]. These lesions are usually located in the mediastinum, testis or the testicular hilus [3, 7]. If TARTs are benign, they can compress the seminiferous tubules and lead to obstructive azoospermia with peritubular fibrosis and irreversible damage to the peritesticular tissue [1, 10]. This can lead to infertility or endocrine defects [3, 10]. A study of 30 CAH, mainly defects in 21-hydroxylase, reported an 86% TART, responsible for spermogram abnormalities in 43% of cases [11].

A deleterious paracrine effect is also suspected for Leydig cells or neighbour germinal cells, due to a potentially toxic effect of local steroids production [1]. Some blocks can finally lead to fertility troubles due to both tumoral invasion and lipid accumulation within steroidogenic cells [4].

TART lesions are mostly echographycally irregular, hypoechogenic, and homogenous, but can also be heterogeneous, or with a round shape, and rarely iso or hyperechogenic [3]. They can contain hyperechogenic elements due to fibrosis or calcifications, especially in adults [3]. In a study recording individuals younger than 18 years old, the size of the lesions was measured between 0.2 and 3.8 cm [3]. TARTs are classically highly vascularized [3, 7]. In MRI, these lesions are T1 hyper or isosignal, and T2 hyposignal, with a clean edge [7]. Imaging follow-up is of high importance as the aspects of ultrasonography may vary over time [12].

These lesions are macroscopically firm, yellow to brown-coloured, round, oval or multilobular [7]. It can be difficult to distinguish TART from mature Leydig cell tumors (LCT), which are the most common stromal testicular neoplasms [1]. It is important to distinguish between these tumors because the treatment is different, whereas the treatment of TART is mainly medical with the prescription of oral drugs, LCT management is surgical. Indeed, TARTs should not be operated except in cases of pain or discomfort due to their high volume [7]. Studies gather interesting histological and genetic markers that can help distinguish one from the other [7].

The patients reported in our paper harbor an extremely rare genetic autosomal recessive disorder with around 40 described families and 30 different mutations [4, 13–17]. There is actually a wide spectrum of different clinical forms within P450Scc defects. In classic form, salt wasting is observed with female genitals for the 46XY subjects. Partial defects are associated with the late onset of adrenal insufficiency or cortisol insufficiency with normal external genitalia, or with various degrees of underandrogenisation. The first description of the late onset of adrenal insufficiency in P450Scc deficiency was published in 2009 [13], where a boy with cryptorchidy and hypospadias presented adrenal insufficiency at 9 years of age. Mild forms were then reported in several families. Those forms seem to be explained by the residual activity of the mutated enzyme, compared to wild-type enzymes according to functional studies. P450Scc deficiency is often grouped with STAR (steroidogenic acute regulatory protein) deficiency under the term of congenial lipoid adrenal hyperplasia (CLAH). STAR allows cholesterol import into the mitochondrial membrane. However, the comparison between P450Scc and STAR deficiencies is controversial as enlarged adrenal glands are not reported in P450Scc deficiency [4].

As far as our patients' mutations are concerned, Goursaud et al. have reported that the functional consequences of these mutations can explain an uncomplete phenotype [8]. Both mutations, c.940G > A or p.Glu314Lys and c.1393C > T or p.Arg465Trp, were found in two families in a compound heterozygous state [8]. Goursaud et al. provided biological proof that p.Arg465Trp completely abolished CYP11A1 activity. Conversely, c.940G > A or p.Glu314Lys seems responsible for the mild phenotype due to its partial splicing impact and a mutated protein that maintains its activity [8]. Maharaj published in 2019 the report of 13 additional families with the p.Glu314Lys mutation and a second rare disruptive or synonymous mutation variant in *CYP11A1*, suggesting that mutations of the gene coding for P450Scc enzyme should be more frequent than previously thought [18].

The diagnosis of the delayed onset of the P450Scc mutation is difficult. Kallali et al. published the case of 3 brothers, among whom one had unilateral orchiectomy at 25 years of age, with the initial conclusion of Leydig cell hyperplasia [4]. The 3 brothers had glucocorticoid deficiency and partial deficiency in mineralocorticoids [4]. Other cases of orchiectomies were reported in patients with TART, leading to the need for endocrinologists to better communicate with urologists to avoid unnecessary surgeries [19, 20].

This observation illustrates the difficulty to diagnose primary adrenal insufficiency in adults, especially with mild phenotypes. On one hand, when a block is already known in an individual presenting CAH, the diagnosis of TART is commonly and easily made with ultrasonography, with no need for biopsy or partial orchiectomy that should indeed be avoided. On the other hand, the new discovery of bilateral testicular lesions in an adult should evoke a TART and lead to minimal endocrinological exploration. The evolution of unoperated TART is classically a regression under medical glucocorticoid treatment.

Consent

The patient and his family had given informed consent for the present paper.

References

[1] N. Charfi, M. Kamoun, M. Feki Mnif et al., "Leydig cell tumor associated with testicular adrenal rest tumors in a patient with congenital adrenal hyperplasia due to 11β-hydroxylase deficiency," *Case reports in urology*, vol. 2012, Article ID 648643, 13 pages, 2012.

[2] S. Naouar, S. Braiek, and R. El Kamel, "Testicular tumors of adrenogenital syndrome: from physiopathology to therapy," *Presse Medicale (Paris, France: 1983)*, vol. 46, no. 6 Pt 1, pp. 572–578, 2017.

[3] Z. Wang, Z. Yang, W. Wang et al., "Diagnosis of testicular adrenal rest tumors on ultrasound," *Medicine*, vol. 94, no. 36, p. e1471, 2015.

[4] W. Kallali, E. Gray, M. Z. Mehdi et al., "Long-term outcome of partial P450 side-chain cleavage enzyme deficiency in three brothers: the importance of early diagnosis," *European Journal of Endocrinology*, vol. 182, no. 3, pp. K15–K24, 2020.

[5] H. Mesa, S. Gilles, M. W. Datta et al., "Immunophenotypic differences between neoplastic and non-neoplastic androgen-producing cells containing and lacking Reinke crystals," *Virchows Archiv*, vol. 469, no. 6, pp. 679–686, 2016.

[6] A. Güven and S. Polat, "Testicular adrenal rest tumor in two brothers with a novel mutation in the 3-beta-hydroxysteroid dehydrogenase-2 gene," *Journal of clinical research in pediatric endocrinology*, vol. 9, no. 1, pp. 85–90, 2017.

[7] M. Engels, P. N. Span, A. E. van Herwaarden, F. C. G. J. Sweep, N. M. M. L. Stikkelbroeck, and H. L. Claahsen-van der Grinten, "Testicular adrenal rest tumors: current insights on prevalence, characteristics, origin, and treatment," *Endocrine Reviews*, vol. 40, no. 4, pp. 973–987, 2019.

[8] C. Goursaud, D. Mallet, A. Janin et al., "Aberrant splicing is the pathogenicity mechanism of the p.Glu314Lys variant in CYP11A1 gene," *Frontiers in Endocrinology*, vol. 9, p. 491, 2018.

[9] R. Mazzilli, A. Stigliano, M. Delfino et al., "The high prevalence of testicular adrenal rest tumors in adult men with congenital adrenal hyperplasia is correlated with ACTH levels," *Frontiers in Endocrinology*, vol. 10, p. 335, 2019.

[10] H. Claahsen-van der Grinten, A. Hermus, and B. Otten, "Testicular adrenal rest tumours in congenital adrenal hyperplasia," *International Journal of Pediatric Endocrinology*, vol. 2009, Article ID 624823, 1 page, 2009.

[11] H. Falhammar, H. F. Nyström, U. Ekström, S. Granberg, A. Wedell, and M. Thorén, "Fertility, sexuality and testicular adrenal rest tumors in adult males with congenital adrenal hyperplasia," *European Journal of Endocrinology*, vol. 166, no. 3, pp. 441–449, 2012.

[12] M. Kocova, V. Janevska, and V. Anastasovska, "Testicular adrenal rest tumors in boys with 21-hydroxylase deficiency, timely diagnosis and follow-up," *Endocrine Connections*, vol. 7, no. 4, pp. 544–552, 2018.

[13] P. Rubtsov, M. Karmanov, P. Sverdlova, P. Spirin, and A. Tiulpakov, "A novel homozygous mutation in CYP11A1Gene is associated with late-onset adrenal insufficiency and hypospadias in a 46, XY patient," *The Journal of Clinical Endocrinology & Metabolism*, vol. 94, no. 3, pp. 936–939, 2009.

[14] T. Sahakitrungruang, M. K. Tee, P. R. Blackett, and W. L. Miller, "Partial defect in the cholesterol side-chain cleavage enzyme P450scc (CYP11A1) resembling nonclassic congenital lipoid adrenal hyperplasia," *The Journal of Clinical Endocrinology & Metabolism*, vol. 96, no. 3, pp. 792–798, 2011.

[15] S. Parajes, A. O. Chan, W. M. But et al., "Delayed diagnosis of adrenal insufficiency in a patient with severe penoscrotal hypospadias due to two novel P450 side-change cleavage enzyme (CYP11A1) mutations (p.R360W; p.R405X)," *European Journal of Endocrinology*, vol. 167, no. 6, pp. 881–885, 2012.

[16] M. K. Tee, M. Abramsohn, N. Loewenthal et al., "Varied clinical presentations of seven patients with mutations

inCYP11A1Encoding the cholesterol side-chain cleavage enzyme, P450scc," *The Journal of Clinical Endocrinology & Metabolism*, vol. 98, no. 2, pp. 713–720, 2013.

[17] V. Kolli, H. Kim, A. Torky et al., "Characterization of the-CYP11A1Nonsynonymous variant p.E314K in children presenting with adrenal insufficiency," *The Journal of Clinical Endocrinology & Metabolism*, vol. 104, no. 2, pp. 269–276, 2019.

[18] A. Maharaj, F. Buonocore, E. Meimaridou et al., "Predicted benign and synonymous variants in CYP11A1 cause primary adrenal insufficiency through miissplicing," *Journal of the Endocrine Society*, vol. 3, no. 1, pp. 201–221, 2019.

[19] J. Sarfati, C. Vatier, I. Keller, J. Guéchot, C. Bellanné-Chantelot, and S. Christin-Maitre, "Severe congenital adrenal hyperplasia presenting as bilateral testicular tumors and azoospermia in the third decade of life," *Journal of the Endocrine Society*, vol. 2, no. 9, pp. 997–1000, 2018.

[20] M. Roy, A. K. Roy, T. Chatterjee, and S. Bansal, "Testicular adrenal rest tumour (TART) or testicular malignancy: a clinical dilemma," *European journal of case reports in internal medicine*, vol. 7, no. 8, Article ID 001669, 2020.

Attenuation of Autoimmune Phenomena in a Patient with Autoimmune Polyglandular Syndrome Type 1

Jill D. Jacobson,[1] Julia R. Broussard,[1] Courtney Marsh,[2] and Brandon Newell[3]

[1]*Division of Endocrinology and Diabetes, Department of Pediatrics, Children's Mercy, University of Missouri-Kansas City School of Medicine, Kansas, MO 64111, USA*
[2]*Division of Reproductive Endocrinology and Infertility, Department of Obstetrics and Gynecology, University of Kansas School of Medicine, Kansas, KS 66160, USA*
[3]*Division of Dermatology, Department of Pediatrics, Children's Mercy Hospital, University of Missouri-Kansas City School of Medicine, Kansas, MO 64111, USA*

Correspondence should be addressed to Jill D. Jacobson; jjacobson@cmh.edu

Academic Editor: Toshihiro Kita

Autoimmune polyglandular syndrome type 1 (APS1) is a progressive life-threatening illness with no known cure. Current treatments involve replacement of the hormone deficiencies that result from autoimmune destruction of multiple endocrine organs. We report on a girl whose disease was progressing rapidly until she began on immunosuppressive agents. A healthy 6-year-old girl with no remarkable medical history presented with new onset hypocalcemic seizures and primary hypoparathyroidism. Howell-Jolly bodies consistent with autoimmune hyposplenism were also noted. Genetic testing revealed compound heterozygosity for 2 disease-associated variants in the autoimmune regulator (AIRE) gene. She later developed elevated liver enzymes, primary adrenal insufficiency, and alopecia totalis. Serologic testing revealed antibodies to 21-hydroxylase, intrinsic factor, and smooth muscle. Hydrocortisone was initiated for adrenal insufficiency. Shortly afterwards, her liver enzymes normalized, and her smooth muscle antibody levels began to decline. Serologic testing performed at age 11 revealed seropositivity for glutamic acid decarboxylase (GAD) antibodies, antinuclear antibodies, and Sjögren syndrome A (SSA) antibodies. At age 12, she was given 2 doses of rituximab. Hair loss rapidly progressed to alopecia totalis and then to alopecia universalis, at which time oral methotrexate treatment was initiated. For the past 7 years while on glucocorticoid and methotrexate treatment, our patient has displayed normalization of 2 antibodies, a lack of progression to additional autoimmune diseases, and experienced reversal of alopecia universalis.

1. Introduction

Autoimmune polyglandular syndrome type 1 (APS1), also known as APECED (autoimmune polyendocrinopathy candidiasis ectodermal dysplasia), is a rare but serious disorder associated with progressive autoimmune destruction of multiple endocrine and nonendocrine organs. APS1 has a high mortality rate. The median age at death ranges from 5 to 34 years, with deaths attributable to endocrinopathies, malignancy, acute hepatitis, and infection [1]. APS1 is caused by biallelic variations of the gene encoding the autoimmune regulator (AIRE), resulting in dysfunction of regulatory T cells, impaired immunologic tolerance to self-antigens with subsequent development of multiple autoimmune conditions [2]. Immunosuppressive therapies have been generally reserved for life-threatening features of APS1. To the best of our knowledge, this is the first case report demonstrating normalization of serology, reversal of an autoimmune condition, and prolonged lack of progression of autoimmune damage in APS1.

2. Case Report

The patient was a previously healthy 6-year-old girl of northern European descent whose only concerns had been enlarged tonsils, chronic constipation, and slow growth. She had no other health problems. There was no family history of endocrine or immunologic diseases. While watching television, she developed a grand mal seizure and became apneic. She was emergently transported to Children's Mercy Hospital. Initial physical examination was unremarkable except for short stature, with weight 20 kg (37.7 percentile) and height 104.6 cm (less than the 1st percentile). Family history revealed that the patient's mother is 162.6 cm tall and father is 177.8 cm tall; midparental height is 167.7 cm (50th percentile).

She was found to have a critically low total calcium of 1.1 mmol/L (normal range 2.2–2.5 mmol/L) and a blood glucose of 3.6 mmol/L (normal range 3.6–6.1 mmol/L). Her phosphorus was elevated at 3.6 mmol/L (1–1.9 mmol/L), and magnesium was low at 0.49 mmol/L (0.66–0.94 mmol/L). Initial iPTH level was low at 7 ng/L (10–89 ng/L), and subsequent iPTH levels remained low. She was diagnosed with primary hypoparathyroidism. She received intravenous calcium chloride and magnesium sulfate. Computed tomography of the head was normal. An extensive endocrine workup revealed that she had Howell-Jolly bodies consistent with autoimmune hyposplenism, a condition frequently seen in APS1 [3]. No other autoimmune deficiencies were noted at that time. Karyotype was 46, XX. Evaluation of 22 q 11 variants was normal. A growth hormone (GH) stimulation test was performed during initial admission. Her peak GH level was 12.8 ng/mL (normal >10 ng/mL).

With the documentation of two unusual autoimmune findings, genetic testing for AIRE gene was performed. The patient was found to be a compound heterozygote for 2 known disease-causing variants. The first was a nucleotide change of C > T in exon 6 of the AIRE gene resulting in the substitution of the normal arginine codon with a stop codon at position 257. This mutation is denoted R257X or Arg257Term. The second mutation was a 13 base-pair deletion in exon 8, beginning in codon leucine 323 and resulting in a change from leucine to serine, followed by a frameshift and premature stop codon 50 residues downstream (denoted c.967 979del13 and p.Leu323SerfsX50). Thus, she was heterozygous for R257X and c.967 979del13. Both are common, independently recurring mutations in APS1 [4]. The 13-base deletion has been published with various nomenclature (c.965 977del13 or p.Cys322fsX5l).

After testing positive for AIRE gene variants, additional serologic testing revealed seropositivity for 21-hydroxylase antibodies (a marker for adrenal autoimmunity) and positivity for intrinsic factor autoantibodies (a marker for atrophic gastritis). Figure 1(a) shows her positive serology over time, along with her immunosuppressive medications. Antibody testing for thyroid disease, type 1 diabetes mellitus, and celiac disease yielded negative results at that time.

At the age of 6 and a half years, a low-dose ACTH stimulation test showed a borderline peak cortisol of 433 nmol/L (normal >500 nmol/L). ACTH stimulation testing was repeated a year later, at which time, she demonstrated a peak cortisol level of 334 nmol/L, in addition to an elevated renin level. Subsequently, hydrocortisone and fludrocortisone replacement therapy were initiated. Figure 1(b) shows the number of autoimmune conditions over time along with her immunosuppressive medications.

Because of persistent short stature, she underwent repeat GH stimulation testing around age 9. Her peak GH level was 11.8 ng/mL, demonstrating GH sufficiency again. However, as her height was below the 3rd percentile, growth hormone therapy was initiated with excellent response. She ultimately achieved an adult height of 161.5 cm, within the range of her midparental height.

Her liver enzymes were modestly elevated at this time. Serologic testing revealed positive smooth muscle antibodies, which are associated with autoimmune hepatitis. At age 10, she developed hypertension and nephrocalcinosis and was placed on thiazide diuretics. At the age of 11 years, serologic testing revealed positive glutamic acid dehydrogenase (GAD), antinuclear antibodies (ANA), and Sjögren syndrome antibodies (SSA). Her thyroid antibodies have remained negative throughout her course. Over time, her smooth muscle antibodies and SSA antibody levels have gradually normalized (Figure 1(c)).

At age 12 years, she began to develop patches of alopecia on her scalp, which was distressing to her. We referred her to rheumatology for aggressive management of her APS1. She was begun on rituximab, monoclonal antibody therapy directed at CD20, a B cell epitope. Unfortunately, soon after she received 2 doses of rituximab, her hair loss progressed rapidly to alopecia totalis and then progressed to alopecia universalis.

The patient was referred to pediatric dermatology, who began with intralesional triamcinolone injections but soon added oral methotrexate. She was begun on 20 mg weekly, but this was increased to 25 mg weekly at age 16, which she continues to date. She was empirically placed on 1 mg folic acid daily and vitamin B12 with the methotrexate therapy. Complete hair regrowth was achieved within a year. Figure 2 denotes progressive hair loss (2(a) and 2(b)) followed by hair regrowth (2(c)). The patient has tolerated the methotrexate well.

At the age of 15, she was referred to gynecology for fertility discussion. Periods had been regular throughout, and gonadotropins were normal. Ovarian antibodies, known to be nonspecific, were measured at that time and were positive. Midcycle LH was 25 IU/L, and FSH was 7.1 IU/L. Anti-Müllerian hormone (AMH) level was 21.3 pmol/L (normal range for AMH 7.5–91.8 pmol/L). Six months later, the AMH level was noted to be 6.9 pmol/L, suggestive of low ovarian reserve [5, 6]. She then underwent fertility preservation. The procedure was highly successful, with 21 eggs harvested and stored. Surprisingly, five months after the retrieval, AMH levels were found to have normalized at 152.4 pmol/L. Her LH and FSH normalized. Her most recent LH is 0.5 IU/L, and her LH is 1.9 IUL. Cycles have remained regular throughout.

At age 18, a bone mineral density study noted focal areas of severely decreased bone mineral density in the distal femurs. Plain films showed ill-defined lucencies with adjacent sclerosis in the distal femurs, which we attribute to metaphyseal dysplasia, a rare bone condition previously described in 2003 in 2 unrelated patients with APS1 [7].

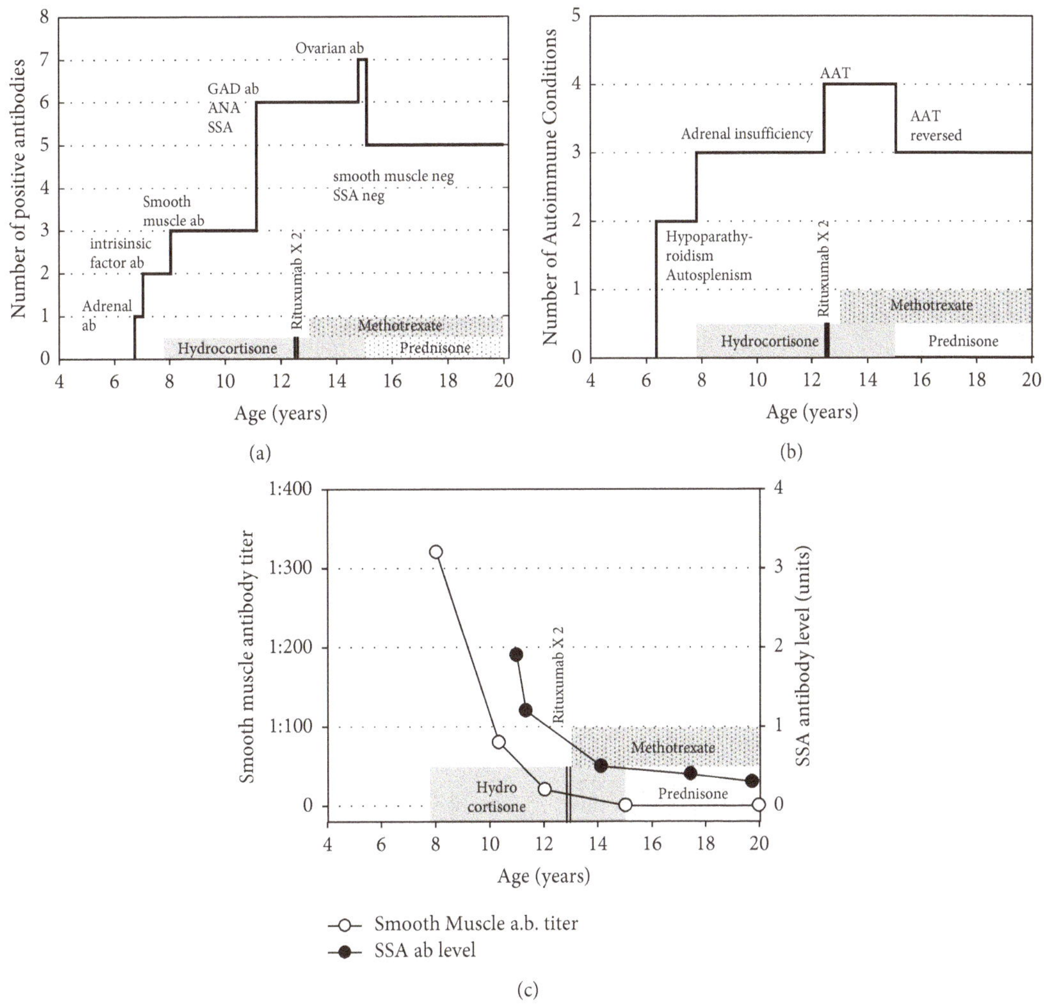

FIGURE 1: Timeline of development of autoantibodies (a), autoimmune processes (b), and smooth muscle and SSA antibodies (c) with time course of known immunosuppressive therapy also shown.

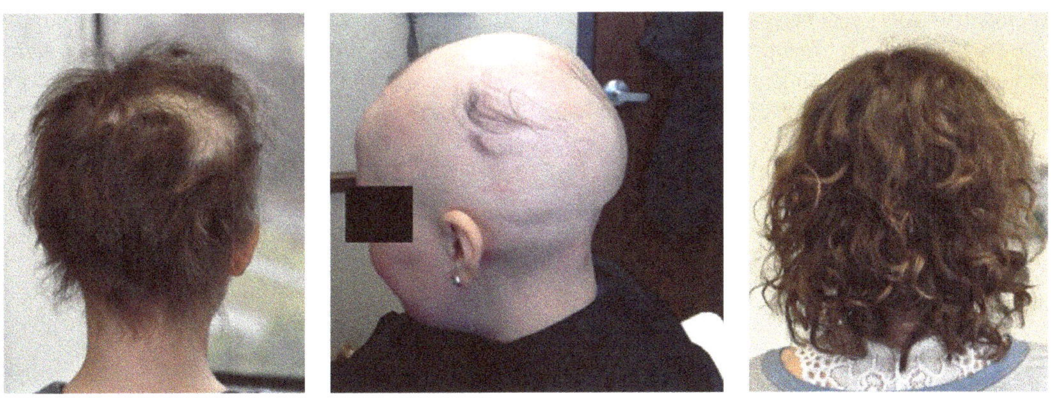

(a) (b) (c)

FIGURE 2: Progression of alopecia: early stages of disease (a), progression of disease (b), improvement in alopecia (c).

Six months later, she suddenly developed profound hypokalemia, which was thought to relate to apparent mineralocorticoid excess that has been described in APS1 [2]. This was managed with spironolactone and a reduction in fludrocortisone. A few weeks later, she experienced sudden mental status changes. She was seen emergently and was thought to be in septic shock. Testing for active COVID-infection was negative, but she had IgG antibodies to COVID-and met the diagnostic criteria for multisystem inflammatory syndrome in children (MIS-C). She required fluids and intensive care support. She recovered uneventfully from MIS-C, although she remains with elevated brain natriuretic peptide.

She is currently doing well as a college student at a major university and undergoes frequent laboratory monitoring.

3. Discussion

Herein, we describe a patient with autoimmune polyglandular syndrome type 1 (APS1) also known as autoimmune polyendocrinopathy candidiasis ectodermal dysplasia (APECED) with molecularly confirmed disease-causing variants in the AIRE gene. She was diagnosed at a young age in the absence of candida infections because of hypoparathyroidism in the presence of Howell-Jolly bodies, suggestive of autosplenism APS1 [3].

Our patient's clinical course is to the best of our knowledge unique. Early in her course, she was developing seropositivity to various antigens autoimmune conditions at a consistent rate of nearly one per year (Figure 1(a)). She was developing autoimmune conditions at nearly the same rate (Figure 1(b)). In the past 7 years, while receiving physiologic glucocorticoids and methotrexate therapy, she has not developed any new autoimmune problems. Moreover, her alopecia universalis has gone into remission, and her smooth muscle and SSA antibodies have normalized (Figure 1(c)). We are not aware of any reports in the literature of such attenuation of APS1.

Current management of APS1 does not generally involve immunosuppressive therapy. The illness tends to fall in the realm of endocrinologists rather than immunologists. Generally, treatment is directed toward replacing the hormones that are deficient as a direct result of the autoimmune processes. Adrenal disease is treated with glucocorticoid and mineralocorticoid replacement. Hypoparathyroidism is treated with oral calcium supplements and activated forms of vitamin D.

A mouse model of APS1 has been developed [8]. Rituximab and anti-CD4 antibody therapy improve APS1 in the mouse model [8], but these therapies have not been translated to humans. We are aware of no active clinical therapeutic trials.

When immunosuppressive therapies have been used, it is often in the setting of life-threatening features of APS1. A recent article outlined the immunosuppressive agents that have been tried in APS1 patients with severe conditions such as interstitial lung disease, autoimmune hepatitis, tubulointerstitial nephritis, pure red cell aplasia, and severe malabsorption [9]. That series included a summary of 13 previously reported patients, and therapies included high-dose glucocorticoids, cyclosporine A, mycophenolate mofetil, rituximab, monoclonal antibodies directed against CD52, macrolide compounds, and methotrexate [1, 9]. Most patients received multidrug therapy. Results were mixed. Only 1 patient, a patient with malabsorption, was treated with methotrexate. Therapy was combined with high-dose steroids, and remission in malabsorption was achieved [10].

A handful of other reports exist in which immunosuppressive agents have been used in APS1. Successful treatment of ocular keratitis with topical cyclosporine has been reported in two patients with APS1 [11]. In another study, 2 of 3 children with autoimmune hepatitis responded well to glucocorticoids and azathioprine [12]. A young boy with APS1 underwent a liver transplant and had a reduction in autoantibodies when he received a regimen of tacrolimus, prednisone, and mycophenolate mofetil [13].

Patients with isolated autoimmune diseases in the absence of APS1 may experience remissions. Isolated alopecia totalis can have a variable, relapsing, or remitting course. The possibility of spontaneous remission exists with this isolated condition for many years after onset. A similar situation exists with ovarian failure. A recent meta-analysis evaluating pregnancies in patients with premature ovarian insufficiency showed a spontaneous pregnancy rate ranging from 2.2 to 14.2% [14].

This study is limited by the difficulty in identifying which immunosuppressive agent may have offered our patient benefit. The two antibodies that normalized began to decline after the initiation of hydrocortisone, a known immunosuppressive agent. Fludrocortisone was initiated simultaneously. Although fludrocortisone has significant glucocorticoid effects, those effects are thought to be minimal at physiologic doses. After the 2 doses of rituximab at age 12, her hair loss acutely accelerated, resulting in a decision to try other forms of immunotherapy. Although hair loss worsened in close temporal proximity to the rituximab injections, it is impossible to say whether the rituximab exacerbated her symptoms or contributed to her later improvement. Based on the timing of the normalization of 2 antibodies prior to beginning on rituximab and methotrexate, it is possible that administration of glucocorticoids even at physiologic doses may have exerted immune benefits. This case may argue for early and repeated testing for adrenal insufficiency in APS1.

She was switched from a short-acting to a long-acting glucocorticoid after she achieved her adult height. We theorized that a long-acting steroid may suppress the immune system more consistently than short-acting ones. She also received small doses of a plant-derived progesterone, which is compounded and administered in troche form in order to titrate the dose. Several studies show that progesterone has glucocorticoid properties [15–17]. To provide steady release of an additional potentially immunosuppressive agent, we recommended low-dose etonogestrel as an implant.

4. Conclusions

We describe a patient with molecularly confirmed APS1 with marked attenuation of her seropositivity and autoimmune phenomena and remission in alopecia universalis while receiving physiologic glucocorticoids and mineralocorticoid, rituximab, and chronic therapy with methotrexate. In APS1, immunosuppressive agents have been used primarily in patients with life-threatening features such as autoimmune hepatitis, pulmonary interstitial disease, or severe malabsorption. As APS1 itself is life-threatening, early consideration of immunosuppressive agents may be warranted. Early testing for adrenal insufficiency may justify early use of glucocorticoids and mineralocorticoids.

Consent

Written informed consent was obtained from the patient for publication of this case report.

Acknowledgments

The authors thank the Children's Mercy Medical Writing Center at Children's Mercy Hospital for editing this manuscript. This study was supported by departmental funds from the Division of Endocrinology and Diabetes.

References

[1] M. Bakrac, V. Jurisic, T. Kostic et al., "Pure red cell aplasia associated with type I autoimmune polyglandular syndrome--successful response to treatment with mycophenolate mofetil: case report and review of literature," *Journal of Clinical Pathology*, vol. 60, no. 6, pp. 717–720, 2007.

[2] J. Perheentupa, "Autoimmune polyendocrinopathy-candidiasis-ectodermal dystrophy," *The Journal of Clinical Endocrinology and Metabolism*, vol. 91, no. 8, pp. 2843–2850, 2006.

[3] T. C. Friedman, P. M. Thomas, T. A. Fleisher et al., "Frequent occurrence of asplenism and cholelithiasis in patients with autoimmune polyglandular disease type I," *The American Journal of Medicine*, vol. 91, no. 6, pp. 625–630, 1991.

[4] M. Heino, P. r. Peterson, J. Kudoh et al., "APECED mutations in the autoimmune regulator (AIRE) gene," *Human Mutation*, vol. 18, no. 3, pp. 205–211, 2001.

[5] K. P. Tremellen, M. Kolo, A. Gilmore, and D. N. Lekamge, "Anti-mullerian hormone as a marker of ovarian reserve," *The Australian and New Zealand Journal of Obstetrics and Gynaecology*, vol. 45, no. 1, pp. 20–24, 2005.

[6] I. A. J. van Rooij, F. J. Broekmans, E. R. te Velde, B. C. Fauser, L. F. Bancsi, F. H. de Jong et al., "Serum anti-Mullerian hormone levels: a novel measure of ovarian reserve," *Human Reproduction*, vol. 17, no. 12, pp. 3065–3071, 2002.

[7] M. Harris, O. Kecha, C. Deal et al., "Reversible metaphyseal dysplasia, a novel bone phenotype, in two unrelated children with autoimmunepolyendocrinopathy-candidiasis-ectodermal dystrophy: clinical and molecular studies," *The Journal of Clinical Endocrinology & Metabolism*, vol. 88, no. 10, pp. 4576–4585, 2003.

[8] M. S. Anderson, E. S. Venanzi, L. Klein et al., "Projection of an immunological self shadow within the thymus by the aire protein," *Science*, vol. 298, no. 5597, pp. 1395–1401, 2002.

[9] K. Kisand and P. Peterson, "Autoimmune polyendocrinopathy candidiasis ectodermal dystrophy," *Journal of Clinical Immunology*, vol. 35, no. 5, pp. 463–478, 2015.

[10] S. Padeh, R. Theodor, A. Jonas, and J. H. Passwell, "Severe malabsorption in autoimmune polyendocrinopathy-candidosis-ectodermal dystrophy syndrome successfully treated with immunosuppression," *Archives of Disease in Childhood*, vol. 76, no. 6, pp. 532–534, 1997.

[11] O. AlAbbasi, M. S. Magliyah, and M. Ahad, "Long term keratits treatment with topical cyclosporin a in autoimmune polyglandular syndrome type 1," *American Journal of Ophthalmology Case Reports*, vol. 21, Article ID 101009, 2021.

[12] T. O. Lankisch, C. P. Strassburg, D. Debray, M. P. Manns, and E. Jacquemin, "Detection of autoimmune regulator gene mutations in children with type 2 autoimmune hepatitis and extrahepatic immune-mediated diseases," *The Journal of Pediatrics*, vol. 146, no. 6, pp. 839-842, 2005.

[13] T. Ulinski, L. Perrin, M. Morris et al., "Autoimmune polyendocrinopathy-candidiasis-ectodermal dystrophy syndrome with renal failure: impact of posttransplant immunosuppression on disease activity," *The Journal of Clinical Endocrinology & Metabolism*, vol. 91, no. 1, pp. 192–195, 2006.

[14] E. Fraison, G. Crawford, G. Casper, V. Harris, and W. Ledger, "Pregnancy following diagnosis of premature ovarian insufficiency: a systematic review," *Reproductive BioMedicine Online*, vol. 39, no. 3, pp. 467–476, 2019.

[15] M. Pineda-Torres, P. Flores-Espinosa, A. Espejel-Nunez et al., "Evidence of an immunosuppressive effect of progesterone uponin vitrosecretion of proinflammatory and prodegradative factors in a model of choriodecidual infection," *BJOG: An International Journal of Obstetrics & Gynaecology*, vol. 122, no. 13, pp. 1798–1807, 2015.

[16] F. Scarpellini, L. Scarpellini, N. Dino, and P. Benvenuto, "Progesterone immunosuppressive levels and luteal steroid profiles in the cycles induced with clomiphene citrate," *Clinical and Experimental Obstetrics & Gynecology*, vol. 20, no. 3, pp. 182–188, 1993.

[17] Y. Xu, H. He, C. Li et al., "Immunosuppressive effect of progesterone on dendritic cells in mice," *Journal of Reproductive Immunology*, vol. 91, no. 1-2, pp. 17–23, 2011.

29

Acute Lymphoblastic Leukemia Presenting as Pituitary Apoplexy: A Case Report and Review of the Literature

Rahul Gupta,[1] **Urmimala Bhattacharjee**,[2] **K. S. Lekshmon**,[2] **Shakun Chaudhary**,[1] **Prashant Sharma**,[2] **Aditya Jandial**,[2] **and Pinaki Dutta**[1]

[1]*Department of Endocrinology, Post Graduate Institute of Medical Education and Research, Chandigarh, India*
[2]*Department of Clinical Hematology and Medical Oncology, Post Graduate Institute of Medical Education and Research, Chandigarh, India*

Correspondence should be addressed to Aditya Jandial; adityapgimer@gmail.com and Pinaki Dutta; drpinakidutta12@gmail.com

Academic Editor: J. Paul Frindik

Thrombocytopenia as a precipitating factor for pituitary apoplexy (PA) is very rare event. There are only five reported cases of PA secondary to thrombocytopenia caused by underlying haematological malignancy. Herein, we report a case of 60-year-old male presenting with acute-onset headache, bilateral vision loss, and ptosis. Computed tomography and magnetic resonance imaging revealed findings indicative of pituitary adenoma with apoplexy. He was noted to have thrombocytopenia, and bone marrow evaluation revealed precursor B-lineage CALLA-positive acute lymphoblastic leukemia. Accordingly, he was started on dexamethasone and vincristine but succumbed to *Acinetobacter baumanii*-related hospital-acquired pneumonia two weeks after initiation of chemotherapy. We performed a literature search and found five cases of pituitary apoplexy secondary to haematological malignancy-related thrombocytopenia. The usual age of presentation was in the 6th to 7th decade, and there was slight male preponderance. The underlying pituitary adenoma was either nonfunctioning or a prolactinoma, and in majority, the apoplexy event occurred after the diagnosis of haematological malignancy. The platelet counts at the time of PA were less than 30×10^9/L in all, and the malignancy subtypes were acute or chronic myeloid leukemia and chronic lymphoid leukemia. The current case highlights the importance of careful evaluation for the cause of thrombocytopenia in a case of PA.

1. Introduction

Pituitary apoplexy (PA) is a clinical syndrome characterized by acute-onset headache caused by sudden hemorrhage and/or infarction. Precipitating factors are identified in only 20 to 40% of the cases [1]. Though the exact precipitating factor remains unidentified in majority, haemodynamic stress, pituitary stimulation test, coagulation disturbances, and thrombocytopenia are few of the reported risk factors [2]. Thrombocytopenia secondary to an underlying haematological malignancy as a precipitating event for apoplexy is uncommon. Here, we present a case of precursor B-cell lineage acute lymphoblastic leukaemia presenting with pituitary apoplexy. The patient provided written informed consent for allowing use of information and publication of images.

2. Case Presentation

A 60-year-old male presented to the emergency department with chief complaints of sudden-onset headache, vision loss in both eyes, and drooping of eyelids for the last two days. On initial evaluation, he was haemodynamically stable, conscious, and fully oriented. Positive findings on examination included bilateral absent light perception, complete external ophthalmoplegia, bilateral ptosis, optic atrophy, and gynaecomastia (Figures 1(a) and 1(b)). A noncontrast computed tomography (NCCT) scan revealed a hyperdense sellar mass (Figure 1(c)), and contrast-enhanced magnetic resonance imaging showed a $3.1 \times 2.7 \times 4.1$ cm sellar mass with the peripheral rim of T1 hyperintensity suggestive of adenoma with an acute to early subacute bleed (Figure 1(d)). The initial pituitary hormone profile was suggestive of

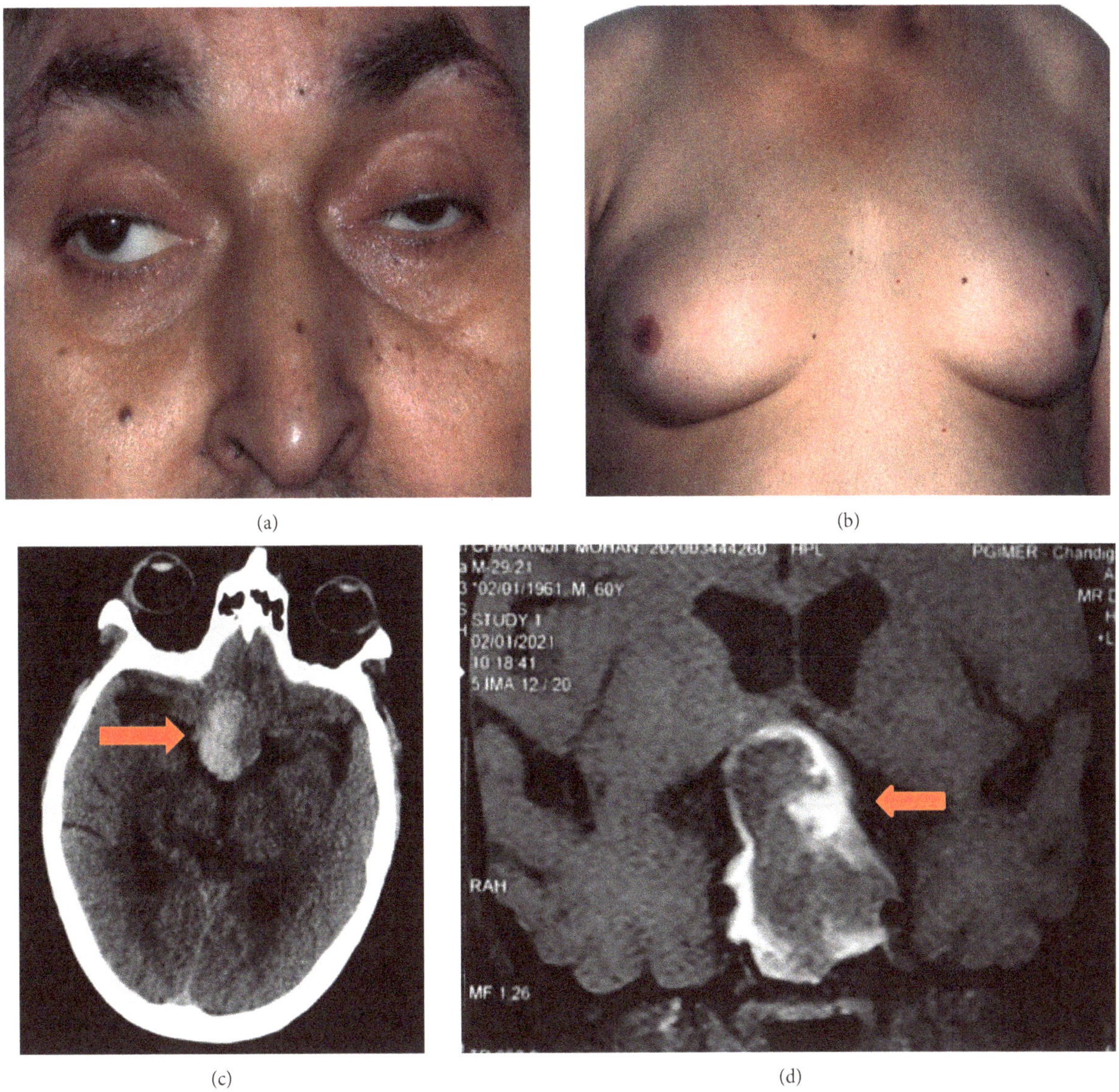

Figure 1: A 60-year-old male presented with sudden-onset severe headache and vision loss. (a) Bilateral ptosis and abducted right eye; (b) bilateral gynaecomastia; (c) axial NCCT head demonstrating a large sellar mass with areas of hyperdensity within suggestive of acute hemorrhage; and (d) coronal noncontrast T1-weighted MRI sellar demonstrating a 3.1 × 2.7 × 4.1 cm pituitary adenoma with peripheral T1 hyperintensity suggestive of acute bleed.

secondary hypothyroidism (T4: 3.79 ug/dl (4.8–12.7); T3: 0.804 ng/ml (0.8–2); and TSH: 7.01 uIU/ml (0.27–4.2)), secondary hypogonadism (LH: 0.270 mIU/ml; testosterone 0.0868 nmol/l (9.9–27.8); and low prolactin 3.01 ng/ml (4.0–15.2)). In view of presumptive diagnosis of apoplexy, he was started on intravenous hydrocortisone before blood sample for cortisol estimation was withdrawn, but had a normal blood pressure, serum electrolytes, and plasma glucose. In view of the pituitary apoplexy score of 6 and presence of bilateral vision loss, he was planned for urgent surgical decompression [3].

He was noted to have pancytopenia on initial complete blood count (Hb: 9.8 gm/dl; TLC: 1.7×10^9/L; DLC: Ne52, Ly42, Mo06%; and Plt: 23×10^9/L) for which bone marrow evaluation was performed. This revealed 70% blast cells that were cytochemically myeloperoxidase negative and on flow cytometry expressed CD19, CD10, CD81, HLA-DR, CD58, and CD38 along with cytoplasmic CD79a, CD22, and nuclear TdT. The blasts were negative for T/NK cell and myeloid lineage markers, as well as for CD86, CD34, and CD123. CD20 was dim to negative. Reverse-transcriptase PCR was negative for *t* (9; 22), *t* (1; 19), and *t* (12; 21). The final hematological diagnosis was precursor B-lineage CALLA-positive acute lymphoblastic leukaemia (Figure 2).

Considering his age, poor performance status, and financial limitation, he was started on dexamethasone 10 mg/m^2 daily and weekly vincristine 1.4 mg/m^2. However, our patient developed *Acinetobacter baumanii*-related hospital-acquired pneumonia two weeks after initiation of chemotherapy and ultimately succumbed due to refractory septic shock.

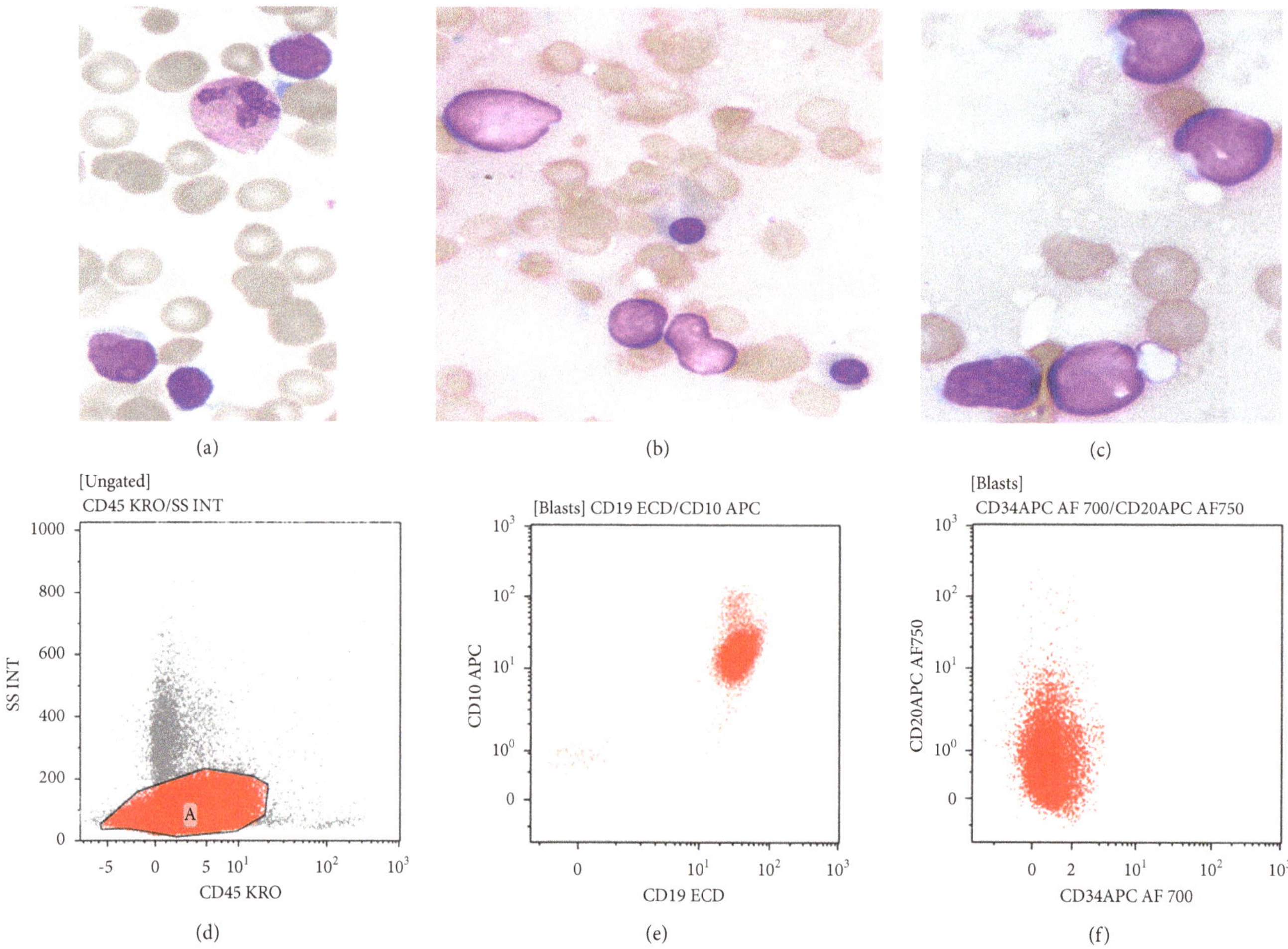

FIGURE 2: Lymphoblasts were rare in the peripheral blood (a) and comprised 70% of all cells in the bone marrow (b, c) (May-Grünwald-Giemsa stain, ×1000). On flow cytometry, they were CD45 negative to dim positive with low side scatter (d) and coexpressed CD19 and CD10 (e) as well as showed dim to negative CD20 expression (f).

3. Review of the Literature

We performed an extensive literature search in PubMed, EMBASE, and SCOPUS using the terms "pituitary, apoplexy, and thrombocytopenia," "pituitary, apoplexy, and leukemia," "apoplexy and thrombocytopenia," and "apoplexy and thrombocytopenia." We came across five cases of pituitary apoplexy associated with haematological malignancy in the English language over a period of 22 years (1996–2018, Table 1). The age at presentation was in the range of 55 years to 72 years. There was slight male preponderance with a male-to-female ratio of 3 : 2. At presentation, headache and vomiting were present in all while visual field abnormalities, opthalmoplegia, altered sensorium, and meningismus were present variably. The lag time from symptom onset to diagnosis varied from 12 hours to 6 weeks. The pituitary adenoma type was either prolactinoma or nonfunctioning, and the associated haematological malignancy was either acute or chronic myeloid leukemia or chronic lymphoid leukemia. In all except one, PA occurred after the diagnosis of haematological malignancy, and the platelet count at the time of PA was less than 30×10^9/L in all. Two of the five cases were managed conservatively and the other three with transsphenoidal surgery (TSS) along with steroids. The resolution of sellar mass was seen in two cases, one managed with TSS while other conservatively (Table 1).

4. Discussion

We report a case of pituitary apoplexy secondary to thrombocytopenia caused by precursor B-cell acute lymphoblastic leukemia.

PA is characterized by sudden hemorrhagic infarction in a pituitary adenoma. This results in an increase in intrasellar pressure leading to a constellation of symptoms that often but not always comprise headache, nausea, vomiting, decreased vision, and diplopia. Rarely, it may lead to meningismus (secondary to extravasation of blood in subarachnoid space), hemiplegia, hypotension, and altered sensorium. True apoplexy (clinical symptoms plus radiological evidence of pituitary hemorrhage) is an uncommon event occurring in 2 to 10% of pituitary adenoma [1]. In a majority of the cases, the event is spontaneous; however, a precipitating cause is identified in 25–30% patients. Various precipitating causes reported include hypertension, hypotension, major surgery, head trauma, radiation, drugs

Table 1: Cases of pituitary apoplexy secondary to underlying haematological malignancy.

Author	N. Wongraparut et al.	Yoshinori Maki et al.	Khaled M. Krisht et al.	L. Silberstein et al.	C. C. Kingdon et al.
Age/gender	72/F	64/F	77/M	55/M	61/M
Pituitary adenoma type	Nonfunctioning	Prolactinoma	Prolactinoma	Nonfunctioning	NA
Haematological malignancy	Acute myeloid leukaemia (subtype M5B)	Chronic myeloid leukaemia	Chronic lymphoid leukaemia	Acute myeloid leukaemia	Chronic lymphoid leukaemia
Diagnosis of apoplexy preceding haematological malignancy	No	No	No	No	Yes
Platelet count	13×10^9/L	29×10^9/L	NA	19×10^9/L	NA
Chemotherapy	High-dose cytarabine	Cabergoline	Warfarin	NA	NA
Clinical presentation	Headache, vomiting, hypotension, b/l visual field deficit, and impairment in visual acuity	Headache, vomiting, hypotension, Rt ptosis, and Lt abducens nerve palsy	Headache, vomiting, left complete ophthalmoplegia, and diminished sensation in V1 and V2	Headache, vomiting, fever, and meningismus	Headache, fever, and altered sensorium
Lag time	12 hours	NA*	48 hours	In hospital (day 6 of chemotherapy)	6 weeks
Hormone dysfunction	Hypothyroidism; hypoprolactinemia		Hypothyroidism; hypocortisolism	Hypothyroidism Hypocortisolism Hypogonadism	NA
Size of pituitary mass	1×1×1 cm	NA	4 × 3.7 × 3.7 cm	NA	NA
Management	TSS# + steroids	TSS + steroids	TSS + steroids	Conservative	Conservative
Resolution of mass size	NA	Yes	NA	Yes	NA
Resolution of					
1. Visual field deficit	NA	NA	NA	NA	NA
2. Visual acuity deficit	Improved	Improved	NA	NA	NA
3.Ocular paresis	NA	Resolved	Improved	NA	NA

*NA: not available; #TSS: transsphenoidal surgery.

(bromocriptne, cabergoline, antiplatelet agents, and anticoagulants), endocrine anterior pituitary stimulation test, and thrombocytopenia [4]. The two major mechanisms by which these factors cause apoplexy are either by causing acute fluctuations in blood pressure or by increasing the bleeding tendency. The pituitary gland being a neuroendocrine organ has a rich venous plexus blood supply network which predisposes it to a hemorrhagic event in response to the abovementioned stressors [4].

Thrombocytopenia leading to PA is a relatively uncommon event, and in a majority of such cases, it is either idiopathic or secondary to an underlying infection such as dengue hemorrhagic fever. To the best of our knowledge, only five cases of PA resulting from a haematological malignancy-induced thrombocytopenia have been reported so far (Table 1) [5–9]. The age of presentation was from the 5th to 7th decade, and they were either prolactinoma or nonfunctioning. In a majority of them, thrombocytopenia was a consequence of chemotherapy for the underlying malignancy and all had a platelet count of less than 30×10^9/L at presentation. Our case had a nonfunctioning pituitary adenoma and presented in the 6th decade with a platelet count of 23×10^9/L. However, it was unusual in that the apoplexy event was the presenting manifestation of an underlying haematological malignancy and highlights the importance of keeping this rare possibility in a case of PA with thrombocytopenia. Furthermore, the possibility of leukemic malignant cell infiltration into the pituitary adenoma cannot be ruled out in the current case, a rare but known event [7]. However, the presence of gynaecomastia suggestive of longstanding hypogonadism and optic atrophy indicates that pituitary adenoma has likely preceded the development of precursor B-cell lineage acute lymphoblastic leukaemia.

Another important issue pertains to the management of PA in the setting of thrombocytopenia. Both medical and surgical treatments are available for management of PA. The aim of surgery is to decrease the intrasellar pressure in order to decompress the optic chiasma and the nerves in cavernous sinus. Except in a scenario of worsening neurological status in whom surgery is indicated, at present, there is no clear recommendation as to the mode of therapy with the best outcome [3]. Furthermore, the presence of thrombocytopenia increases the perioperative risk of hemorrhagic complications. Though there are no clear recommendations for preoperative platelet count for neurosurgical procedures, the platelet count should be more than 100×10^9/L [10]. In regard to long-term outcomes following endoscopic endonasal surgery, improvement in visual field and cranial nerve paresis is seen in 70 to 90% of the cases while hypopituitarism persists in majority [11–13]. Hence, one needs to balance the risk of perioperative hemorrhagic complications with that of uncertain long-term benefits of surgery in a case of PA with thrombocytopenia. In our patient, persistent thrombocytopenia despite platelet transfusion, intact sensorium, an improving external ophthalmoplegia, and vision in response to dexamethasone made us decide in favour of medical management. In this regard, a comprehensive evaluation by a team comprising of endocrinologists, haematologists, and neurosurgeons is of utmost importance for timely diagnosis and optimal patient outcome.

5. Conclusions

In a case of pituitary apoplexy associated with thrombocytopenia, a systematic evaluation for the cause of the latter is required. The selection of the management modality in such cases should balance the risk of perioperative hemorrhagic complications with that of uncertain long-term benefits of surgery, and such cases are likely to be better managed by a multidisciplinary team.

Disclosure

Rahul Gupta and Urmimala Bhattacharjee are co-first authors.

References

[1] R. N. Nawar, D. AbdelMannan, W. R. Selman, and B. M. Arafah, "Analytic review: pituitary tumor apoplexy: a review," *Journal of Intensive Care Medicine*, vol. 23, no. 2, pp. 75–90, 2008.

[2] C. Briet, S. Salenave, J.-F. Bonneville, E. R. Laws, and P. Chanson, "Pituitary apoplexy," *Endocrine Reviews*, vol. 36, no. 6, pp. 622–645, 2015.

[3] S. Rajasekaran, M. Vanderpump, S. Baldeweg et al., "UK guidelines for the management of pituitary apoplexy," *Clinical Endocrinology*, vol. 74, no. 1, pp. 9–20, 2011.

[4] S. Murad-Kejbou and E. Eggenberger, "Pituitary apoplexy: evaluation, management, and prognosis," *Current Opinion in Ophthalmology*, vol. 20, no. 6, pp. 456–461, 2009.

[5] N. Wongpraparut, N. Pleanboonlers, P. Suwattee et al., "Pituitary apoplexy in a patient with acute myeloid leukemia," *Pituitary*, vol. 3, no. 2, pp. 113–116, 2000.

[6] Y. Maki, Y. Kurosaki, K. Uchino, R. Ishibashi, M. Chin, and S. Yamagata, "Pituitary apoplexy in long-term cabergoline user during thrombocytopenia due to chemotherapy for chronic myelocytic leukemia," *World Neurosurgery*, vol. 120, pp. 290–295, 2018.

[7] K. M. Krisht, C. A. Palmer, and W. T. Couldwell, "Combined chronic lymphocytic leukemia and prolactinoma: a rare occurrence in a patient presenting with pituitary apoplexy," *Journal of Neurosurgery*, vol. 119, no. 4, pp. 924–928, 2013.

[8] L. Silberstein, C. Johnston, A. Bhagat, L. Tibi, and J. Harrison, "Pituitary apoplexy during induction chemotherapy for acute myeloid leukaemia," *British Journal of Haematology*, vol. 143, no. 2, p. 151, 2008.

[9] C. Kingdon, P. Sidhu, and J. Cohen, "Pituitary apoplexy secondary to an underlying abscess," *Journal of Infection*, vol. 33, no. 1, pp. 53–55, 1996.

[10] D. Li, T. Glor, and G. A. Jones, "Thrombocytopenia and neurosurgery: a literature review," *World Neurosurgery*, vol. 106, pp. 277–280, 2017.

[11] D. J. Pangal, K. Chesney, Z. Memel et al., "Pituitary apoplexy case series: outcomes after endoscopic endonasal transsphenoidal surgery at a single tertiary center," *World Neurosurgery*, vol. 137, pp. e366–e372, 2020.

[12] M. Zoli, L. Milanese, M. Faustini-Fustini et al., "Endoscopic endonasal surgery for pituitary apoplexy: evidence on a 75-case series from a tertiary care center," *World Neurosurgery*, vol. 106, pp. 331–338, 2017.

[13] J. A. Gondim, L. A. F. de Albuquerque, J. P. Almeida et al., "Endoscopic endonasal surgery for treatment of pituitary apoplexy: 16 years of experience in a specialized pituitary center," *World Neurosurgery*, vol. 108, pp. 137–142, 2017.

Rare Association between Two Genetic Conditions: Turner Syndrome and Neurofibromatosis Type 1

R. El Qadiry, K. Danaoui, H. Nassih, A. Bourrahouat, and I. Ait Sab

Pediatric B Department, Mother-Child Pole, Mohammed VI University Hospital, Marrakesh, Morocco

Correspondence should be addressed to R. El Qadiry; rabiy.elqadiry@gmail.com

Academic Editor: Toshihiro Kita

Turner's syndrome (TS) is a sex chromosome disorder due to loss of either all or part of the X chromosome, in some or all the cells of the body. Neurofibromatosis type 1 (NF-1) is a multisystemic genetic disorder that is only rarely observed in association with Turner syndrome. Only six cases of Turner syndrome associated with NF-1 have been reported in the literature. In this study, we report the first case with TS and NF-1 in a Moroccan child. *Case Report*. A 16-year-old female was born of a nonconsanguineous marriage. In her family history, her mother had multiple café-au-lait spots with Lisch nodules on ophthalmologic examination. She was diagnosed with TS (karyotype: 45, X) due to short stature and characteristic features. The diagnosis of NF-1 was made according to the presence of four diagnostic criteria of the National Institute of Health Consensus Development Conference. *Conclusion*. Coexistence of NF-1 with TS is rare. We consider that this may be the seventh case report of TS associated with NF-1.

1. Introduction

Turner's syndrome (TS) occurs due to loss of either all or part of the X chromosome, in some or all the cells of the body with an incidence of at least 1 in 2500 live births. Short stature is a cardinal finding in all girls with TS [1].

Neurofibromatosis type 1 (NF-1) is an autosomal dominant disorder due to loss-of-function mutations in the tumor suppressor NF-1 gene. It is characterized particularly by café-au-lait spots and fibromatous tumors of the skin [2].

NF-1 is rarely observed in association with Turner syndrome. Only six cases of TS associated with NF-1 have been reported in the literature. In this study, we report the first case with TS and NF-1 in a Moroccan child.

2. Case

A 16-year-old female was admitted to our department for evaluation of short stature and delayed puberty. She was born of a nonconsanguineous marriage, after an uncomplicated pregnancy via vaginal delivery. Psychomotor development was delayed. There was a positive history of congenital lymphedema and recurrent acute otitis media with normal hearing assessment. In her family history, her mother had multiple café-au-lait spots (Figure 1) with Lisch nodules on ophthalmologic examination.

The patient's weight was 21 kg (greater than 4 SD) and her height was 120 cm (greater than 4 SD). The physical examination revealed a webbed neck, shielded chest, a low posterior hair line, and scoliosis (Figure 2). She had stage 1 for both breast and pubic hair development on Tanner staging. Dermatological examination revealed more than 10 café-au-lait spots with diameter >0.5 cm, axillary and inguinal freckling (Figure 3). The patient did not have any neurofibroma. The mucous membranes were not affected. The rest of the clinical examinations were normal.

Investigations were ordered to confirm Turner syndrome as well as neurofibromatosis type 1. The primary laboratory profile included a complete blood count, fasting blood sugar, blood urea nitrogen and creatinine, liver function test, and lipid profile and was normal. Her FSH was 154.90 IU/l and LH was 27.4 IU/l. A karyotype analysis was done because the Turner stigmata revealed 45, X0.

The pertinent paraclinical studies, including echocardiography, celiac serology, and thyroid function test, were normal. Ultrasonography of the abdomen showed agenesis

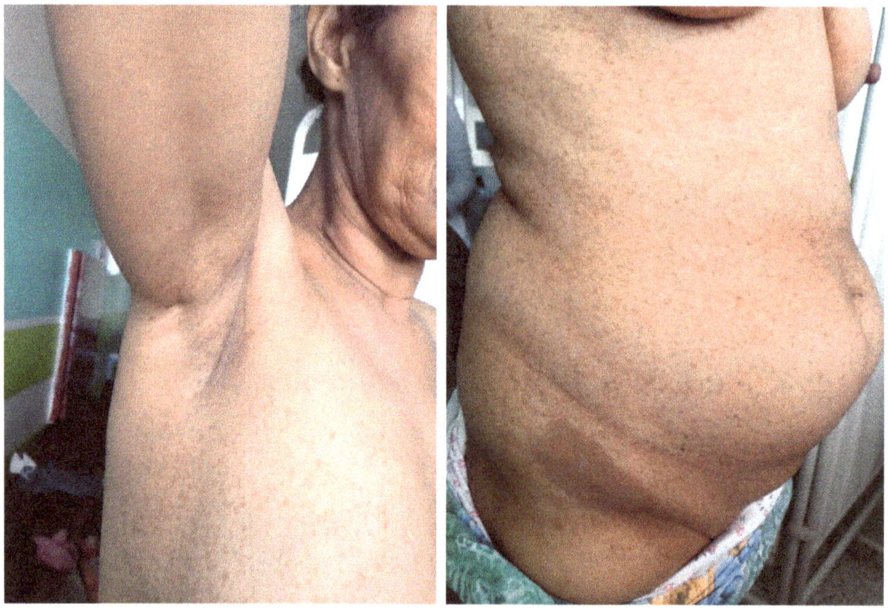

Figure 1: Hyperpigmented skin macules with multiple café-au-lait spots, axillary, and inguinal freckling in her mother.

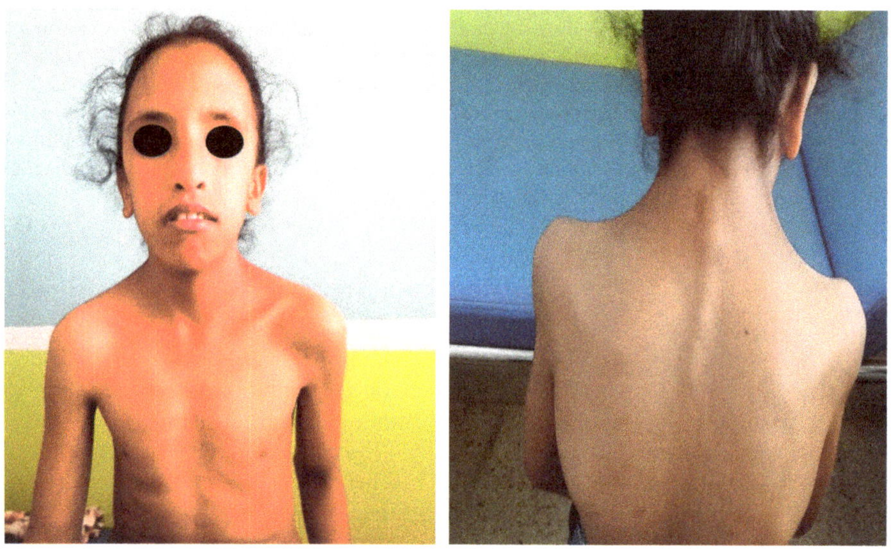

Figure 2: Characteristic appearance with webbed neck, shielded chest, and a low posterior hair line.

of gonads with hypoplastic uterus. Kidneys, ureters, and bladder were normal. Skeletal maturation, evaluated by a left wrist X-ray according to the technique of Greulich and Pyle, was 15 years. Serum IGF-1 level was within normal limits. A brain and pituitary MRI to exclude pituitary lesions or structural abnormalities showed normal results. Her eyes showed Lisch nodules without clinical visual involvement during ophthalmologic examinations (Figure 4).

A final diagnosis of Turner syndrome with neurofibromatosis type 1 was made according to the presence of four diagnostic criteria of the National Institute of Health Consensus Development Conference.

Because the patient had an advanced bone age (15 years) and the high risk of malignancy development, GH therapy was not administered. Hence, she was treated with estrogen replacement therapy, with periodic evaluations.

3. Discussion

There is a well-known association between NF-1 and Noonan syndrome-like manifestations, but there are a few cases reporting an association between NF-1 and Turner syndrome. Our patient is the seventh reported with clinical features of both NF-1 and TS.

Neurofibromatosis type 1 (NF-1) is the most common among the forms of neurofibromatosis (NF). Clinically, NF-1 is characterized by the presence of multiple (>6) café-au-lait spots and at least one of the following diagnostic criteria of the National Institute of Health Consensus Development Conference: axillary or groin freckling, Lisch nodules, optic glioma, cutaneous or subcutaneous neurofibromas, or first-degree relative with an NF-1 diagnosis. Our patient presents four signs of NF-1 [3].

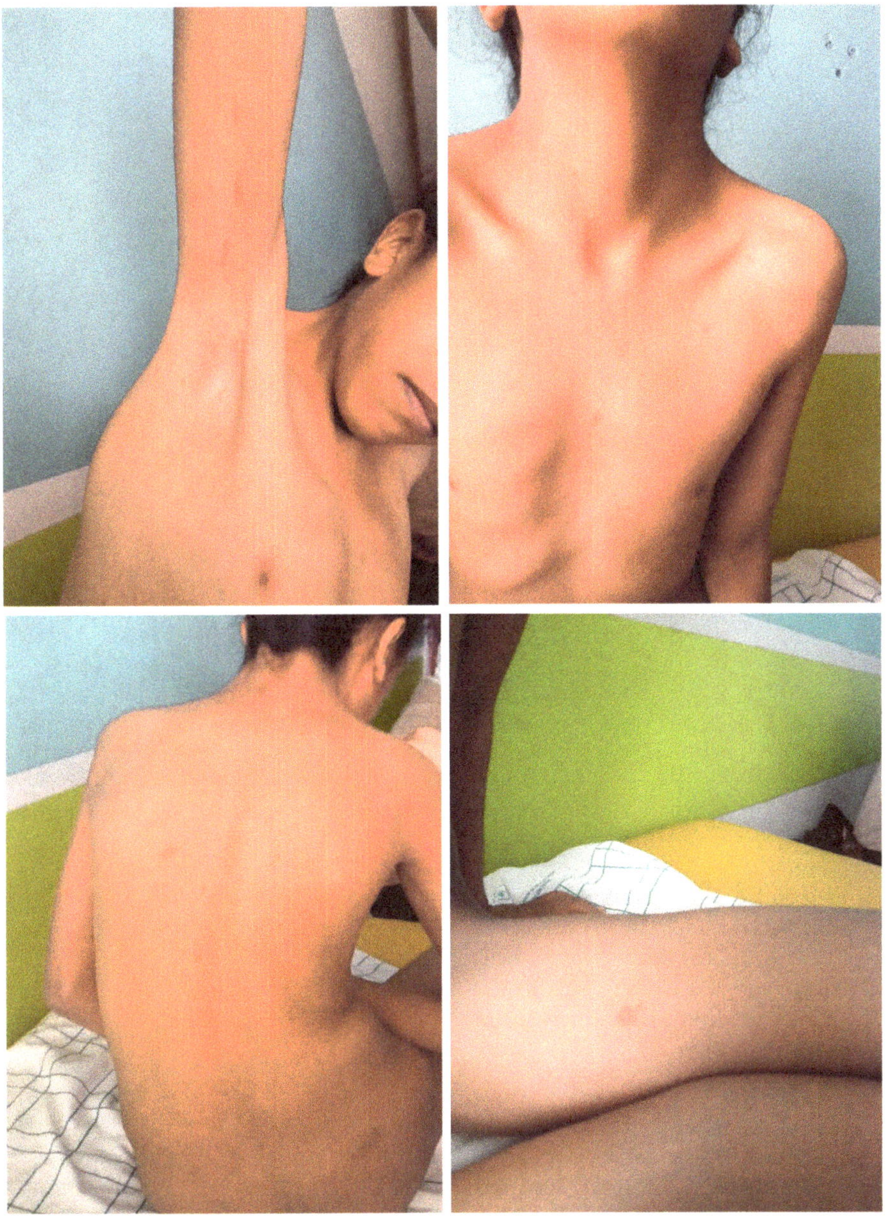

FIGURE 3: Hyperpigmented skin macules with multiple café-au-lait spots and axillary freckling in our patient.

NF-1 represents a major risk factor for development of malignancy, particularly malignant peripheral nerve sheath tumors and optic gliomas, and malignancy is an important component of the NF-1 phenotype and one of the few potentially fatal complications [4].

NF-1 is often associated with endocrine abnormalities and short stature. These abnormalities have been generally attributed to the presence of suprasellar or other brain lesions, which may cause growth hormone (GH) deficiency (GHD), scoliosis, and other skeletal problems that may interfere with normal skeletal development. In our patient, these risk factors were explored, and there was no GHD or intracranial lesion, except for mild scoliosis [5].

Turner syndrome is defined by a combination of phenotypic features that vary throughout a patient's life. The most common presentation for TS is short stature. The guidelines recommend screening if the girl has an unexplained short stature. Due to characteristic features like webbing of neck, low hair line, widely spaced nipple, and lack of breast development with elevated follicle-stimulating hormone levels with short stature, Turner syndrome was suspected and confirmed in our patient [6].

Earlier diagnosis of Turner syndrome has been shown to give the best chance for effective treatment and thus good clinical outcomes. It allows the timely introduction of recombinant human growth hormone (rhGH) to improve the height prior to estrogen therapy. Unfortunately, the diagnosis in our patient is made at the age of sixteen years; the time gap to initiate rhGH therapy is missed [6].

Finally, there has been a long-standing concern about the safety of GH treatment in NF-1 patients. It has been pointed out that rhGH treatment, at the dose recommended in GH

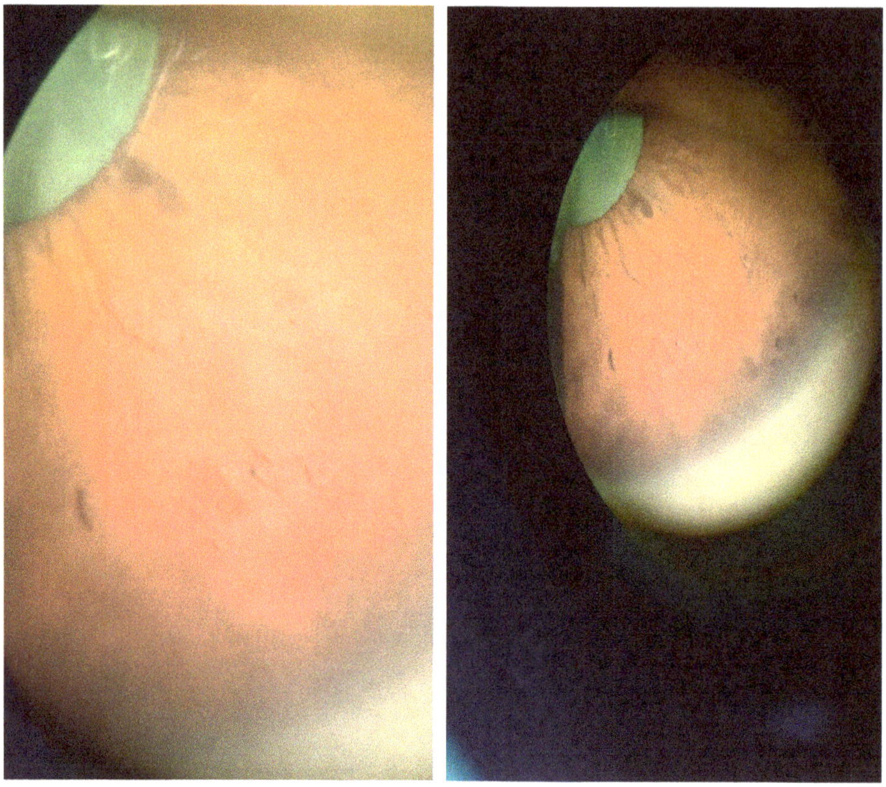

Figure 4: Lisch nodules without clinical visual involvement on ophthalmologic examination.

deficiency, is well tolerated and does not influence the incidence of intracranial tumor development in NF-1 patients. Although these observations on a large number of patients are reassuring, there remains the problem of the high dose of rhGH recommended in Turner syndrome with inherent risk of malignancy [7].

4. Conclusion

Coexistence of NF-1 with TS is rare. Thus, these disorders may be overlapping. We therefore emphasize that each patient with Turner-like symptoms should be carefully examined for café-au-lait macules. The decision to treat with GH a condition such as NF-1, generally associated with inherent risk of malignancy, is challenging, especially in our context.

References

[1] N. Gengel and I. Marshall, "Rare presentation of neurofibromatosis and turner syndrome in a pediatric patient," *Pediatric Reports*, vol. 9, no. 2, p. 6810, 2017.

[2] C. Sayah, M. Benmahmoud, S. Ait Yahia, and Z. Soualili, "Neurofibromatosis type 1 (NF1): case report and review of literature," *Journal of Childhood & Developmental Disorders*, vol. 2, no. 3, p. 3, 2016.

[3] M. L. Iezzi, G. Varriale, L. Zagaroli, M. Greco, S. Lasorella, and A. Verrotti di Pianella, "Growth hormone deficit as a first clinical manifestation of early diffuse cerebral glioma in patient with neurofibromatosis," *Annals of Clinical and Laboratory Research*, vol. 5, p. 1, 2017.

[4] B. R. Korf, "Malignancy in neurofibromatosis type 1," *The Oncologist*, vol. 5, no. 6, pp. 477–485, 2000.

[5] R. Vassilopoulou-Sellin, M. J. Klein, and J. K. Slopis, "Growth hormone deficiency in children with neurofibromatosis type 1 without suprasellar lesions," *Pediatric Neurology*, vol. 22, no. 5, pp. 355–358, 2000.

[6] L. Apperley, U. Das, R. Ramakrishnan et al., "Mode of clinical presentation and delayed diagnosis of turner syndrome: a single centre UK study," *International Journal of Pediatric Endocrinology*, vol. 2018, no. 1, p. 4, 2018.

[7] S. J. Howell, P. Wilton, A. Lindberg, and S. M. Shalet, "Growth hormone and neurofibromatosis," *Hormone Research*, vol. 53, no. Suppl 1, pp. 70–76, 2000.

Pregnancy in a Transgender Male: A Case Report and Review of the Literature

Ayesha Hassan,[1] Jessica Perini,[2] Amna Khan,[3] and Apoorva Iyer[1]

[1]*Department of Internal Medicine, West Virginia University Hospital, Morgantown, WV, USA*
[2]*Department of Endocrinology and Metabolism, West Virginia University Hospital, Morgantown, WV, USA*
[3]*Avalon University of Medicine, Youngstown, OH, USA*

Correspondence should be addressed to Ayesha Hassan; ayesha.hassan@hsc.wvu.edu

Academic Editor: Suat Simsek

Introduction. Pregnancy in transgender men is an area of increasing study due to data showing that pregnancy can occur in this population despite the reduction in fertility that generally accompanies treatment with gender-affirming hormone therapies. *Case.* In this case, we describe a healthy 21-year-old transgender man who was able to achieve pregnancy without reproductive assistance after stopping his testosterone therapy for 2 months. *Discussion.* Our case is important as it highlights how little is known in regards to gender-affirming hormone therapy on fertility. While testosterone is known to reduce fertility by inducing anovulation and altering ovarian histology, its long-term effects on conception rates and pregnancy are largely unknown. Some studies demonstrate that transgender men, treated with gender-affirming hormone therapy (GAHT), including testosterone, have similar oocyte quantity and quality, as well as similar ovarian reserve, when compared to cisgender women, suggesting that resumption of fertility may be possible after cessation of GAHT. Long-term outcomes for the pregnancy and the offspring of those who have been treated with GAHT are unknown. *Conclusion.* Recent studies have shown that pregnancy is possible for transgender men who desire biological children and have received gender-affirming hormonal therapy without fertility-preserving measures. Further research is needed to help determine rates of fertility, the likelihood of recovery of fertility, conception rates, and long-term pregnancy outcomes. Such information would help guide physicians in providing education and counseling to their transgender patients regarding reproductive options.

1. Introduction

Gender-affirming hormone therapy (GAHT) in transgender men lowers fertility rates. Nevertheless, many transgender individuals are able to achieve pregnancy. Transgender male pregnancy is a topic that is becoming increasingly prevalent in medical literature. However, many areas pertaining to this topic still require further study.

2. Case Presentation

A 21-year-old transgender man who had been prescribed gender-affirming hormone therapy for over two years presented to his follow-up appointment at 17 weeks pregnant. Past medical history included ADHD, asthma, and gender dysphoria. Home medications included albuterol and weekly intramuscular depo-testosterone 100 mg injections, which he had been taking consistently for 2 years prior to conceiving. The gynecological history was unremarkable, and menses had stopped one month after starting testosterone therapy. Testosterone measurements on routine labs performed every 3 to 6 months over the preceding 2 years for the purpose of monitoring testosterone levels had consistently shown levels within the mid-normal range for men.

The patient had stopped his testosterone therapy 2 months prior to conceiving, with the intention of trying to become pregnant. He had a menstrual period one month after discontinuing his testosterone therapy, and the following month a pregnancy test was positive. Pregnancy was achieved through vaginal intercourse with the patient's healthy cismale partner.

TABLE 1

Gender-affirming therapy	Dosing Frequency	Advantages	Disadvantages
Intramuscular testosterone	Every 1 or 2 weeks	Better compliance than topical due to less frequent dosage	Fluctuating testosterone levels, injection complications
Subcutaneous testosterone	Bi-weekly or weekly	Better compliance than topical, with a shorter needle than IM forms	Fluctuating testosterone levels, not approved in USA
Testosterone gel	Daily	Ease of application, and less variation in testosterone levels	Slower masculinization than IM or SC, potential transfer with contact
Testosterone patch	Daily	Ease of application, and less variation in testosterone levels	Skin irritation, and lower testosterone levels than gel

Prior to starting GAHT, the patient had been counseled about reduced fertility with hormone therapy and was given a referral to reproductive endocrinology; however, at that time, he had not desired future pregnancy and did not undergo any fertility-preserving measures.

Neither the patient nor his partner received any reproductive assistance, and the patient underwent pregnancy without any significant complications and successfully delivered a healthy baby girl via *C*-section.

3. Discussion

Our case report is important because minimal and conflicting data exist regarding fertility, conception rates, and pregnancy in transgender men. Our case report questions the commonly held belief that transgender male pregnancy is highly difficult in people receiving GAHT who have not received fertility preservation. Although many transgender men use gender-affirming hormone therapy to masculinize body parts and align their physical appearance more with their gender identity, the majority retain their uterus and ovaries [1, 2]. One of the effects of GAHT is the cessation of menstrual cycles, which generally occurs within the first few months of medication use. It is not known to what degree fertility can be restored after the cessation of GAHT.

Exogenous testosterone therapy, a mainstay of treatment for transgender men, is associated with reduced fertility rates. Testosterone therapy reduces fertility by negative feedback to the hypothalamus and pituitary, suppressing LH and FSH, thereby inhibiting ovulation and leading to amenorrhea. One study showed that testosterone rapidly induces hypothalamic-pituitary-gonadal suppression and induces anovulation. This study also showed, however, that individuals can break through their hormonal suppression, even after long-term use, and experience dysfunctional ovulation [3] Table 1.

Testosterone Formulations Hembree W. C., Cohen-Kettenis P. T., Gooren L., et al. Endocrine treatment of gender-dysphoric/gender-incongruent persons: an Endocrine Society* clinical practice guideline. J Clin Endocrinol Metab 2017; 102:1.

Long-term testosterone therapy has also been associated with altered ovarian histology [4]. One study done in 2010 looked at the ovarian morphology of 112 transgender men who had undergone hysterectomy with bilateral oophorectomy. All had been treated with testosterone therapy for at least 6 months. Evaluation of the ovaries revealed collagenization of the outer cortex, luteinization of stroma cells, stromal hyperplasia, and multifollicular ovaries, typical of polycystic ovarian morphology [5]. Due to these potential effects of GAHT, fertility-preserving measures, such as ovarian tissue cryopreservation, are offered to transgender male patients who desire future pregnancy.

While testosterone has historically been thought to significantly reduce fertility rates, recent studies have shown that conception after receiving long-term exogenous testosterone is possible. A study done in 2019 compared the success of assisted reproductive technology in transgender men who stopped testosterone for 4 months to ciswomen, and showed similar oocyte quality and quantity in both groups after receiving ovarian stimulation [6].

While the effect of long-term testosterone therapy on fertility is not known, transgender men who have received 1 year of testosterone therapy appear to have preserved functional ovarian reserve. These individuals have normal anti-Mullerian hormone levels and preserved antral follicle counts, indicating that they still have ovarian reserve and preserved ovarian function [7].

4. Conclusion

Many areas pertaining to the effects of gender-affirming therapy on long-term fertility still require further research. Many studies have shown conflicting data regarding the possibility of pregnancy after receiving gender-affirming therapy. While it was previously thought that conception after receiving hormonal therapy was nearly impossible, many recent studies, including ours, have refuted this claim. Transgender patients should be counseled about fertility-preserving measures prior to hormonal therapy due to the lack of clear data about the effects of long-term hormonal therapy on fertility. New data, however, does provide hope to transgender people who desire biological children and did not undergo fertility preservation therapies prior to starting GAHT. This is exciting and positive news for doctors as well as for patients, as recent data has shown that many transgender individuals do desire to have biological children [7, 8].

Furthermore, increasing evidence that pregnancy is possible in transgender individuals highlights the importance of counseling these patients about contraception to avoid an unwanted pregnancy. Unplanned pregnancies have occurred in transgender male patients, and contraception is often an area overlooked by many health care professionals when treating transgender patients [9].

Our study also highlights the importance of counseling patients on gender-affirming hormone therapy to recognize pregnancy if it occurs, as many medications used to affirm gender have teratogenic side effects. High levels of testosterone during pregnancy have been associated with fetal growth restriction and cardiovascular and metabolic syndrome in the baby and mother [10]. Exogenous testosterone can also be associated with urogenital abnormalities in female fetuses [11]. It is important to discontinue testosterone therapy during pregnancy to avoid these complications.

There has been an increase in studies regarding transgender individuals, with increasing societal acceptance of these individuals. An area that is increasingly being studied and documented in medical literature is transgender pregnancy. Despite this, many areas pertaining to this require further study, such as the long-term effect of testosterone therapy on fertility rates, adverse effects of testosterone on the fetus, and the average time to conception in transgender males.

Very little systemic data exists overall regarding this topic, and further study would not only be greatly beneficial in aiding physicians in providing better care for these patients, but also in aiding patients in making important decisions related to their fertility. This case highlights that transgender male pregnancy is possible and also reflects areas pertaining to this topic that require further study.

References

[1] C. Unger, "Hormone therapy for transgender patients," *Translational Andrology and Urology*, vol. 5, no. 6, pp. 877–884, 2016.

[2] A. Hoffkling, J. Obedin-Maliver, and J. Sevelius, "From erasure to opportunity: a qualitative study of the experiences of transgender men around pregnancy and recommendations for providers," *BMC Pregnancy and Childbirth*, vol. 17, no. 332, p. 332, 2017.

[3] R. Taub, S. Ellis, G. Neal-Perry, A. Magaret, S. Prager, and E. Micks, "The effect of testosterone on ovulatory function in transmasculine individuals," *American Journal of Obstetrics and Gynecology*, vol. 223, no. 2, pp. 229–e8, 2020.

[4] P. Cheng, A. Pastuszak, J. Myers, I. Goodwin, and J. Hotaling, "Fertility concerns of the transgender patient," *Translational Andrology and Urology*, vol. 8, no. 3, pp. 209–218, 2019.

[5] M. Grynberg, R. Fanchin, G. Dubost et al., "Histology of genital tract and breast tissue after long-term testosterone administration in a female-to-male transsexual population," *Reproductive BioMedicine Online*, vol. 20, no. 4, pp. 553–558, 2010.

[6] A. Leung, D. Sakkas, S. Pang, K. Thornton, and N. Resetkova, "Assisted reproductive technology outcomes in female-to-male transgender patients compared with cisgender patients: a new Frontier in reproductive medicine," *Fertility and Sterility*, vol. 112, no. 5, pp. 858–865, 2019.

[7] I. Yaish, K. Tordjman, H. Amir et al., "Functional ovarian reserve in transgender men receiving testosterone therapy: evidence for preserved anti-müllerian hormone and antral follicle count under prolonged treatment," *Human Reproduction*, vol. 36, no. 10, pp. 2753–2760, 2021.

[8] A. Light, J. Obedin-Maliver, J. Sevelius, and J. Kerns, "Transgender men who experienced pregnancy after female-to-male gender transitioning," *Obstetrics & Gynecology*, vol. 124, no. 6, pp. 1120–1127, 2014.

[9] L. Abern and K. Maguire, "Contraception knowledge in transgender individuals: are we doing enough?" *Obstetrics & Gynecology*, vol. 131, p. 655, 2018.

[10] K. Sathishkumar, R. Elkins, V. Chinnathambi, H. Gao, G. D. Hankins, and C. Yallampalli, "Prenatal testosterone-induced fetal growth restriction is associated with down-regulation of rat placental amino acid transport," *Reproductive Biology and Endocrinology*, vol. 9, no. 1, p. 110, 2011.

[11] F. Thornton and K. Mattatall, "Pregnancy in transgender men," *Canadian Medical Association Journal*, vol. 193, no. 33, p. E1303, 2021.

32

Spontaneous Adrenal Hemorrhage with Mild Hypoadrenalism in a Patient Anticoagulated with Apixaban for Antiphospholipid Syndrome: A Case Report and Literature Review

Jia Wei Tan,[1] **Anant Shukla**,[1] **Jiun-Ruey Hu**,[2] **and Sachin K. Majumdar**[1,3]

[1]*Department of Internal Medicine, Yale New Haven Health, Bridgeport Hospital, Bridgeport, CT, USA*
[2]*Section of Cardiovascular Medicine, Department of Internal Medicine, Yale School of Medicine, New Haven, CT 06510, USA*
[3]*Department of Endocrinology, Yale New Haven Health, Bridgeport Hospital, Bridgeport, CT, USA*

Correspondence should be addressed to Jia Wei Tan; jia.tan094@gmail.com

Academic Editor: Wayne V. Moore

Background. Adrenal hemorrhage (AH) is a serious endocrine complication of antiphospholipid syndrome (APLS). *Case Presentation.* We report a 45-year-old man who presented with several deep venous thromboses and was initially treated with apixaban, who later developed bilateral AH. Laboratory findings were consistent with cortisol deficiency yet preserved aldosterone physiology. He was diagnosed with APLS and treated with warfarin. After 8 months of follow-up, he remained on cortisol replacement with no evidence of recovery. We reviewed PubMed/MEDLINE indexed articles from 1950 to 2022 for cases of AH in APLS patients on anticoagulation. Six cases of patients on direct oral anticoagulants (DOACs) were reported. *Discussion.* The unique vasculature of the adrenal glands creates a "functional vascular dam" in the zona reticularis, which is susceptible to thrombosis in situ and hemorrhage. DOACs may further increase the risk of AH. *Conclusion.* Depending on the degree of adrenal involvement in AH, patients can present with partial or complete primary adrenal insufficiency. More data are needed to characterize adrenal function after AH, and the safety of DOAC versus warfarin in patients with APLS warrants further studies.

1. Introduction

Primary adrenal insufficiency (PAI) is a rare and life-threatening complication of antiphospholipid syndrome (APLS). The pathophysiology of PAI is considered due to thrombosis from the underlying coagulopathy, with possible transformation into hemorrhagic infarction [1]. The destruction of the adrenal cortex secondary to thrombosis and/or hemorrhage can progress rapidly; however, the degree to which it may affect adrenal function can vary.

The use of a new generation of direct-acting oral anticoagulants (DOACs) has largely replaced warfarin in the management of hypercoagulable state. DOACs have predictable anticoagulation effects and do not require dose monitoring, unlike warfarin. The convenience of DOACs leads to a surge in their use. However, to date, there is not an adequately powered randomized control trial establishing DOAC safety in APLS.

Our aim is to present a case of AH in APLS on DOAC and review the existing literature to inform subsequent management.

2. Case Report

2.1. Case Presentation. A 45-year-old man without significant past medical history presented with a left lower extremity deep vein thrombosis (DVT) and pulmonary embolism (PE). He had no personal or family history of previous trauma, bleeding, or clotting events. He was discharged on apixaban.

Three days later, he was readmitted with bilateral flank pain. Abdominal CT (Figure 1) showed bilateral adrenal gland edema. He was hemodynamically stable. Due to persistent right flank pain and concern for ileus, an abdominal CT was repeated revealing enlarging adrenal glands

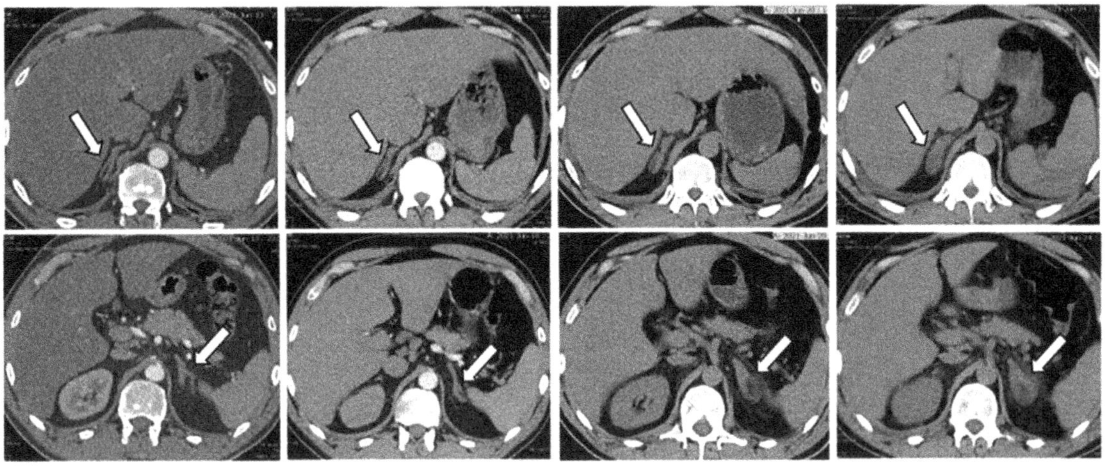

Figure 1: Evolution of the right (first row) and left (second row) adrenal gland enlargement.

concerning for AH (Figure 1). He subsequently complained of asthenia. Further tests revealed a reduced morning cortisol of 1.4 μg/dL (reference (ref): 6.0–18.4 μg/dL) and an elevated morning ACTH of 149 pg/mL (ref: 7.2–63.3 pg/mL). Plasma dehydroepiandrosterone sulphate (DHEA-S) was reduced at 39 mcg/dL (ref: 70–495 mcg/dL), and epinephrine and norepinephrine were undetectable. Plasma aldosterone in the morning was undetectable and renin activity was 0.76 ng/ml/h (ref: 0.25–5.82 ng/mL/h). He was started on stress dose steroids and discharged on maintenance hydrocortisone without reinitiating anticoagulation.

Two weeks later, he represented with a right lower extremity DVT. The APLS panel that was sent from prior admission resulted and revealed an anti-beta2 glycoprotein 1 IgG of 201 U/ml (ref: <7.0 U/mL) and anti-cardiolipin IgG of 56.4 GPL (ref: 0.0–23 GPL). He had a dilute Russell's viper venom (dRVV) normalized ratio of 3.08 (ref: ≤1.20) and silica clotting time (SCT) normalized ratio of 3.06 (ref: ≤ 1.20). Partial thrombin time (PTT) 1 : 1 mixing studies were performed. PTT at 0 seconds (s) was 36.2 s (ref: 22.0–35.0 s) and 38.7 s after 60 s, indicating the presence of lupus anticoagulant. Anti-nuclear antibody (ANA) titer was 1 : 40, and the anti-double stranded DNA antibody test was negative. Laboratory workup for other causes of thrombosis, including inherited and acquired thrombophilias, anatomical vascular obstruction, paroxysmal nocturnal hemoglobinuria (PNH), heparin-induced thrombocytopenia (HIT), and myeloproliferative neoplasms (MPN), was negative.

Warfarin was started with an international normalized ratio (INR) target range of 2-3. Hydrocortisone was continued at a total daily dose of 30 mg. Since discharge, with up to 8 months of follow-up, his morning cortisol levels prior to taking hydrocortisone have been low at 4.4–4.9 μg/dL and ACTH has remained high at 92–137 pg/mL, but aldosterone has been variable at <1 to 9 ng/dL, and renin has been normal at 0.35 ng/mL/h, while DHEA-S remains low. This suggests that what transpired was a microthrombi-associated intra-adrenal hemorrhage involving the zona fasciculata and possibly reticularis with preservation of the glomerulosa.

2.2. Methods. We reviewed all publications that reported the development of AH from 1989 to 2022. We searched MEDLINE and PubMed with the following phrases: "adrenal insufficiency," "adrenal hemorrhage," "addison disease," "antiphospholipid syndrome," "APLS," "novel oral anticoagulants," "direct-acting oral anticoagulants," "rivaroxaban," "apixaban," "edoxaban," "dabigatran," "coumadin," "warfarin," "vitamin K antagonist oral anticoagulants," and "heparin." References of retrieved articles were also examined for the key terms. Cases were analyzed with specific reference to patient demographics, clinical, laboratory, treatment, and outcome. Reports of non-APLS patients were excluded from the analysis.

2.3. Results. At the time of this writing, we found 8 cases [2–9] of AH in patients with APLS on anticoagulation (Table 1). Six out of 8 patients were on DOACs. The remaining 2 cases of AH were patients on warfarin, and their presenting INRs were supratherapeutic. All of the 8 patients were discharged on warfarin. Six out of 8 patients (75%) of these patients required corticosteroids and aldosterone at discharge. Long-term adrenal function is unknown.

3. Discussion

Adrenal hemorrhage (AH) is rare, with an estimated 15% mortality rate [10]. Risk factors for AH include anticoagulation therapy, recent surgery, tumor metastasis, corticotropin stimulation, adrenal tumor, physiological stress (trauma and burns), severe sepsis, and APLS [1].

The incidence of adrenal insufficiency in APLS is 0.4% [11]. In a series of 69 APLS patients with adrenal involvement who underwent CT and/or MRI, 57% had AH, whereas 10% had adrenal infarction, and 10% had adrenal enlargement. Adrenal involvement was bilateral in 77% of the patients [1].

Although APLS is a hypercoagulable state, biopsy (autopsy in 16 patients) in 22 APLS patients with adrenal insufficiency revealed hemorrhagic infarction with vessel

Table 1: Case reports of patients with adrenal hemorrhage while on anticoagulation for APLS.

Reference / Gender	Comuth et al. [2] Female	Lavoipierre [3] Male	Arosemena et al. [4] Male	Sanford et al. [5] Male	Bakhsh et al. [6] Female	DiCenso et al. [7] Male	Aneke and Gunendran [8] Female	Godfrey et al. [9] Female
Age (years)	63	47	46	42	40	46	53	68
Triple positive	Yes	Yes	NA	NA	NA	NA	NA	NA
Prior warfarin use	No	No	No	Yes	No	Yes	Current	Current
Type of DOAC	Rivaroxaban	Apixaban	Rivaroxaban	Apixaban	Rivaroxaban	Rivaroxaban	Warfarin	Warfarin
Duration of AC prior to admission	5 months	2 months	Few months	1 month	2 weeks	Unknown	7 years	Unknown
Clinical manifestations	LUQ abdominal pain, vomiting	Abdominal pain, livedo reticularis	Abdominal pain, nausea, weight loss	Fever, right flank pain	Severe RUQ pain, nausea	Abdominal pain, syncope	Nausea, vomiting, fever, rigors, R flank pain	Bilateral loin pain, vomiting, fever, confusion
Laboratory findings	K of 4.2 mmol/L and Na of 137 mmol/L		Na of 121 mmol/L, K of 5.4 mmol/L	NA	Renal function test reported normal	Na of 121 mmol/L, K of 5.5 mmol/L, random cortisol of 0.8 mcg/dL (22 nmol/L)	Na of 122, cortisol of 1.4 mcg/dL (40 nmol/L)	Na of 132, cortisol of 1.7 mcg/dL (48 nmol/L)
CT findings	Dilatation of both adrenal glands	Bilateral adrenal hematomas	Bilateral adrenal hemorrhage	Right-sided adrenal hemorrhage	Enlargement of the right adrenal gland	Thickening of the adrenal glands	Bilateral adrenal hemorrhage	Bilateral heterogenous adrenal pathology
MRI findings	Unknown	Unknown	T1 signal in the region of bilateral adrenal glands	Unknown	Unknown	T1 hyper-intensity of the bilateral adrenal glands	No	No
ACTH stimulation	Positive	Positive	NA	NA	NA	NA	NA	NA
Treatment	Methylpred 40 mg IV-switched to HC (dose/duration unknown)	HC + fludrocortisone	HC 50 mg q 6 hr + fludrocortisone 0.1 mg daily	Unknown	Methylpred 1.5 mg/kg	HC 50 mg IV every 8 hours	IV HC	IV HC 100 mg q 6 h->switched to oral HC + fludrocortisone
Medication upon discharge	Unknown	HC + fludrocortisone	HC 15 mg in AM and 10 mg in PM fludro 0.1 mg daily	Unknown	Unknown	HC + fludrocortisone	Oral HC-reducing doses to reach target dose: 10 mg AM, 5 mg noon, 5 mg night	HC + fludrocortisone
Anticoagulation upon discharge	Dalteparin 15.000 IE daily-switched to warfarin after a month (unknown target INR)	Warfarin	Warfarin (unknown target INR)	Warfarin (target INR 2.5–3.5)	Warfarin (target INR 2–2.5)	Unknown	Fondaparinux-switched back to warfarin after 5 days	Unknown

N/A: not applicable, DOAC: direct oral anticoagulant, Na: sodium, K: potassium, LUQ: left upper quadrant, Methylpred: methylprednisolone, HC: hydrocortisone, and IV: intravenous.

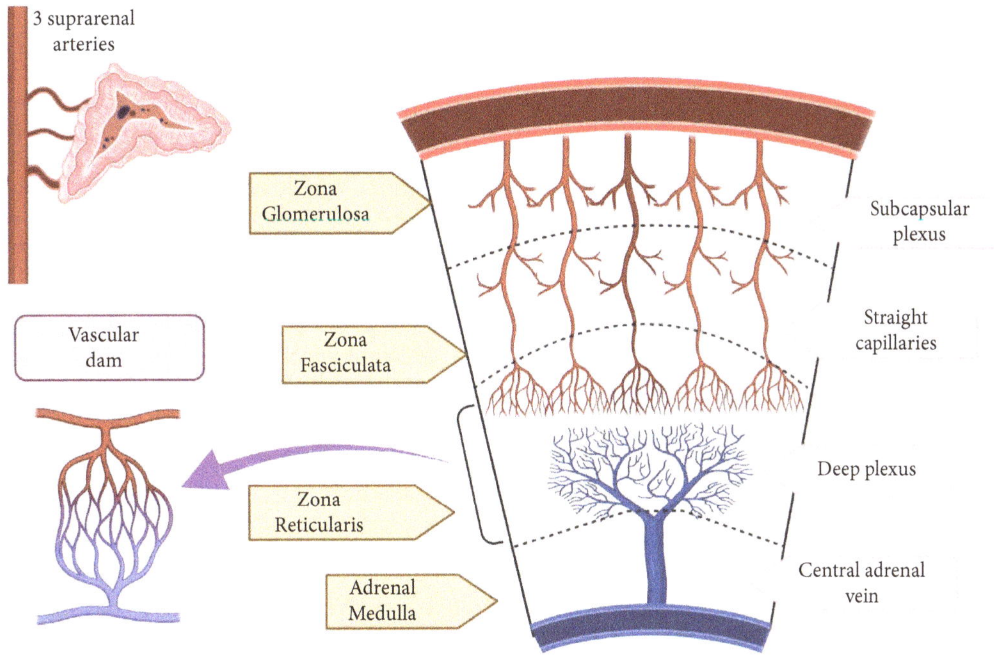

Figure 2: Adrenal gland circulation illustrating the abrupt transition from multiple arteries into capillary plexus, forming the "vascular dam" that increases risk of thrombotic hemorrhagic infarction.

thrombosis as the most frequent finding, present in 55% of patients. This is followed by adrenal hemorrhage in 27%, adrenal infarction in 5%, and normal appearance in 9% of patients [1]. These findings support the notion that in most of the cases of PAI in APLS, the primary event is adrenal vein thrombosis followed by hemorrhagic transformation.

The central pathophysiology of adrenal vein thrombosis is based on its unique vascular anatomy (Figure 2). The adrenal gland is highly vascular, with three main arteries but only one vein. The adrenal arteries branch into capillaries that form a vascular plexus around the zona reticularis. The abrupt transition of the artery-capillary plexus is referred to as a "vascular dam." Venous stasis and hypercoagulability in this region can promote thrombosis, infarction, and subsequent hemorrhage. The capillary plexus eventually empties into medullary sinusoids that form a single central vein.

Additionally, the musculature of the vein is arranged eccentrically and composed of thick longitudinal muscle bundles. This favors the formation of thrombi in pockets of local stasis emerging from their contraction. The zona reticularis may be more severely affected compared to zona glomerulosa and fasciculata that are located further away from the vascular dam.

In our case, the diagnosis of adrenal hemorrhage was discovered on CT imaging incidentally showing adrenal congestion with evidence of mild hemorrhage. The diffuse thickening of the glands and adrenal enlargement has been reported as a precursor of adrenal hemorrhage [10, 12–14]. A high index of suspicion is needed, and any clinical indicators of acute adrenal insufficiency should prompt immediate measurement of cortisol and ACTH. Additional laboratory tests may be helpful to support the diagnosis of adrenal insufficiency and include DHEAS, aldosterone, and renin activity. It is not clear what the role of catecholamine measurement would be in these circumstances, but epinephrine production may be most noticeable as it is secreted from the medulla and depends on intra-adrenal cortisol for its synthesis. Norepinephrine may be of less value since it is also produced extra adrenally. What remains uncertain is whether recovery of adrenal function is possible in cases such as ours where there is evidence of partially preserved adrenal function.

The choice of anticoagulant in APLS may be relevant to the risk of developing AH, yet only a few case reports are available and thus one can only hypothesize that warfarin may confer less risk of AH in comparison to DOACs. It has also been reported that APLS patients developed catastrophic APLS (CAPS) after switching to DOAC from warfarin [15, 16]. Notably, they were all triple-positive APLS. AH also occurred in non-APLS patients taking DOACs [17–19].

Currently, the evidence for secondary prevention of thrombotic events in patients with APLS using DOACs is mixed [20]. Our patient had triple-positive APLS developed VTE during DOAC treatment. The risk of thrombosis with DOACs use may be stratified by the patient's APLS antibody status. In a recent retrospective study, the rate of venous thromboembolism or bleeding events with DOAC (apixaban or rivaroxaban) use among single-positive APLS patients is not significantly different from those treated with warfarin [21]. The European League Against Rheumatism (EULAR) suggests against DOAC use in triple-positive APLS [22]. Warfarin should remain the as the reference anticoagulation until further evidence regarding the safety of DOACs in APLS is available.

There is a lack of information on the course of adrenal recovery when AH occurs, particularly when there is evidence of partial preservation of function, when aldosterone appears preserved with mild to moderate deficiencies in cortisol, adrenal androgens, and possibly catecholamines. Therefore, close follow-up with periodic assessment of the HPA axis and empiric steroid replacement therapy is reasonable, and long-term outcome reporting should be encouraged to obtain prognostic information.

4. Conclusion

This case highlights that hypoadrenalism can be one of the complications of APLS, and the risk of AH might be heightened with DOAC use. Patients may have partially preserved adrenal function depending on the extent of adrenal involvement in AH, and biochemical and imaging evaluation is important for diagnostic and perhaps prognostic purposes. Hormonal replacement should be guided by clinical and biochemical findings as is typically done for the management of adrenal insufficiency with periodic assessment for recovery. Until further evidence is available for DOAC use in APLS, warfarin should be the first-line anticoagulation treatment.

Abbreviations

AH: Adrenal hemorrhage
PAI: Primary adrenal insufficiency
MPN: Myeloproliferative neoplasms.
DOAC: Direct oral anticoagulant
APLS: Antiphospholipid syndrome
CAPS: Catastrophic antiphospholipid syndrome
EULAR: European league against rheumatism
HPA: Hypothalamus pituitary axis
DVT: Deep vein thrombosis
PE: Pulmonary embolism
ACTH: Adrenocorticotropic hormone

Disclosure

This case was presented as an abstract and poster presentation at the Endocrine Society meeting in Atlanta, GA, 2022.

References

[1] G. Espinosa, E. Santos, R. Cervera et al., "Adrenal involvement in the antiphospholipid syndrome: clinical and immunologic characteristics of 86 patients," *Medicine (Baltimore)*, vol. 82, no. 2, pp. 106–118, 2003.
[2] W. Comuth, J. J. Christiansen, A. M. Bloch-Münster, and S. Husted, "Bilateral adrenal gland hemorrhage in a patient treated with rivaroxaban," *Blood Coagulation and Fibrinolysis*, vol. 28, no. 1, pp. 102–104, 2017.
[3] V. Lavoipierre, M. Talbot, C. Soubrier et al., "Bilateral adrenal hemorrhage under apixaban in primary antiphospholipid syndrome," *La Revue de Medecine Interne*, vol. 41, no. 7, pp. 489–492, 2020.
[4] M. A. Arosemena, A. Rodriguez, and H. Ediriweera, "Bilateral adrenal haemorrhage secondary to rivaroxaban in a patient with antiphospholipid syndrome," *BMJ Case Reports*, vol. 13, no. 7, p. e234947, Article ID e234947, 2020.
[5] Z. Sanford, A. Nanjundappa, F. H. Annie, and S. Embrey, "Adrenal hemorrhage in a patient anticoagulated with apixaban with antiphospholipid syndrome," *Cureus*, vol. 11, no. 7, p. e5108, 2019.
[6] E. A. Bakhsh, R. A. Alkhathami, S. Mukaddam, and O. Alarfaj, "Bilateral adrenal hemorrhage in APLS (anti-phospholipid syndrome) patient on Novel Anticoagulant: a case report," *European Journal of Medical Case Reports*, vol. 1, no. 1, pp. 48–51, 2017.
[7] D. M. DiCenso, C. A. Penaherrera, and A. Ayala, "SUN-192 spontaneous adrenal hemorrhage in a patient with antiphospholipid syndrome on rivaroxaban: a potentially fatal complication," *Journal of the Endocrine Society*, vol. 4, no. Supplement_1, 2020.
[8] I. A. Aneke and T. Gunendran, "The role of vitamin K in the non-operative management of bilateral adrenal hemorrhage on a background of antiphospholipid syndrome and coagulopathy: a case report," *Journal of Surgical Case Reports*, vol. 2021, no. 10, p. rjab440, Article ID rjab440, 2021.
[9] R. L. Godfrey, J. Clark, and B. Field, "Bilateral adrenal haemorrhagic infarction in a patient with antiphospholipid syndrome," *Case Reports*, vol. 2014, no. nov19 1, p. bcr2014207050, Article ID bcr2014207050, 2014.
[10] M. Di Serafino, R. Severino, V. Coppola et al., "Nontraumatic adrenal hemorrhage: the adrenal stress," *Radiology Case Reports*, vol. 12, no. 3, pp. 483–487, 2017.
[11] R. Cervera, J. C. Piette, J. Font et al., "Antiphospholipid syndrome: clinical and immunologic manifestations and patterns of disease expression in a cohort of 1, 000 patients," *Arthritis & Rheumatism*, vol. 46, no. 4, pp. 1019–1027, 2002.
[12] G. X. V. Tan and T. Sutherland, "Adrenal congestion preceding adrenal hemorrhage on CT imaging: a case series," *Abdom Radiol (NY)*, vol. 41, no. 2, pp. 303–310, 2016.
[13] R. Galatola, M. Gambardella, C. Mollica et al., "Precocious ischemia preceding bilateral adrenal hemorrhage: a case report," *Radiology Case Reports*, vol. 15, no. 6, pp. 803–807, 2020.
[14] S. A. Warriach, M. Mustafa, D. O'Keeffe, and M. Watts, "Unusual case of antiphospholipid syndrome presenting as adrenal insufficiency," *BMJ Case Reports*, vol. 13, no. 3, p. e233631, Article ID e233631, 2020.
[15] R. Stammler, P. Legendre, P. Cacoub, P. Blanche, J. C. Piette, and N. Costedoat-Chalumeau, "Catastrophic antiphospholipid syndrome following the introduction of rivaroxaban," *Lupus*, vol. 29, no. 7, pp. 787–790, 2020.
[16] M. P. Crowley, M. J. Cuadrado, and B. J. Hunt, "Catastrophic antiphospholipid syndrome on switching from warfarin to rivaroxaban," *Thrombosis Research*, vol. 153, pp. 37–39, 2017.
[17] M. Alidoost, R. Soomro, A. Gubeladze et al., "Rivaroxaban related bilateral adrenal hemorrhage: a rare complications of direct oral anticoagulants–a case reports," *Am J Case Rep*, vol. 20, pp. 1607–1611, 2019.
[18] B. Zampetti, R. Attanasio, and R. Cozzi, "Hyponatremia after anticoagulant treatment: a rare cause of adrenal failure," *Endocrinology, Diabetes & Metabolism Case Reports*, vol. 2018, p. 18-0101, 2018.

[19] B. A. Ly and L. Quintero, “Adrenal insufficiency from unilateral adrenal hemorrhage in a patient on rivaroxaban thromboprophylaxis,” *AACE Clinical Case Reports*, vol. 5, no. 1, pp. e70–e72, 2019.

[20] B. Kakadia, G. A. Suero-Abreu, R. Daci, and R. K. Then, “Would you use novel oral anticoagulants (NOACs) for thromboprophylaxis in patients with an underlying hypercoagulable state? A literature review through a case report,” *BMJ Case Reports*, vol. 13, no. 10, p. e237238, Article ID e237238, 2020.

[21] A. Liu, K. V. Rupani, and L. Naymagon, “Direct oral anticoagulants versus warfarin in patients with single antibody-positive anti-phospholipid syndrome,” *European Journal of Haematology*, vol. 109, no. 1, pp. 69–74, 2022.

[22] M. G. Tektonidou, L. Andreoli, M. Limper et al., “EULAR recommendations for the management of antiphospholipid syndrome in adults,” *Annals of the Rheumatic Diseases*, vol. 78, no. 10, pp. 1296–1304, 2019.

33

Ectopic ACTH Syndrome Emerging 5 Years after the Diagnosis of Neuroendocrine Tumor

Minghao Liu,[1] **Diane Hamele-Bena**,[2] **John Ausiello**,[3] **and Gabrielle Page-Wilson**[1]

[1]*Endocrinology Division, Department of Medicine, Columbia University Medical Center, 650 West 168th St., Room 2012, New York, NY 10032, USA*
[2]*Department of Pathology and Cell Biology, Columbia University Medical Center, Physicians and Surgeons Building, Room 404, 630 W 168th St., New York, NY 10032, USA*
[3]*Endocrinology Division, Department of Medicine, Columbia University Medical Center, Harkness Pavilion, 9th floor, 180 Fort Washington Ave., New York, NY 10032, USA*

Correspondence should be addressed to Minghao Liu; ml3931@cumc.columbia.edu

Academic Editor: John Broom

Ectopic ACTH syndrome (EAS) arising years after the diagnosis of a neuroendocrine tumor (NET) is exceedingly rare. We describe a case of EAS occurring five years after the diagnosis of a metastatic lung NET in a 61-year-old woman. She presented with severe hypokalemia but was not overtly Cushingoid on exam. Serum cortisol was 61mcg/dL after an overnight 1mg dexamethasone suppression test (<1.8mcg/dL) and urinary free cortisol was 7544 mcg/24h (<45mcg/24h), establishing the diagnosis of Cushing's syndrome. Plasma levels of peptides which have been associated with EAS, Agouti-related peptide (AgRP) and the ACTH precursors POMC (31-kDa) and pro-ACTH (22-kDa), were elevated. Metyrapone was initiated, but hypercortisolism persisted and the patient succumbed to pneumonia shortly after presentation. Retrospective examination of biopsy tissues showed rare ACTH immunoreactivity at the time of initial diagnosis, followed by staining in a greater proportion of cells as the disease progressed, consistent with EAS arising years after the diagnosis of NET. Given the increase in mortality associated with EAS, this unusual case highlights the importance of early detection and raises the possibility that early immunohistochemical stains for ACTH and measurements of ACTH precursors may facilitate the identification of NETs at high risk for EAS.

1. Introduction

Neuroendocrine tumors (NETs) arise from cells that have the ability to synthesize and secrete various peptides and amines, some of which may be metabolically active and give rise to distinct paraneoplastic syndromes. Lung NETs have an annual incidence of 0.2-2.0 per 100,000 and 1% of these cases are complicated by ectopic ACTH syndrome (EAS), a rare condition characterized by tumoral ACTH production, hypercortisolism, and increased mortality [1, 2]. While EAS is classically associated with small-cell lung carcinomas and carcinoids, it can be a paraneoplastic complication of neuroendocrine carcinoma (NEC), an aggressive form of NET [3]. We describe a rare case of a lung neuroendocrine carcinoma complicated by EAS five years after the tumor diagnosis. Tumoral ACTH immunoreactivity was retrospectively noted on the initial diagnostic biopsy specimen and plasma POMC concentrations were elevated at onset of EAS.

2. Case Presentation

A 61-year-old woman with Hashimoto's thyroiditis was hospitalized for new-onset hypokalemia two weeks following initiation of hydrochlorothiazide. Five years earlier, the patient had been diagnosed with a metastatic lung neuroendocrine tumor, while imaging for chronic cough revealed a lung lesion, subcarinal lymph node, and liver nodule. Follow-up PET scan had shown FDG avidity at those sites without brain involvement. Subcarinal node biopsy showed malignant cells with neuroendocrine features including nuclear molding,

Table 1: Laboratory values on admission.

Laboratory Test	Patient's Value	Reference Range
Sodium (mmol/L)	147	137-145
Potassium (mmol/L)	2.6	3.5-5.1
Bicarbonate (mmol/L)	37	19-27
Creatinine (mg/dL)	0.67	0.50-0.95
AST (units/L)	46	10-37
ALT (units/L)	78	9-50
Alkaline Phosphatase (units/L)	260	40-129
Hemoglobin A1c (%)	6.0%	<5.7%
TSH (mIU/L)	0.22	0.41-4.81
Free T4 (ng/dL)	0.63	0.83-1.90
Total T3 (ng/dL)	56.4	78-158

"salt and pepper" chromatin, and apoptosis. Immunohistochemical staining was positive for chromogranin, synaptophysin, and CD56, with an initial Ki67 index <5%. Plasma chromogranin A was 120 ng/mL (0-95 ng/mL). Morning cortisol and ACTH were normal at 9.3 mcg/dL (5.0-25.0 mcg/dL) and 19 pg/mL (6-58 pg/mL), respectively. Treatment with temozolomide and capecitabine was initiated with near resolution of the liver metastasis and stable disease was achieved for 2 years. However, disease progression characterized by new dedifferentiated metastases (Ki-67 index > 20%) to the liver, vertebra, brain (parietal region), shoulder soft tissue, ovary, and orbits subsequently occurred. Sequential treatment with radioembolization of hepatic metastases, octreotide, gamma knife, everolimus, and lanreotide was pursued over the course of 3 years.

On the day of admission, the patient presented from home with diffuse pain, chronic fatigue, and weakness. She denied fevers, chills, weight changes, and easy bruisability and had no history of recent fractures. Exam revealed an ill-appearing woman with a BMI of 27.8 and normal vital signs. She was not overtly Cushingoid; there was no facial plethora, supraclavicular/dorsocervical fullness, acanthosis, hirsutism, striae, or ecchymoses. Proximal muscle weakness, trace pretibial edema, and 1+ reflexes without delayed relaxation were noted. Laboratory evaluation demonstrated hypokalemia, metabolic alkalosis, mild hypernatremia, elevated hemoglobin A1c, transaminitis, elevated alkaline phosphatase, and hypothyroidism (Table 1). Morning cortisol was 48 mcg/dL (4.8-19.5) and was 61 mcg/dL after a 1 mg dexamethasone suppression test (<1.8). ACTH was 141 pg/mL (6-58) and urinary free cortisol was 7544 mcg/24h (<45). MRI showed multiple new orbital and brain metastasis, including a new 0.97 x 0.74 cm sellar/suprasellar lesion involving the pituitary stalk. The patient was found to have diabetes insipidus and treated with nightly desmopressin.

Although pituitary Cushing's was a possible diagnosis when considering a sellar/suprasellar lesion and a high plasma ACTH level in isolation, the patient had several features that pointed away from Cushing's disease and towards EAS: she had rapid onset of symptoms, severe hypokalemia, and an extremely high urinary free cortisol level (7544 mcg/24h). Furthermore, the appearance of the sellar/suprasellar lesion late in the timeline after spread of the lung NET to other regions of the body, the lesion's involvement of the pituitary stalk, and the patient's diabetes insipidus all strongly suggested that it was a metastasis of the NET. We did not perform inferior petrosal sinus sampling because of low clinical suspicion for Cushing's disease and because the patient was too ill to undergo this procedure.

Given high suspicion for EAS, plasma POMC and AgRP were measured as part of a Columbia University Medical Center IRB-approved research protocol in patients with ACTH-dependent Cushing's syndrome [4]. POMC was measured using an immunoradiometric assay (IRMA) that detects POMC (31-kDa) and pro-ACTH (22-kDa) but not ACTH or other ACTH precursors, as previously described [5], and AgRP was measured by ELISA [4]. POMC level was 80 fmol/mL (7-32 fmol/mL) and AgRP level was 884 pg/mL (42-118 pg/mL), supporting the diagnosis of EAS [4].

Hydrochlorothiazide was discontinued but hypokalemia requiring 120-200 mEq of daily potassium chloride repletion persisted until spironolactone was uptitrated to 50mg twice daily. Home levothyroxine was increased from 50 to 75mcg daily. Ketoconazole was deferred in the setting of diffuse hepatic metastases. Metyrapone was initiated and aggressively uptitrated, but hypercortisolism persisted and the patient died from multifocal pneumonia shortly after presentation.

Retrospective histologic examination of the subcarinal lymph node and liver biopsy specimens from the time of initial NET diagnosis confirmed ACTH immunoreactivity (Ventana Medical Systems: AB2335961) in rare malignant cells (Figure 1). A progressive increase in the number of malignant cells displaying strong ACTH immunoreactivity was observed in subsequent biopsy specimens obtained at least 3.5 years after diagnosis. While AgRP immunoreactivity (R&D Systems: AB355537) was absent from the initial tumor specimens, rare cells with AgRP immunoreactivity were observed in later biopsy specimens.

3. Discussion

This case demonstrates the rare occurrence of ectopic ACTH syndrome five years after the diagnosis of a lung neuroendocrine tumor. While EAS is known to be a potential paraneoplastic complication of a diverse array of NETs, several features of this case are unique. EAS is usually associated with typical carcinoids or small cell lung cancers [1]. While it has been observed with other tumors including pheochromocytomas, pancreatic islet-cell tumors, medullary thyroid carcinomas, and prostate carcinomas, its occurrence in the setting of non-small-cell lung cancer is exceedingly rare [6]. There are case reports of EAS complicating large cell neuroendocrine carcinoma of the lung [7] and lung adenocarcinoma. However, the primary malignancy in this case was an aggressive lung neuroendocrine carcinoma with neither small cell, large cell, nor glandular cell features. The tumor was initially diagnosed as a neuroendocrine tumor with a low proliferative index. However, three and a half years into her course, the tumor exhibited more aggressive characteristics including a high mitotic count and an elevated Ki-67 index. Given that the proliferative index is scored on only a

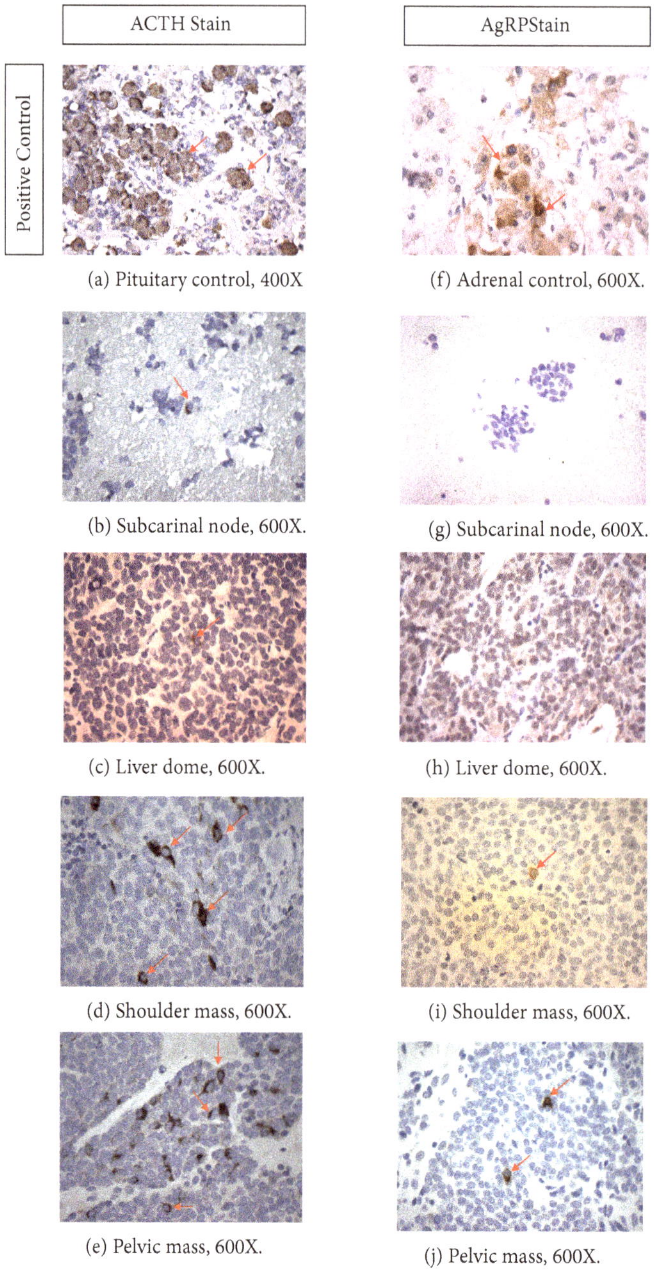

FIGURE 1: *Histopathology and immunohistochemistry of metastatic NEC biopsy specimens*: (a) Positive control: ACTH staining in normal pituitary tissue. Stained cells (red arrows) have brown cytoplasm. (b) Rare ACTH-positive cells in the subcarinal node that provided the initial diagnosis of NET and in (c) liver dome biopsied 3.5 years later. Increase in staining intensity and number of cells staining positive for ACTH in (d) shoulder mass and (e) pelvic mass, biopsied 4 and 4.5 years after initial diagnosis, respectively. (f) Positive control: AgRP staining in normal adrenal tissue. No staining for AgRP in specimens biopsied earlier in the disease course: (g) subcarinal node and (h) liver dome. Specimens biopsied later: (i) shoulder mass and (j) pelvic mass: show rare cells staining for AgRP.

small portion of the tumor specimen, it is possible that the original pathologic assessment was inadequate. Alternatively, the original NET may have progressed over time to a high-grade neuroendocrine carcinoma.

The second noteworthy feature of this case is the markedly delayed occurrence of EAS. The temporal onset of EAS in patients with neuroendocrine tumors is categorized as synchronous, diagnosed within the 3-month period before or after tumor diagnosis; metachronous, diagnosed greater than 3 months after tumor diagnosis; or cyclic [1]. In the majority of cases, EAS occurs synchronously and it is not uncommon for patients to present with paraneoplastic EAS before a cancer diagnosis is made [8]. There is little available data about the temporal onset of EAS specifically in patients with lung neuroendocrine tumors. However, in a large cohort of 918 thoracic and gastroenteropancreatic NETs evaluated by

Kamp et al., which included 51 lung/bronchial NETs, paraneoplastic Cushing's was identified metachronously in only 4 of the 29 cases associated with EAS [1]. The duration between the onset of hypercortisolism and the initial NET diagnoses was not reported. In our extensive review of the literature, we identified only two reported cases of metachronous EAS associated with lung NET. In the first case, EAS was diagnosed 12 years after the initial diagnosis of a malignant bronchial carcinoid and heralded recurrent disease [9]. In the second case, the delayed occurrence of EAS was documented 3 years after the diagnosis of malignant carcinoid or small-cell carcinoma of the lung in the setting of new brain metastases [10]. The occurrence of paraneoplastic EAS is most prevalent among NET patients with advanced (stage IV) disease. This clinical feature can complicate the diagnosis because many of the pathognomonic features of hypercortisolism may be obscured by cancer-related symptoms and chemotherapy-associated side effects.

Regular screening for Cushing's may have improved our patient's outcome, but given the rarity of EAS and the potential for its delayed occurrence, routine surveillance for EAS in all NETs is not likely to be cost effective. The ability to preemptively identify NET patients at high risk for EAS may facilitate the timely diagnosis and treatment of this morbid paraneoplastic complication. In this case report, the plasma cortisol and ACTH levels were normal when the initial NET diagnosis was made. However, the diagnostic tumor specimen was immunoreactive for ACTH, which may have heralded the tumor's potential for ACTH synthesis. Over time, there was an increase in tumoral ACTH staining followed by the eventual onset of EAS, which suggests that, while rare, it is possible for NETs to transform from clinically silent to hormonally functional tumors even years after their diagnosis. The mechanisms underlying this transformation may parallel those observed when silent corticotroph adenomas transform into functioning corticotroph adenomas, in part by increasing levels of the processing enzymes that mediate the conversion of POMC to ACTH [11]. While it is also possible that the development of Cushing's syndrome reflects an overall increase in the burden of ACTH immunoreactive tumor, a lack of concordance between tumor size and ACTH levels has been previously observed in EAS [3].

To date, specific biochemical markers indicative of NET's potential for clinically relevant ACTH secretion have not been comprehensively validated. However, elevations in POMC, the peptide precursor to ACTH, have been associated with occult and overt EAS [4]. Most nonpituitary tissues transcribe a short POMC mRNA that is not translated, but unmethylation of an upstream promoter allows ectopic ACTH-producing tumors to transcribe a longer mRNA that is translated into POMC protein [12]. However, in EAS, tumoral dedifferentiation is often associated with aberrant posttranslational processing of POMC, resulting in high circulating concentrations of unprocessed POMC peptide and ACTH precursors [13]. Consistent with these observations, we confirmed elevated plasma POMC (31-kDa) and pro-ACTH (22-kDa) concentrations in this case.

In addition, we observed a markedly elevated AgRP level in this patient. AgRP is most well known as a hypothalamic neuropeptide that stimulates appetite and inhibits energy expenditure by inhibiting the effect of alpha-MSH at melanocortin receptors. Plasma AgRP has been shown to reflect hypothalamic AgRP; it rises with fasting, falls with refeeding, and is inversely associated with BMI [14–17]. While AgRP is regulated by leptin, it is also regulated by cortisol in both animals and humans. Cortisol stimulates AgRP, which may partially explain why the AgRP is high in this case despite the patient having a BMI that is not low [17]. Another likely explanation for the elevated AgRP is the production of AgRP by the metastatic lung NET. AgRP is known to be expressed in tissues other than the hypothalamus including the lungs, adrenals, kidneys, and gonads [18, 19]. Furthermore, elevated plasma levels of AgRP have been observed in EAS and such elevations may be associated specifically with NETs arising from the lungs and the adrenals [4, 18]. Our patient's metastatic lung NEC was focally immunoreactive for AgRP, providing strong support for the tumoral origin of this circulating peptide. Studies establishing concordance between elevations in plasma AgRP and NET AgRP immunoreactivity are needed to support the clinical use of AgRP as a biomarker for EAS. However, the elevations in plasma POMC and AgRP in this case highlight the potential utility of these neuropeptides as tumor markers.

Delayed EAS occurring years after a cancer diagnosis is rare. However, it is imperative for providers to be aware of this potential complication because timely diagnosis and treatment can improve survival. The presence of ACTH immunoreactivity in diagnostic NET biopsy specimens may facilitate the early identification of patients at the highest risk of developing EAS. The presence of elevations in circulating neuroendocrine peptides, particularly POMC, may also serve as a specific marker of a NET's potential for ectopic ACTH secretion.

Additional Points

(i) Polyclonal Adrenocorticotropin Antibody, Ventana Medical Systems Cat# 760-2708, RRID:AB_2335961, http://antibodyregistry.org/search.php?q=AB_2335961. (ii) Human AgRP Affinity Purified Polyclonal Antibody, R and D Systems Cat# AF704, RRID:AB 355537, http://antibodyregistry.org/search.php?q=AB_355537. (iii) POMC levels were assessed using an immunoradiometric assay (IRMA) based on two monoclonal antibodies: the capture antibody is directed towards ACTH and the detection antibody is directed against γMSH. Thus, this IRMA detects the only two peptides containing both epitopes: POMC (31-kDa) and pro-ACTH (22-kDa). It does not detect other ACTH precursors. The antibodies for the IRMA are obtained from Dr. Anne White's lab (University of Manchester, Salford, UK) and the assay is performed as her group previously described [5].

Acknowledgments

This work has been supported by the Robert Wood Johnson Foundation, Harold Amos Medical Faculty Development Program, Grant no. 71591 (Gabrielle Page-Wilson) and the NIH, Department of Health and Human Services, Public Health Service, Grant no. T32 DK 007271 (Minghao Liu).

References

[1] K. Kamp, R. A. Alwani, E. Korpershoek, G. J. H. Franssen, W. W. De Herder, and R. A. Feelders, "Prevalence and clinical features of the ectopic ACTH syndrome in patients with gastroenteropancreatic and thoracic neuroendocrine tumors," *European Journal of Endocrinology*, vol. 174, no. 3, pp. 271–280, 2016.

[2] A. H. Limper, P. C. Carpenter, B. Scheithauer, and B. A. Staats, "The Cushing syndrome induced by bronchial carcinoid tumors," *Annals of Internal Medicine*, vol. 117, no. 3, pp. 209–214, 1992.

[3] I. Ilias, D. J. Torpy, K. Pacak, N. Mullen, R. A. Wesley, and L. K. Nieman, "Cushing's syndrome due to ectopic corticotropin secretion: twenty years' experience at the national institutes of health," *The Journal of Clinical Endocrinology & Metabolism*, vol. 90, no. 8, pp. 4955–4962, 2005.

[4] G. Page-Wilson, P. U. Freda, T. P. Jacobs et al., "Clinical utility of plasma POMC and AgRP measurements in the differential diagnosis of ACTH-dependent Cushing's syndrome," *The Journal of Clinical Endocrinology & Metabolism*, vol. 99, no. 10, pp. E1838–E1845, 2014.

[5] S. R. Crosby, M. F. Stewart, J. G. Ratcliffe, and A. White, "Direct measurement of the precursors of adrenocorticotropin in human plasma by two-site immunoradiometric assay," *The Journal of Clinical Endocrinology & Metabolism*, vol. 67, no. 6, pp. 1272–1277, 1988.

[6] G. Kaltsas, I. I. Androulakis, W. W. De Herder, and A. B. Grossman, "Paraneoplastic syndromes secondary to neuroendocrine tumours," *Endocrine-Related Cancer*, vol. 17, no. 3, pp. R173–R193, 2010.

[7] C.-S. Lin, N.-S. Yao, M.-F. Cheng, and S.-H. Lin, "Ectopic ACTH syndrome associated with large-cell neuroendocrine carcinoma of the lung," *The American Journal of the Medical Sciences*, vol. 334, no. 6, pp. 487–489, 2007.

[8] L. C. Pelosof and D. E. Gerber, "Paraneoplastic syndromes: an approach to diagnosis and treatment," *Mayo Clinic Proceedings*, vol. 85, no. 9, pp. 838–854, 2010.

[9] T. Isawa, K. Okubo, K. Konno, M. Oshibe, and S. Kidokoro, "Cushing's syndrome caused by recurrent malignant bronchial carcinod. Case report with 12 years' observation," *The American Review of Respiratory Disease*, vol. 108, no. 5, pp. 1200–1204, 1973.

[10] K. Sakamoto, H. Masuzaki, N. Fujimura et al., "A case of Cushing syndrome caused by ACTH producing atypical lung carcinoid tumor," *Nippon Naibunpi Gakkai Zasshi*, vol. 68, no. 8, pp. 743–751, 1992.

[11] A. Ben-Shlomo and O. Cooper, "Silent corticotroph adenomas," *The Pituitary Society*, vol. 21, no. 2, pp. 183–193, 2018.

[12] J. Newell-Price, "Proopiomelanocortin gene expression and DNA methylation: Implications for Cushing's syndrome and beyond," *Journal of Endocrinology*, vol. 177, no. 3, pp. 365–372, 2003.

[13] M. Terzolo, G. Reimondo, A. Alì et al., "Ectopic ACTH syndrome: Molecular bases and clinical heterogeneity," *Annals of Oncology*, vol. 12, no. 2, pp. S83–S87, 2001.

[14] G. Page-Wilson, K. Meece, A. White et al., "Proopiomelanocortin, agouti-related protein, and leptin in human cerebrospinal fluid: correlations with body weight and adiposity," *American Journal of Physiology-Endocrinology and Metabolism*, vol. 309, no. 5, pp. E458–E465, 2015.

[15] C. Gustavsson, U. Andersson Hall, A. Pelanis et al., "Cerebrospinal fluid levels of insulin, leptin, and agouti-related protein in relation to BMI in pregnant women," *Obesity*, vol. 24, no. 6, pp. 1299–1304, 2016.

[16] G. Page-Wilson, K. T. Nguyen, D. Atalayer et al., "Evaluation of CSF and plasma biomarkers of brain melanocortin activity in response to caloric restriction in humans," *American Journal of Physiology-Endocrinology and Metabolism*, vol. 312, no. 1, pp. E19–E26, 2017.

[17] G. Page-Wilson, J. B. Peters, S. K. Panigrahi et al., "Plasma agouti-related protein and cortisol levels in cushing disease: evidence for the regulation of agouti-related protein by glucocorticoids in humans," *The Journal of Clinical Endocrinology & Metabolism*, vol. 104, no. 3, pp. 961–969, 2019.

[18] M. M. Ollmann, B. D. Wilson, Y.-K. Yang et al., "Antagonism of central melanocortin receptors in vitro and in vivo by agouti-related protein," *Science*, vol. 278, no. 5335, pp. 135–138, 1997.

[19] J. R. Shutter, M. Graham, A. C. Kinsey, S. Scully, R. Lüthy, and K. L. Stark, "Hypothalamic expression of ART, a novel gene related to agouti, is up-regulated in obese and diabetic mutant mice," *Genes & Development*, vol. 11, no. 5, pp. 593–602, 1997.

34

Acute Secondary Adrenal Insufficiency Misdiagnosed as Acute Cholecystitis

Moslem Sedaghattalab[1] **and Amir Hossein Doustimotlagh**[2]

[1]*Department of Internal Medicine, Yasuj University of Medical Sciences, Yasuj, Iran*
[2]*Medicinal Plants Research Center, Yasuj University of Medical Sciences, Yasuj, Iran*

Correspondence should be addressed to Amir Hossein Doustimotlagh; amirhosseindoustimotlagh@gmail.com

Academic Editor: J. Paul Frindik

Hypopituitarism refers to insufficient secretion of the pituitary hormones. Patients with acute adrenocorticotropic hormone (ACTH) deficiency may be presented with fatigue, dizziness, orthostatic hypotension, hypoglycemia, nausea, vomiting, or nonspecific abdominal pain. This study described an unusual case of hypopituitarism in a patient who presented with general abdominal pain, abdominal tenderness, nausea, vomiting, hypotension, and hypoglycemia. At first, the patient was admitted with the diagnosis of acute cholecystitis, but after treatment of hypopituitarism and adrenal insufficiency, his symptoms resolved completely, without the need for surgery. Hypopituitarism and secondary adrenal insufficiency should be considered in the differential diagnosis of the patients who present with acute abdomen, hypotension, or hypoglycemia.

1. Introduction

The pituitary gland is divided into anterior and posterior lobes. Anterior pituitary hormones include TSH (thyroid stimulating hormone), LH (luteinizing hormone), FSH (follicles-stimulating hormone), ACTH (adrenocorticotropic hormone), GH (growth hormone), and prolactin. ADH (antidiuretic hormone) is produced by the hypothalamus and travels to the posterior pituitary gland through the pituitary stalk [1]. Hypopituitarism refers to insufficient secretion of the aforementioned pituitary hormones. Diagnosis of hypopituitarism is confirmed via measurement of the levels of those hormones [2].

Causes of hypopituitarism include pituitary cell destruction (accounts for more than 95% of cases), by pituitary adenoma [3], hypothalamic tumors (meningiomas and craniopharyngiomas), surgical or radiation therapy of the pituitary adenoma, and infiltrative lesions such as histiocytosis and hereditary hemochromatosis [4]. Sheehan's syndrome (postpartum pituitary apoplexy) is a common cause of hypopituitarism in women in developing countries [5, 6]. Patients with ACTH deficiency may present with fatigue, dizziness, orthostatic hypotension, hypoglycemia, nausea, vomiting, or nonspecific abdominal pain [7, 8]. In this study, an unusual case of hypopituitarism and secondary adrenal insufficiency was described in a patient who presented with acute abdomen.

2. Case Report

A 70-year-old woman presented to emergency ward with general abdominal pain, nausea, and vomiting. She also had a history of hypothyroidism. Medication was levothyroxine. Her siblings had minor thalassemia.

On examination, the body temperature, blood pressure, heart rate, respiratory rate, and oxygen saturation were 36°C, 80/60 mm Hg, 100 beats/min, 22 breaths/min, and 90%, respectively. The patient was pale (Figure 1). Abdominal examination revealed tenderness in right upper quadrant and positive Murphy's sign. All other examinations were normal. Body mass index was 23 (kg/m^2).

The patient was admitted in general surgery ward with impression of acute cholecystitis, and internal medicine consult was requested for managing hypotension and

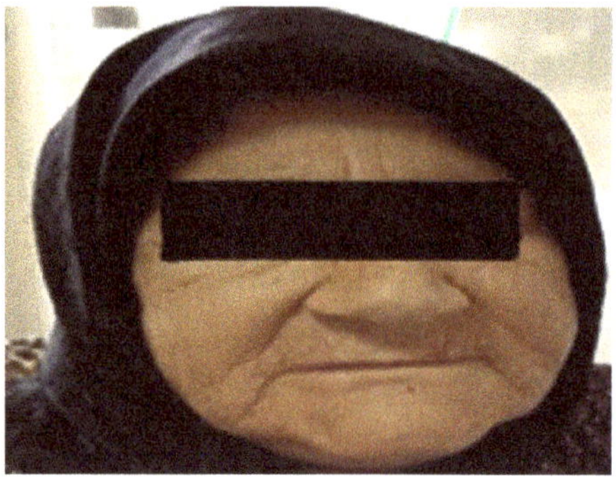

Figure 1: Alabaster-colored pale skin of patient seen in secondary adrenal insufficiency.

hypoglycemia. The patient's history of hypothyroidism, abdominal pain, hypotension, and hypoglycemia suggested adrenal insufficiency as the main cause of her symptoms and signs.

The hemoglobin was 8 (g/dL), the platelet counts 160 (10^9/L), and the white blood cell counts 8.2 (10^{12}/L). The alanine aminotransferase was 13 (IU/L), aspartate aminotransferase 35 (IU/L), alkaline phosphatase 280 (IU/L), albumin 4.5 (g/dL), total bilirubin 2.7 (mg/dL), conjugated bilirubin 0.7 (mg/dL), erythrocyte sedimentation rate (ESR) 24.5 (mm/h), serum iron 165 (μg/dL), total iron binding capacity (TIBC) 191 (μg/dL), PH (potential of hydrogen) 7.25, CO_2 (carbon dioxide) 30 (mm Hg), HCO_3 (bicarbonate) 13 (mEq/L), sodium 144 (mEq/L), potassium 3.8 (mEq/L), blood sugar 40 (mg/dL), blood urea nitrogen (BUN) 28 (mg/dL), creatinine 1.7 (mg/dL), LH 0.5 (IU/L), FSH 0.3 (IU/L), cortisol 2 (μg/dL), ACTH 0.2 (pg/L), and thyroid stimulating hormone (TSH) 2.1 (mU/L). Other laboratory tests, such as partial thromboplastin time, prothrombin time, and lipase, were normal.

Abdominal ultrasonography revealed gallstones and positive Murphy's sign. A computerized tomography (CT) scan of the chest and abdomen revealed linear atelectasis of right lower lobe of the lung and gallstone without any evidence of acute cholecystitis. The patient refused to do hypophysis MRI because of elevated creatinine and the risk of nephrogenic systemic fibrosis.

Treatment with hydrocortisone, normal saline, and dextrose water was initiated, and the patient's symptoms resolved completely without need to surgery.

Two months after initial presentation and treatment, our patient had no morbidity relating to acute abdomen, and treatment with hydrocortisone and levothyroxine is continuing. She had no any visual complaint before treatment and during follow-up time.

3. Discussion

ACTH deficiency leads to secondary adrenal insufficiency, in which cortisol secretion from adrenal gland reduces, but mineralocorticoid production is preserved; this is contrary to primary adrenal insufficiency, in which both cortisol and mineralocorticoid production are reduced. Secondary adrenal insufficiency is characterized by weakness, anorexia, fatigue, nausea, vomiting, and occasionally, hypoglycemia [9].

Patients with chronic adrenal insufficiency present with nonspecific symptoms, such as loss of energy and fatigue. Acute adrenal insufficiency is more frequently observed in primary adrenal insufficiency, and patients may present with hypotension, nausea, vomiting, fever, features of acute abdomen with abdominal tenderness, stupor, and coma. Adrenal crisis can be triggered by surgery or other stresses such as intercurrent illness [9].

In this study, an unusual case of hypopituitarism and secondary adrenal insufficiency was described in a patient who presented with general abdominal pain, abdominal tenderness, nausea, vomiting, hypotension, and hypoglycemia. She had metabolic acidosis and acute kidney injury due to hypotension and tissue hypoperfusion.

The history of hypothyroidism in addition to reduced gonadotropin levels and ACTH level suggested involvement of all axes of hypophysis.

At first, the patient was admitted in general surgery ward with diagnosis of acute cholecystitis, but after treatment with hydrocortisone, normal saline, and dextrose water, the patient's symptoms resolved completely without any need to surgery. Although unusual, hypopituitarism and secondary adrenal insufficiency should be considered in differential diagnosis of patients presenting with acute abdomen, hypotension, or hypoglycemia.

4. Conclusion

Acute adrenal insufficiency and features of acute abdomen more frequently observed in patients with primary adrenal insufficiency in which both cortisol and mineralocorticoid production are reduced; however, in this case, it happened in secondary adrenal insufficiency [9, 10]. Then, secondary adrenal insufficiency and hypopituitarism should be considered in the differential diagnosis of the patients who present with acute abdomen, hypotension, or hypoglycemia.

Consent

Informed consent was obtained for publication of this case report.

Authors' Contributions

Moslem Sedaghattalab collected data, analyzed, and discussed the study. Amir Hossein Doustimotlagh reviewed and edited the article.

Acknowledgments

The authors thank Habibeh Bayatmanesh who helped us with editing this manuscript.

References

[1] M. Skugo and A. Hamrahian, "Pituitary anatomy," in *Cleveland Clinic: Current Clinical Medicine*, Cleveland Clinic Foundation, Cleveland, OH, USA, 2010.

[2] M. Antonopoulou, R. Sharma, A. Farag, M. A. Banerji, and J. G. Karam, "Hypopituitarism in the elderly," *Maturitas*, vol. 72, no. 4, pp. 277–285, 2012.

[3] S. Lamberts, W. de Herder, and A. van der Lely, "Pituitary insufficiency," *The Lancet*, vol. 352, no. 9122, pp. 127–134, 1998.

[4] N. M. Appelman-Dijkstra, N. E. Kokshoorn, O. M. Dekkers et al., "Pituitary dysfunction in Adult patients after cranial radiotherapy: systematic review and meta-analysis," *Journal of Clinical Endocrinology & Metabolism*, vol. 96, no. 8, pp. 2330–2340, 2011.

[5] L. Curtò and F. Trimarchi, "Hypopituitarism in the elderly: a narrative review on clinical management of hypothalamic–pituitary–gonadal, hypothalamic–pituitary–thyroid and hypothalamic–pituitary–adrenal axes dysfunction," *Journal of Endocrinological Investigation*, vol. 39, no. 10, pp. 1115–1124, 2016.

[6] A. S. Bates, W. Van't Hoff, P. J. Jones, and R. N. Clayton, "The effect of hypopituitarism on life expectancy," *Journal of Clinical Endocrinology and Metabolism*, vol. 81, no. 3, pp. 1169–1172, 1996.

[7] C. W. Burke, "Adrenocortical insufficiency," *Clinics in Endocrinology and Metabolism*, vol. 14, no. 4, pp. 947–976, 1985.

[8] W. Arlt and B. Allolio, "Adrenal insufficiency," *The Lancet*, vol. 361, no. 9372, pp. 1881–1893, 2003.

[9] W. Arlt, "Disorders of the adrenal cortex," in *Harrison's Principles of Internal Medicine, 19th Eddition*, D. L. Longo, D. L. Kasper, J. L. Jameson, A. S. Fauci, S. L. Hauser, and J. Loscalzo, Eds., p. 2324, McGraw-Hill, New York, NY, USA, 2015.

[10] R. L. Rushworth, D. J. Torpy, and H. Falhammar, "Adrenal crisis," *New England Journal of Medicine*, vol. 381, no. 9, pp. 852–861, 2019.

The Utility of Immunohistochemistry in Differentiating Metastatic Primary Squamous Cell Carcinoma of the Thyroid from a Primary Lung Squamous Cell Carcinoma

Nern Hoong Kao ,[1] Chien Sheng Tan,[2] and Adrian Jit Hin Koh[1]

[1]*Department of General Surgery, Changi General Hospital, 2 Simei Street 3, Singapore 529889*
[2]*Department of Histopathology, Changi General Hospital, 2 Simei Street 3, Singapore 529889*

Correspondence should be addressed to Nern Hoong Kao; kao.nern.hoong@singhealth.com.sg

Academic Editor: Osamu Isozaki

Primary squamous cell carcinoma of the thyroid gland (PSCCTh) and anaplastic thyroid carcinoma with extensive squamous differentiation are rare entities which pose a diagnostic challenge in determining the primary site when presented as metastases. The difficulty in confirming a thyroid primary is further compounded by the aggressive nature of these tumours which frequently present at advanced stages. We present a case in which the patient presented with a thyroid mass and a lung mass simultaneously. The risk of misinterpreting the site of primary tumour as lung is greatly increased because squamous cell carcinoma of lung is much more common than its thyroid counterpart. This case highlights the effectiveness of PAX-8 stain in determining the primary site of tumour when squamous cell carcinoma is found in both lung and thyroid gland.

1. Introduction

Primary squamous cell carcinoma of the thyroid (PSCCTh) is a rare malignancy of the thyroid gland. According to Yang et al., PSCCTh accounts for only approximately 0.1% of all primary thyroid carcinomas [1]. A review of the SEER database yielded only 243 cases between the period of 1973–2015.

PSCCTh is an aggressive disease and holds a dismal prognosis with a median survival of six to nine months regardless of the modality of treatment received [1, 2]. However, patients with disease limited to the thyroid gland alone tend to have a better disease free survival [1, 3]. It is therefore imperative that PSCCTh be diagnosed early so as to initiate treatment as early as possible due to the aggressiveness of this disease.

Patients with PSCCTh commonly present with an enlarging anterior neck mass (60%). The patients may also develop dyspnea or dysphagia (20%) or with a change in their voice (15%). These patients tend to be after their 6th decade of life and were more likely to be female [2]. Unfortunately, at the time of diagnosis, most patients were found with either locally advanced disease (76%), nodal (50%) or distant metastases (28%) [1].

Metastasis to the thyroid gland from lung squamous cell carcinoma is uncommon but likely to be more common than PSCCTh with lung metastases. The case presentation highlights the potential pitfall of misdiagnosing the lung tumour as a second primary, given the similarity between both tumours on morphology. In this context, PAX-8 immunohistochemical stain plays a vital role in determining the primary origin of squamous cell carcinoma.

2. Aim

Here, we present a rare case of metastatic PSCCTh masquerading as metastatic squamous cell carcinoma of the lung.

3. Case Presentation

A 69-year-old Chinese male presented via the emergency department with a one day history of mild shortness of breath. Upon closer interview, he also complained of a progressively enlarging left neck mass which had more than doubled in size

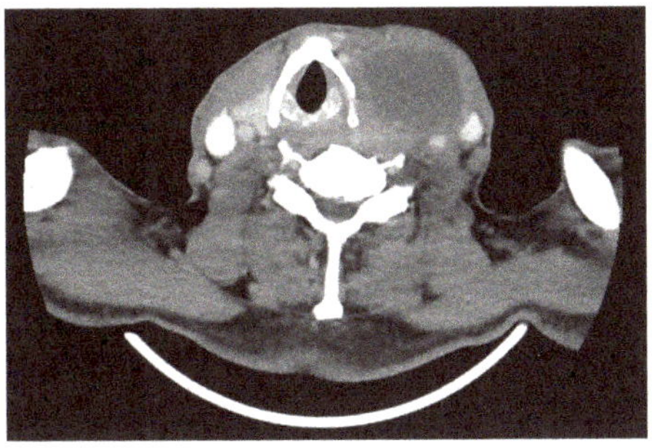

FIGURE 1: CT scan (axial) showing a large hypoechoic nodule with ill-defined nodular margins. This is suggestive of a solid-cystic nodule in the left thyroid.

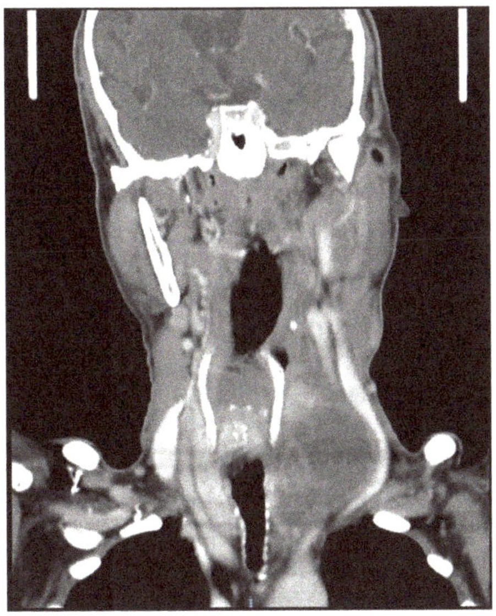

FIGURE 2: CT scan (coronal) showing gross deviation of the common carotid artery. The lack of fat plane suggests involvement of the carotid. The trachea is deviated but is not narrowed.

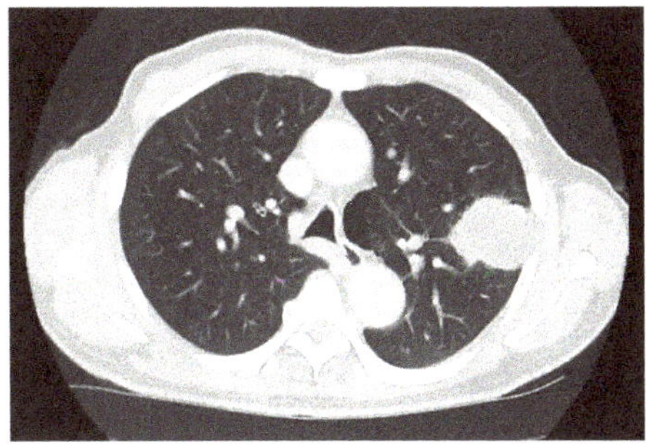

FIGURE 3: CT scan (axial) showing a 4.3 × 3.4 cm spiculated hyperechoic lesion in the left upper lobe abutting the pleura.

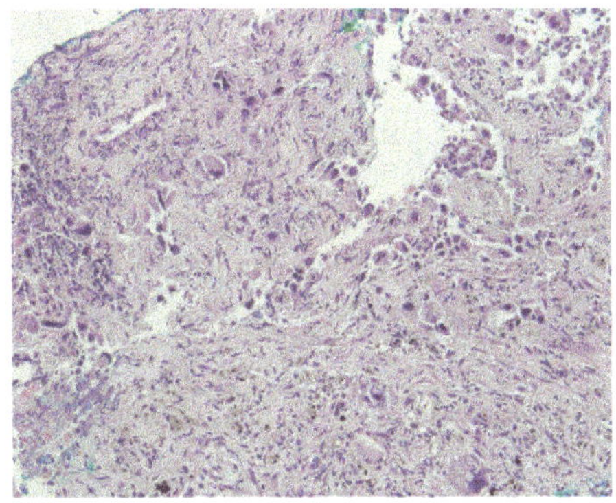

FIGURE 4: Lung parenchyma infiltrated by poorly differentiated carcinoma with squamoid features. Prominent background desmoplasia is noted.

over the period of six weeks. He did not note any stridor, hoarseness or dysphagia. The patient was a smoker of 50 pack years but did not consume alcohol. He had history of mild chronic obstructive pulmonary disease but otherwise did not have a family history of thyroid disorders. Physical examination showed a large (7 cm) left anterior neck mass which moved with swallowing. The mass was not tender and there was no retrosternal extension. There were no enlarged cervical lymph nodes or evidence of airway obstruction.

Blood tests performed showed a normal thyroid function with free thyroxine (fT4) at 12.85 pmol/L and thyroid-stimulating hormone at 0.619 μIU/L. The white blood cell count (WBC) was also elevated at 21.6×10^9/L. This was predominantly neutrophilic with an absolute neutrophil count of 17.9×10^9/L. However, the other inflammatory markers were not significantly raised with a C-Reactive Protein (CRP) of 62 mg/L and a Pro-Calcitonin of 0.13 μg/L.

Contrast-enhanced CT scan (Figure 1) showed a 6.4 × 5.6 × 4.9 cm solid-cystic nodule arising from the left thyroid lobe and encasing the left common carotid artery. The trachea was deviated to the right but there was otherwise no airway narrowing (Figure 2). There were also several subcentimeter necrotic lymph nodes within the left cervical region. In addition, the CT scan also revealed a 4.3 × 3.4 cm spiculated mass in the left upper lobe of the lung as well as several other smaller subcentimeter lung nodules (Figure 3). A contrasted CT abdomen and pelvis did not show any intra-abdominal pathology. These radiological findings raised the possibility of synchronous tumours.

The patient underwent a bedside fine needle aspiration (FNAC) of which copious amount of pus was aspirated and concurred on cytology. In view of this finding, the authors were swayed towards the possibility of tuberculosis.

An ultrasound-guided FNAC of the solid component of the nodule was arranged. This showed atypical squamous cells highly suspected for squamous cell carcinoma (Figure 4). No thyroid epithelial cells or anaplastic cells were seen in the cytology specimen. This finding contradicted the clinical impression of a common primary thyroid cancer. Acid fast bacilli (AFB) smears were negative.

The patient also underwent a CT guided biopsy of the lung lesion. Histology showed poorly differentiated carcinoma with squamous differentiation. Immunohistochemistry staining (Figure 5) showed diffuse reactivity to p40, CK7 and paired box 8 (PAX-8) and were negative for Napsin A and thyroid transcription factor-1 (TTF-1). This was suggestive of a thyroid primary rather than a primary lung squamous cell cancer.

In view of this, the patient was diagnosed as primary squamous cell carcinoma of the thyroid with nodal and lung

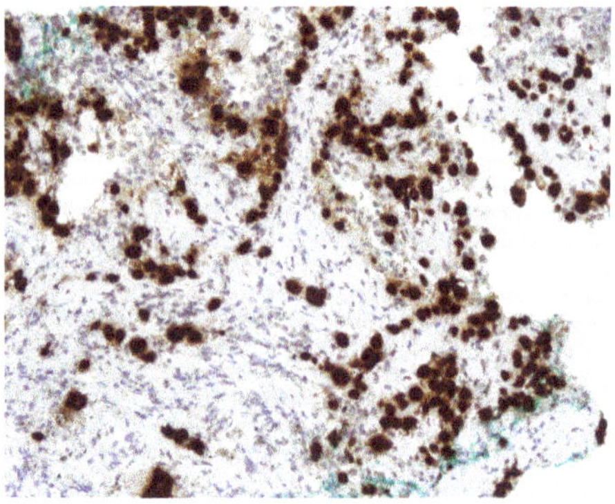

FIGURE 5: Tumour cells are diffusely immunoreactive to P40 stain. This finding is indicative of squamous differentiation. Diffuse P40 staining in tumour cells is in keeping with squamous cell carcinoma.

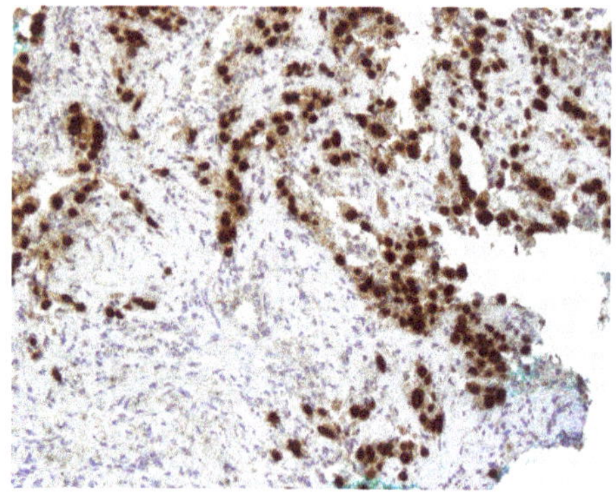

FIGURE 6: Tumour cells are also diffusely immunoreactive to PAX-8 stain. Coexpression of P40 and PAX-8 is supportive of a thyroid primary.

metastases. As most patients with advanced disease succumb to airway obstruction, the patient was offered an elective tracheostomy. However, he declined all treatment and opted for best supportive care. The patient passed away six weeks later.

4. Discussion

The clinical presentation with the rapid rate of growth was initially suggestive of anaplastic thyroid cancer. This was further conflicted by the presence of a large lung tumour and the presence of atypical squamous cells in the thyroid FNAC. The constellation of findings raised the possibility of a lung squamous cell carcinoma metastasizing to the thyroid gland or synchronous tumours. FNAC was not helpful in this case and it was not until tissue biopsy of the lung lesion was obtained that we could achieve the diagnosis. In a meta-analysis performed by Cho et al., FNAC had limited value in identifying PSCCTh. Only 27% of patients diagnosed with PSCCTh had prior FNAC results that showed SCC or suspicious for SCC.

Tissue obtained from a biopsy or from a thyroidectomy specimen is more useful for diagnosis. The role of immunohistochemistry in assessing a metastatic tumour of unknown primary is well established. In this case, tissue obtained from the lung biopsy was invaluable as it stained positive for PAX-8 which was suggestive of a thyroid origin. It was unlikely to be a lung primary as the tissue was negative for Napsin A and TTF-1. Other microscopic features would include the presence of keratin or intercellular bridge structures within the thyroidal tissue [4, 5]. Suzuki et al. showed the rate of presence of PAX-8 to be as high as 91% in PSCCTh [6]. PAX-8 is a paired-box gene important in the embryogenesis of the thyroid gland, kidney, parathyroid gland, and Mullerian structures (Figure 6). It is markedly associated with thyroid gland organogenesis, thus the usefulness in identifying the most probable primary site in this case. Other useful markers include thyroglobulin (62.5%), p53 (50%), and TTF-1 (37.5%) [7].

One key point is the need to exclude local invasion of the thyroid from SCC of adjacent structures such as the larynx. This should be suspected should the specimen test negative for PAX-8. Imaging such as CT scans are a useful adjunct for this purpose. In a systematic review by Syed et al., there were no specific radiological features to aid in the diagnosis of PSCCTh. However, CT scans are useful to exclude other potential sources of SCC with thyroid metastases or causing direct invasion of the thyroid gland. PSCCTh was also found to be more likely to encase the oesophagus rather than invade into the oesophagus. This is helpful in excluding an oesophageal primary invading into the thyroid as there would still be a fat plane seen around the oesophagus. CT scans were also found to be useful in assessing the severity of airway compression [8].

The success of treatment largely depends on being able to achieve R0 resection. Disease free survival is further improved if adjuvant radiotherapy or radiochemotherapy is given [9, 10]. However, radiotherapy and/or chemotherapy alone without surgical treatment holds a dismal outcome as PSCCTh is relatively radioresistant [7, 11]. Multiple studies have also shown PSCCTh to be poorly responsive to chemotherapy [8]. PSCCTh is similar to anaplastic thyroid carcinoma and does not uptake iodine. There is no role for radioactive iodine ablation or thyroid suppression. Recent development in the area of immunotherapy based on programmed cell death ligand 1 inhibitors (PD-L1) might prove to be a viable option for a small number of patients with tumour showing high expression of PD-L1 on immunohistochemistry studies [12].

5. Conclusion

Primary squamous cell carcinoma of the thyroid gland with a dominant metastatic tumour could pose a diagnostic challenge due to its rarity and indistinguishable morphological features from other primary squamous cell carcinomas. In such clinical settings, PAX-8 immunohistochemical stain could prove to be useful in determining the primary origin of squamous cell carcinoma.

References

[1] S. Yang, C. Li, X. Shi et al., "Primary squamous cell carcinoma in the thyroid gland: a population-based analysis using the SEER database," *World Journal of Surgery*, vol. 43, no. 5, pp. 1249–1255, 2019.

[2] J. K. Au, J. Alonso, E. C. Kuan, A. Arshi, and M. A. St. John, "Primary squamous cell carcinoma of the thyroid: a population-based analysis," *Otolaryngology–Head and Neck Surgery*, vol. 157, no. 1, pp. 25–29, 2017.

[3] J. K. Cho, S.-H. Woo, J. Park, M.-J. Kim, and H.-S. Jeong, "Primary squamous cell carcinomas in the thyroid gland: an individual participant data meta-analysis," *Cancer Medicine*, vol. 3, no. 5, pp. 1396–1403, 2014.

[4] W. J. Simpson and J. Carruthers, "Squamous cell carcinoma of the thyroid gland," *The American Journal of Surgery*, vol. 156, no. 1, pp. 44–46, 1988.

[5] C. Kleer, T. J. Giordano, and M. J. Merino, "Squamous cell carcinoma of the thyroid: an aggressive tumour associated with tall cell variant of papillary thyroid carcinoma," *Modern Pathology*, vol. 13, no. 7, pp. 742–746, 2000.

[6] A. Suzuki, M. Hirokawa, N. Takada et al., "Diagnostic significance of PAX8 in thyroid squamous cell carcinoma," *Endocrine Journal*, vol. 62, no. 11, pp. 991–995, 2015.

[7] F. Booya, T. J. Sebo, J. L. Kasperbauer, and V. Fatourechi, "Primary squamous cell carcinoma of the thyroid: report of ten cases," *Thyroid*, vol. 16, pp. 89–93, 2006.

[8] M. I. Syed, M. Stewart, S. Syed et al., "Squamous cell carcinoma of the thyroid gland: primary or secondary disease?," *The Journal of Laryngology & Otology*, vol. 125, no. 1, pp. 3–9, 2011.

[9] F. Struller, M. Senne, C. Falch, A. Kirschniak, A. Konigsrainer, and S. Muller, "Primary squamous cell carcinoma of the thyroid: case report and systematic review of the literature," *International Journal of Surgery Case Reports*, vol. 37, pp. 36–40, 2017.

[10] A. Wygoda, T. Rutkowski, B. Szczesniak-Klusek, J. Mrochem-Kwarciak, M. Jędrzejewska, and K. Składowski, "Primary squamous-cell thyroid carcinoma – a successful treatment with five-year follow-up," *Endokrynologia Polska*, vol. 68, no. 5, pp. 592–596, 2017.

[11] A. K. Sarda, S. Bal, M. K. Arunabh Singh, and M. M. Kapur, "Squamous cell carcinoma of the thyroid," *Journal of Surgical Oncology*, vol. 39, no. 3, pp. 175–178, 1988.

[12] S. Ulisse, C. Tuccilli, S. Sorrenti et al., "PD-1 Ligand Expression in Epithelial Thyroid Cancers: Potential Clinical Implications," *International Journal of Molecular Sciences*, vol. 20, no. 6, p. 1405, 2019.

36

Nonmosaic Isodicentric Y Chromosome: A Rare Cause of Azoospermia— From Genetics to Clinical Practice

Jolijn Van Cauwenberghe,[1] Sigri Beckers,[2] and Peter Coremans[3]

[1]Antwerp University Hospital, Department of Diabetology-Endocrinology, Wilrijkstraat 10, 2650 Edegem, Belgium
[2]Antwerp University Hospital, Department of Genetics, Wilrijkstraat 10, 2560 Edegem, Belgium
[3]AZ Nikolaas, Department of Diabetology-Endocrinology, Moerlandstraat 1, 9100 Sint-Niklaas, Belgium

Correspondence should be addressed to Jolijn Van Cauwenberghe; jolijn.vancauwenberghe@uza.be

Academic Editor: Suat Simsek

Azoospermia is diagnosed when no spermatozoa can be detected after centrifugation of seminal fluid on at least two separate occasions. A number of genetic disorders can be related to nonobstructive azoospermia, and in up to 15% of azoospermic males, a genetic disorder is diagnosed. A 36-year-old male with nonobstructive azoospermia was referred to our department of diabetes and endocrinology due to an aberrant testicular biopsy. The biopsy showed a disrupted spermatogenesis with a maturation arrest at the spermatocyte level in most tubuli seminiferi while others showed a Sertoli cell-only syndrome. Screening for Y chromosome microdeletions on peripheral blood using molecular analysis detected a terminal deletion of AZFbc. The result of karyotyping and fluorescence in situ hybridization (FISH) described an isodicentric Y chromosome with karyotype 46,X,idic(Y)(q11.22). Based on this case and the current available literature, we conclude that performing a testicular biopsy in patients with a nonmosaic idic(Y)(q) is not meaningful and that the prognosis on infertility is poor. Biological fatherhood is extremely unlikely in these patients, and proper counselling should be provided.

1. Introduction

Ten to 15% of males with infertility are found to have a complete absence of spermatozoa in the ejaculate, called azoospermia [1]. Azoospermia is diagnosed when no spermatozoa can be detected after centrifugation of seminal fluid on at least two separate occasions. Azoospermia can be caused by endocrine abnormalities, intrinsic spermatogenesis disorders, or posttesticular causes [2].

A genetic cause can be found in up to 15% of males with azoospermia [3]. Sex chromosomal abnormalities, diagnosed through karyotyping, are one of the most common genetic abnormalities and include numerical and structural abnormalities. Two-thirds of chromosomal abnormalities in infertile men are caused by the well-known numerical disorder Klinefelter syndrome (47,XXY) [4, 5]. Furthermore, microdeletions of the azoospermia factor region (*AZF* gene) on the Y chromosome are another important type of genetic aberration that can be found in approximately 10% of nonobstructive azoospermic males [6]. These microdeletions are divided into deletions of AZFa, AZFb, and AZFc or combined deletions and can be detected using polymerase chain reaction (PCR) techniques. The clinical consequences are determined by the site and length of the deletion [6].

Isochromosome Y (iso(Y)) and isodicentric chromosome Y (idic(Y)) are structural Y chromosome aberrations that are associated with male infertility and nonobstructive azoospermia [6–10]. An idic(Y) is formed due to an aberrant homologous crossing over between opposite arms of a palindrome during spermatogenesis. This can result in a duplication of the short arm and proximal long arm and a deletion of a part of the long arm and is referred to as idic(Y)(q). Chromosomes affected in this way contain two centromeres and are often unstable during mitosis. Therefore, most cases described are mosaics with a 45,X cell line

[7, 10–12]. A broad range of phenotypes are reported in these cases, ranging from male to abnormal female or individual with ambiguous genitalia [13]. Knowledge about this specific chromosomal aberration is important considering the great impact on the possibility of assisted reproductive technology (ART) [1, 14].

We describe a patient with nonmosaic isodicentric Y chromosome (46,X,idic(Y)(q11.22)) presenting with nonobstructive azoospermia. Informed consent was obtained.

2. Case Report

A 36-year-old male was referred because of an aberrant testicular biopsy. The biopsy showed disrupted spermatogenesis with maturation arrest at the spermatocyte level in most tubuli seminiferi (Figure 1), while others showed a Sertoli cell-only syndrome. The referring urologist performed the biopsy in the context of primary infertility with confirmed azoospermia on the semen sample. There was no history of cryptorchidism, mumps, orchitis, testicular cancer, radiation, surgery or testicular trauma, nor a family history of infertility. The only medication our patient took was levothyroxine for hypothyroidism. There was no history of drug use or abuse. On physical examination, we found a man of normal constitution with normal virilization. Scrotal palpation detected the presence of bilateral vas deferens and small testicular volumes of 6 to 8 millilitres using an orchidometer. Ultrasonography of both testes confirmed the small testis ($2 \times 1.4 \times 3.7$ cm left and $2.2 \times 1.4 \times 3.4$ cm right), and there were no suspicious lesions to withhold. Blood tests showed an elevated follicle-stimulating hormone (14.50 U/l, normal value: 0.7–10.8 U/l) with a normal luteinizing hormone (5.0 U/l, normal value 2.0–5.3 mU/l) and low normal testosterone (302.0 ng/dl, normal value 300–1000 ng/dl). Prolactin levels were normal (7.7 μg/L, normal value 1.6–18.8 μg/L). Screening for Y chromosome microdeletions on peripheral blood using molecular analysis detected a terminal deletion of AZFbc. The result of karyotyping and fluorescence in situ hybridization (FISH) on cultured peripheral lymphocytes described an isodicentric Y chromosome with karyotype 46,X,idic(Y)(q11.22) (Figure 2). These results implicate the impossibility of biological fatherhood for this patient, and we, therefore, referred our patient and the partner to a multidisciplinary fertility clinic for further counselling.

3. Discussion

In azoospermic males, genetic testing is strongly advised considering that a genetic disorder can be diagnosed in up to 15 percent of the cases [14]. To ensure proper counselling for patients confronted with infertility, a correct genetic diagnosis is essential. In addition, expensive and invasive diagnostic tests and treatments can be avoided. This case describes a rare genetic disorder associated with nonobstructive azoospermia: the isodicentric Y chromosome. Although data are lacking for the general population, in infertile men with an abnormal Y chromosome, idic(Y) occurs in 15–30% [15]. An idic(Y) is formed due to an aberrant homologous crossing over between opposite arms of a palindrome during spermatogenesis. This can result in a duplication of the short arm and proximal long arm and a deletion of a part of the long arm and is referred to as idic(Y)(q). The q11 region of the long arm of the Y chromosome is susceptible as a breakpoint for this aberrant crossing over due to the presence of AT-rich regions which are fragile sites for breaking. In addition, the q11.2 region contains a direct repeat [16] (Figures 3 and 4).

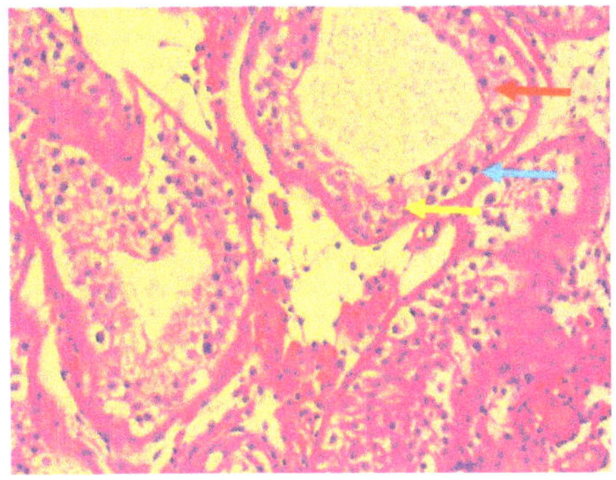

FIGURE 1: Testicular biopsy with maturation arrest at the spermatocyte level. Red arrow = spermatocyte. Blue arrow = spermatogona. Yellow arrow = Sertoli cell.

The vast majority of reported idic(Y)(q) cases (55–100%) present as mosaics with a 45,X cell line due to the instability during mitosis [7, 8, 10–12]. This mosaicism provides a broad range of phenotypes, from phenotypically normal males to even phenotypical females [12]. There is a known variability in the distribution of idic(Y) in different tissues, with higher variability in gonadal tissue. The sex differentiation is believed to be depending on this mosaicism in gonadal tissue [16].

The case we describe showed a 46,X,idic(Y)(q11.22) karyotype without mosaicism, and in contrast to most published cases, we performed a complete work-up (physical examination, hormonal evaluation, and testis biopsy) (Figure 3.) We made a comparison with 12 published cases of infertile men with nonmosaic idic(Y)(q) in order to provide guidance for clinical practitioners confronted with similar patients (Table 1). The majority of the patients had small testes, and all but one case had azoospermia on a repeated semen sample. The one case, described by Antonelli et al., showed spermatocytes on the cytomorphological sediment in the sperm sample, which cannot be used in ART. To the best of our knowledge, testicular histology was reported for only six cases of infertile men with nonmosaic idic(Y)(q). All these cases showed a severe disruption of spermatogenesis with maturation arrest and/or Sertoli cell-only histology. In the diagnostic evaluation of the azoospermic males, current guidelines state that a diagnostic testicular biopsy is indicated in men with normal testicular size and normal reproductive hormones in order to distinguish between obstructive and a nonobstructive azoospermia. In

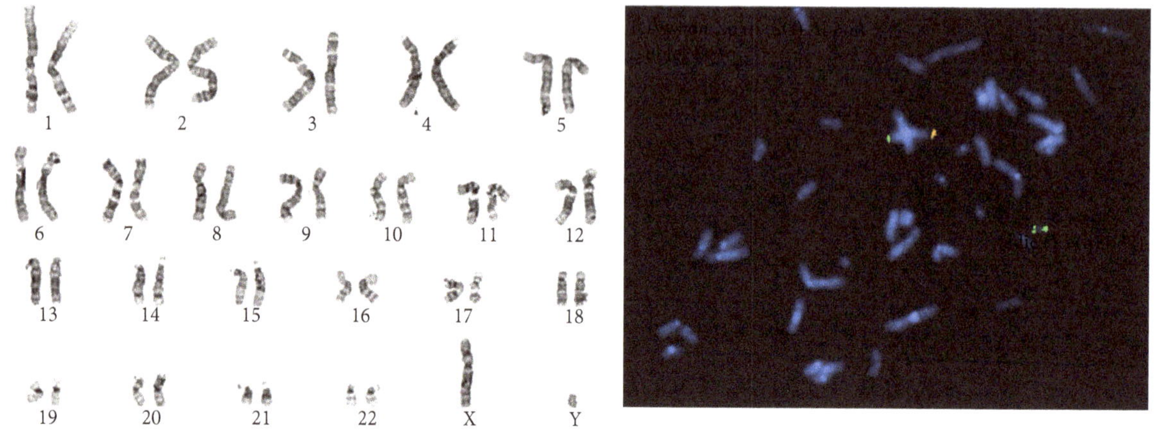

(a) (b)

FIGURE 2: Karyotyping and fluorescence in situ hybridization (FISH) analyses. (a) Conventional chromosome analysis of cultured peripheral lymphocytes identified an idic(Y)(q11.22) chromosome. (b) FISH analysis was performed using probes for the telomeric regions of both the X and Y chromosomes. Green signals indicate the pter-region of the X and Y chromosomes (Abbott TelVysion Xp/Yp probe). Red signals indicate the qter-region of the X and Y chromosomes (in-house subtelomeric XqYq probe). FISH analysis demonstrated that the aberrant Y chromosome contained 2 signals for the Yp subtelomeric probe and absence of the Yq subtelomeric probe. This confirmed the presence of an idic(Y)(q).

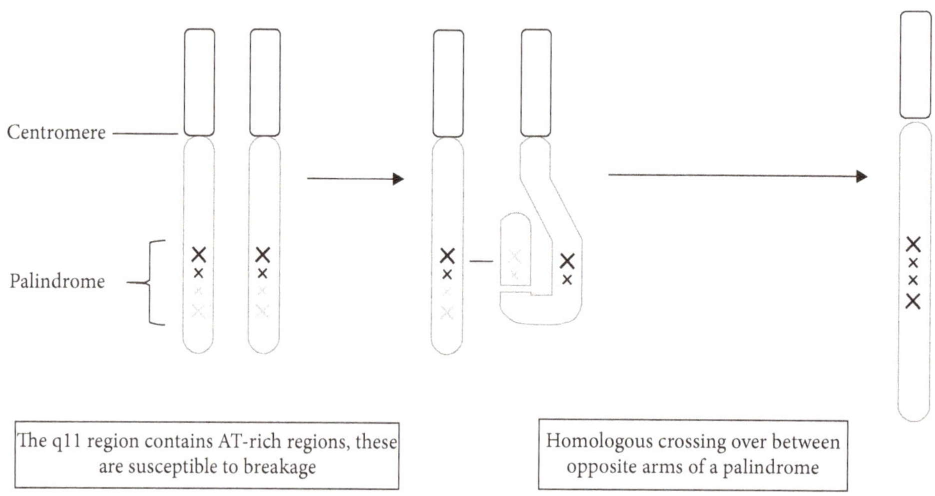

FIGURE 3: Schematic representation of aberrant homologous crossing over between opposite arms of a palindrome during spermatogenesis with the formation of an isodicentric Y chromosome.

azoospermia with high FSH, a testicular biopsy can determine the presence of a normal or abnormal spermatogenesis, although it does not provide accurate prognostic information [14, 17]. Since the genetic testing provides a clear diagnosis of nonobstructive azoospermia, a testicular biopsy in patients with idic(Y)(q) is not meaningful. This invasive technique should, therefore, not be performed before genetic testing is completed in patients with nonobstructive azoospermia.

Furthermore, both Mascarenhas et al. and Takeda et al. performed a testicular sperm extraction (TESE) and micro-TESE, respectively, in a nonmosaic idic(Y)(q) male without success, meaning there were no spermatozoa retrieved [6, 7]. All these data show the poor prognosis of fertility in patients with nonmosaic idic(Y)(q). As there were no spermatozoa on testicular biopsy and micro-TESE in the described cases up till now, the use of ART seems limited, and biological fatherhood is extremely unlikely in patients with a nonmosaic idic(Y)(q).

In infertile men with mosaic idic(Y)(q), the prognosis for infertility is less clear. Overall, all infertile men with idic(Y)(q) present with a nonobstructive azoospermia [8–10]. Nevertheless, one of the mosaic idic(Y)(q) cases reported by Antonelli et al. showed a low number of spermatocytes on the semen sample ($<0.1\ 10^6$/ml). [10] Furthermore, Kim et al. report a normal spermatogenesis on testicular biopsy in an azoospermic male with mosaic idic(Y)(q) [8]. Thus, despite the low chance of success, ART

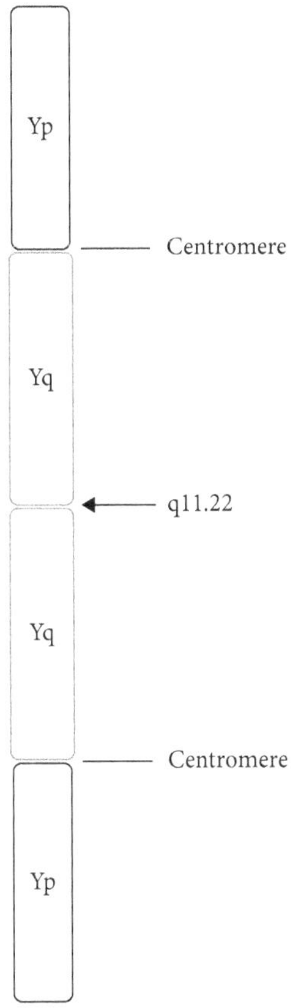

FIGURE 4: Schematic representation of isodicentric Y chromosome idic(Y)(q11.22). The breakpoint (arrow) is located at q11.22 (long arm), with a duplication of short arm, centromere, and proximal long arm and loss of all distal long arm material.

TABLE 1: Summary of idic(Y)(q) cases described in the literature.

	idic(Y)	Testicular volume (ml)	Semen	Hormone levels			Testicular biopsy	AZF microdeletion	TESE
				FSH	LH	Testosterone			
Current case	46,X,idic(Y)(q11.22)	8	AZ	Elevated	Normal	Normal	MA + SCO	AZF bc	
Kalantari et al. [9]	46,X,idic(Y)(q11.22)	—	AZ	—	—	—	MA + SCO	AZF bc	
	46,X,idic(Y)(q11.22)	—	AZ	—	—	—	MA + SCO	AZF bc	
	46,X,idic(Y)(q11.22)	—	AZ	—	—	—	MA + SCO	AZF bc	
Kim et al. [8]	46,X,idic(Y)(q11.2)	11	AZ	Normal	Normal	Normal	MA	AZF bc	
	46,X,idic(Y)(q11.21)	5	AZ	Low	Low	Normal	—	AZF abc	
	46,X,idic(Y)(q11.222)	12	AZ	Normal	Normal	Normal	—	AZF bc	
	46,X,idic(Y)(q11.2)	2	AZ	Normal	Normal	Normal	—	AZF abc	
	46,X,idic(Y)(q12)	3	AZ	Normal	—	Normal	MA	Normal	
Antonelli et al. [10]	46,X,idic(Y)(q11.2)	Normal[1]	AZ	Normal	Normal	Normal	—	AZF bc	
	46,X,idic(Y)(q12)	Normal[1]	Spermatocytes	Normal	Normal	Normal	—	Normal	
Takeda et al. [7]	46,X,idic(Y)(q11.2)	7	—	Elevated	Normal	Normal	SCO	—	No spermatozoa[2]
Mascarenhas et al. [6]	46,X,idic(Y)(q11.21)	—	AZ	Elevated	—	—	—	—	No spermatozoa

AZ = azoospermia; MA = maturation arrest; SCO = Sertoli cell-only; TESE = testicular sperm extraction. [1]No detailed testicular volume reported; [2]micro-TES.

cannot be completely excluded in infertile men with mosaic idic(Y)(q).

4. Conclusions

To the best of our knowledge, this is only the second case of a nonmosaic idic(Y)(q) that had an extensive evaluation. Based on our case report and the available literature, we conclude that performing a testicular biopsy in patients with a nonmosaic idic(Y)(q) is futile. Furthermore, the prognosis on infertility is poor. It seems that retrieval of spermatozoa is impossible, and therefore, biological fatherhood is extremely unlikely in these patients. Proper counselling for patients and their partners should be provided.

References

[1] S. C. Esteves, "Clinical management of infertile men with nonobstructive azoospermia," *Asian Journal of Andrology*, vol. 17, no. 3, pp. 459–470, 2015.

[2] M. Cocuzza, C. Alvarenga, and R. Pagani, "The epidemiology and etiology of azoospermia," *Clinics*, vol. 68, no. S1, pp. 15–26, 2013.

[3] N. Pandiyan and A. M. Jequier, "Genetics: mitotic chromosomal anomalies among 1210 infertile men," *Human Reproduction*, vol. 11, no. 12, pp. 2604–2608, 1996.

[4] Y. Naasse, H. Charoute, B. El Houate et al., "Chromosomal abnormalities and Y chromosome microdeletions in infertile men from Morocco," *BMC Urology*, vol. 15, p. 95, 2015.

[5] Practice Committee of the American Society for Reproductive Medicine, "Management of nonobstructive azoospermia: a committee opinion," *Fertility and Sterility*, vol. 110, no. 7, pp. 1239–1245, 2018.

[6] M. Mascarenhas, S. Thomas, M. S. Kamath et al., "Prevalence of chromosomal abnormalities and Y chromosome microdeletion among men with severe semen abnormalities and its correlation with successful sperm retrieval," *Journal of Human Reproductive Sciences*, vol. 9, no. 3, pp. 187–193, 2016.

[7] T. Takeda, S. Iwatsuki, T. Hamakawa et al., "Chromosomal anomalies and sperm retrieval outcomes of patients with nonobstructive azoospermia: a case series," *Andrology*, vol. 5, no. 3, pp. 473–476, 2017.

[8] J.-W. Kim, S.-Y. Park, H.-M. Ryu et al., "Molecular and clinical characteristics of 26 cases with structural Y chromosome aberrations," *Cytogenetic and Genome Research*, vol. 136, no. 4, pp. 270–277, 2012.

[9] H. Kalantari, S. Asia, M. Totonchi et al., "Delineating the association between isodicentric chromosome Y and infertility: a retrospective study," *Fertility and Sterility*, vol. 101, no. 4, pp. 1091–1096, 2014.

[10] A. Antonelli, L. Marcucci, R. Elli et al., "Semen quality in men with Y chromosome aberrations," *International Journal of Andrology*, vol. 34, no. 5pt1, pp. 453–460, 2011.

[11] C. M. Tuck-Muller, H. Chen, J. E. Martínez et al., "Isodicentric Y chromosome: cytogenetic, molecular and clinical studies and review of the literature," *Human Genetics*, vol. 96, no. 1, pp. 119–129, 1995.

[12] L. Y. F. Hsu, "Phenotype/karyotype correlations of Y chromosome aneuploidy with emphasis on structural aberrations in postnatally diagnosed cases," *American Journal of Medical Genetics*, vol. 53, no. 2, pp. 108–140, 1994.

[13] M. DesGroseilliers, M. Beaulieu Bergeron, P. Brochu, E. Lemyre, and N. Lemieux, "Phenotypic variability in isodicentric Y patients: study of nine cases," *Clinical Genetics*, vol. 70, no. 2, pp. 145–150, 2006.

[14] Practice Committee of American Society for Reproductive Medicine in Collaboration with Society for Male Reproduction and Urology, "Evaluation of the azoospermic male," *Fertility and Sterility*, vol. 90, no. 5, pp. S74–S77, 2008.

[15] M. Codina-Pascual, M. Oliver-Bonet, J. Navarro et al., "FISH characterization of a dicentric Yq (p11.32) isochromosome in an azoospermic male," *American Journal of Medical Genetics Part A*, vol. 127a, no. 3, pp. 302–306, 2004.

[16] M. B. Bergeron, P. Brochu, E. Lemyre, and N. Lemieux, "Correlation of intercentromeric distance, mosaicism, and sexual phenotype: molecular localization of breakpoints in isodicentric Y chromosomes," *American Journal of Medical Genetics Part A*, vol. 155, no. 11, pp. 2705–2712, 2011.

[17] G. R. Dohle, S. Elzanaty, and N. J. van Casteren, "Testicular biopsy: clinical practice and interpretation," *Asian Journal of Andrology*, vol. 14, no. 1, pp. 88–93, 2012.

37

Clinical Features and Outcomes of Dipeptidyl Peptidase-4 Inhibitor-Associated Bullous Pemphigoid (DPP4i-Associated BP) in Thai Patients

Yotsapon Thewjitcharoen,[1] **Ekgaluck Wanothayaroj**,[1] **Chattip Thammawiwat**,[1] **Sriurai Porramatikul**,[1] **Chuleekorn Vorayingyong**,[2] **Soontaree Nakasatien**,[1] **Sirinate Krittiyawong**,[1] **Kumutnart Chanprapaph**,[3] **and Thep Himathongkam**[1]

[1]*Diabetes and Thyroid Center, Theptarin Hospital, Bangkok, Thailand*
[2]*Department of Dermatology, Theptarin Hospital, Bangkok, Thailand*
[3]*Division of Dermatology, Department of Medicine, Ramathibodi Hospital, Bangkok, Thailand*

Correspondence should be addressed to Yotsapon Thewjitcharoen; kamijoa@hotmail.com

Academic Editor: Osamu Isozaki

The use of dipeptidyl peptidase-4 inhibitors (DPP4i) appears to be associated with a small but significantly elevated risk of bullous pemphigoid (BP). Although the pathogenic mechanism of DPP4i-associated BP remains unclear, this adverse event is reported with multiple gliptins, suggesting a class effect. However, previous studies from various countries showed that vildagliptin had been implicated in most cases. The aim of this study was to illustrate a case series of DPP4i-associated BP in Thai patients. We conducted a retrospective study from consecutive cases of BP in people with type 2 diabetes mellitus (T2DM) from January 2008, the year in which the first DPP4i was introduced in Thailand, until December 2019. During the study period, 10 BP patients with T2DM were identified. A total of 5 DPP4i-associated BP (3 on vildagliptin, 1 on linagliptin, and 1 on sitagliptin) were found. All patients were male with a mean age at BP development of 80.4 years (73–86 years). All patients had a long-standing duration of diabetes (median duration 34 years), and mean A1C was 7.5 ± 1.4%. The median time to BP development after the introduction of DPP4i was 64 months (range 20–128 months). The severity of BP was classified as mild in 2 cases. In all cases, the association between the drug intake and BP onset was classified as "possible" according to the Naranjo causality scale. All of the patients continued taking DPP4i after BP diagnosis, and one patient died of lung cancer 18 months after BP diagnosis. Only 2 patients could achieve complete remission at least 2 months after stopping DPP4i. Our case series demonstrated a potential link between DPP4i and the development of BP, which mainly occurred in very elderly male patients. The latency period from an introduction of DPP-4i could be several years, and the clinical course after DPP4i discontinuation varied. Clinicians prescribing DPP4i should be aware of this association and consider stopping this medication before a refractory disease course ensues.

1. Introduction

Bullous pemphigoid (BP) is an uncommon acquired autoimmune disease that occurs mainly in elderly patients with multiple comorbidities and is a relatively rare condition (21–66 cases per a million people in European studies) [1]. However, the incidence of BP is increasing, and recent several studies confirmed that dipeptidyl peptidase-4 inhibitors (DPP4i), which is a common class of antidiabetic medication among elderly patients due to its safety profiles, had been associated with BP [2–5]. A group of Japanese researchers suggested that DPP4i-associated BP displays unique clinical and immunological features with a predominate of the noninflammatory phenotype, and autoantibodies target distinct epitopes on BP180 [6]. However, these findings need to be confirmed in other ethnicities.

Available data from the pharmacovigilance database and cohort studies worldwide had emerged to reveal that various

DPP4is, especially vildagliptin, are a potential trigger agent for the development of BP [7–11]. However, most case series on DPP4i-associated BP had been reported from Japan and with subsequently large database from Western countries illustrating the same potential association. More accumulated case series in other ethnicities are required to better understand the clinical features and outcomes of this rare adverse event from a commonly used antidiabetic medication for people with type 2 diabetes mellitus (T2DM). The aim of this study was to illustrate a case series of DPP4i-associated BP in Thai patients from Theptarin Hospital, one of the largest diabetes centers in Bangkok. The clinical outcomes were also reported after discontinuation of DPP4i.

2. Materials and Methods

We conducted a retrospective study from consecutive cases of BP in people with T2DM from January 2008, the year in which the first DPP4i was introduced in Thailand, to December 2019 to assess whether the use of DPP4i in T2DM is potentially related to the occurence of BP. The clinical characteristics, latency period, Naranjo adverse drug reaction probability scale, and clinical outcomes were evaluated. The Naranjo scale is a validated rating scale to determine the likelihood of whether an adverse event is actually due to the drug rather than a result of other factors [12]. This scoring system is composed of 10 questions with 3 possible answers (yes/no/do not know) and 4 adverse events categories (doubtful, possible, probable, and definite).

The diagnosis of BP was based on typical or consistent clinical features, compatible histological findings, and/or positive immunopathological studies, including direct and indirect immunofluorescence microscopy and enzyme-linked immunosorbent assays (ELISA) for BP180 and BP230. BP180 is a transmembrane glycoprotein, which connects intracellular (BP230) and extracellular hemidesmosome proteins. Due to the high specificity of both tests, serum anti-BP180 IgG and anti-BP230 IgG have been used in establishing the diagnosis of BP [13]. We also assessed BP severity by determining whether steroids were administered systemically and whether patients were hospitalized. After the withdrawal of DPP4i, complete remission was defined as no treatment or receiving minimal therapy for at least 2 months [14]. Minimal therapy is defined as less than or equal to 0.1 mg/kg/day of prednisone or 20 g/week of topical clobetasol propionate. This study was approved by the Institutional Review Board committee of Theptarin Hospital (EC No.6-2019).

3. Results

Between January 2008 and December 2019, a total of 26 BP patients were identified. Among these, 10 patients had T2DM and 5 of whom were under DPP4i treatment (3 on vildagliptin, 1 on linagliptin, and 1 on sitagliptin) as shown in Figure 1. During this period, a total of 3,678 T2DM were first prescribed with various DPP4is and were followed up regularly at our hospital. Therefore, the estimated incidence of DPP4i-associated BP was 1.4 cases per 1,000 DPP4i-treated patients. All patients were male, and the mean age at BP development was 80.4 years (73–86 years). All patients had a long-standing duration of diabetes (median duration of 32 years), and mean A1C was 7.5 ± 1.4%. The median time to BP development after the introduction of DPP4i was 64 months (range 20–128 months). The severity of BP was classified as mild in 2 cases. In all cases, the association between the drug intake and BP onset was classified as "possible" according to the Naranjo causality scale. The median follow-up period after the diagnosis of BP was 32 months (range 7–35 months).

All of the patients continued taking DPP4i after BP diagnosis. DPP4i withdrawal was attempted in all cases except Case no. 1 who passed away of lung cancer at 13 months after the diagnosis of BP. The details and outcomes of each case are illustrated in the followings sections and are summarized in Table 1.

4. Case Reports

4.1. Case 1. An 87-year-old man with T2DM, hypertension, and chronic kidney disease (eGFR 55 ml/min/1.73 m^2) presented with erythematous vesiculobullous lesions on both the legs after 40 months of treatment with glipizide, metformin, and linagliptin. His other medications included candesartan, rosuvastatin, and folic acid. Skin biopsies were taken, and the diagnosis of bullous pemphigoid was suspected. No direct immunofluorescence (DIF) method or serological tests were performed to further confirm the diagnosis. Topical treatment of clobetasol propionate 0.05% ointment was given without oral steroid. All of his medications were maintained after the diagnosis of bullous pemphigoid. Skin lesions were partially improved after topical steroid treatment only. At 6 months later, he had been diagnosed with nonsmall cell lung carcinoma accidentally from routine chest X-ray imaging. The patient had been under palliative treatments for 12 months, until he passed away from obstructive pneumonia.

4.2. Case 2. A 74-year-old man with poorly controlled T2DM, hypertension, dyslipidemia, ischemic heart disease, heart failure, and predialysis end stage renal disease presented with erythematous bullous lesions in the back in December 2017 and then progressed to lower extremities within 3 months. He had been treated with several DPP4i in the past 10 years, starting from sitagliptin in 2008–2014, linagliptin 2014–2016, and finally vildagliptin since October 2016 (15 months before eruption of skin lesions). Other medications included metformin, pioglitazone, empagliflozin, valsartan, spironolactone, simvastatin, ezetimibe, and clopidogrel. Skin biopsies confirmed the diagnosis of bullous pemphigoid with the positive DIF method. Topical treatment of clobetasol propionate 0.05% ointment and oral prednisolone 20 mg per day were given. No mucosal involvement was found. All of his medications were maintained after the diagnosis of bullous pemphigoid. Skin lesions were improved after oral prednisolone and then gradually tapered to 5 mg per day within 6 months. Vildagliptin was discontinued in July 2018 due to progression of

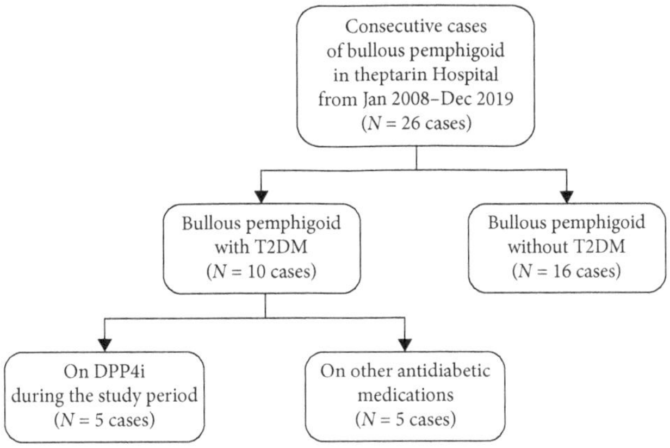

FIGURE 1: Flow selection of studied patients.

TABLE 1: Summary of clinical characteristics and outcomes in our case series of DPP4i-associated bullous pemphigoid.

Case no.	Age/sex	Type of DPP4i	Latency period (months)	Dechallenge	Final outcomes
1	87/M	Linagliptin	40	No	Died from CA lung
2	74/M	Vildagliptin	128	Yes, after the onset of BP 8 months	Stable with oral prednisolone 5 mg/day
3	85/M	Vildagliptin	64	Yes, after the onset of BP 24 months	Complete remission for 5 months, and then, he died from sudden cardiac arrest
4	84/M	Sitagliptin	65	Yes, after the onset of BP 15 months	Complete remission for 4 months, and then, relapsed
5	72/M	Vildagliptin	20	Yes, after the onset of BP 2 months	BP gradually progressed, and then, he died from sudden cardiac arrest

renal failure requiring hemodialysis. Current, his BP lesions are stable with oral prednisolone 5 mg per day, and his glycemic control is treated with multiple daily insulin injections. In summary, the clinical course of BP was easily controlled after stopping vildagliptin; however, remission could not be achieved.

4.3. Case 3. An 85-year-old man with T2DM and dyslipidemia presented with gradual eruption of erythematous vesiculobullous lesions at his forearms and then spread to all over the body within 1 month. No mucosal involvement was found. The diagnosis of severe bullous pemphigoid was confirmed with typical histological findings, positive DIF, and positive serum anti-BP180 and anti-BP230. He had been hospitalized and treated with intravenous steroid and oral azathioprine 150 mg/day. His medications included glicazide, metformin, vildagliptin, and simvastatin. Vildagliptin was started for 64 months before the diagnosis of BP and was still continued for 24 months after the diagnosis. After the potential association between DPP4i and bullous pemphigoid was widely reported in 2018, vildagliptin was discontinued in October 2018. His BP maintenance treatment with oral prednisolone could be tapered from 15 mg to 2.5 mg per day within 2 months after stopping vildagliptin. Oral azathioprine also was stopped without further eruption of skin lesions. Unfortunately, the patient passed away from sudden cardiac arrest at the age of 88 years.

4.4. Case 4. An 84-year-old man with underlying T2DM, dyslipidemia, ischemic heart disease, and complete remission of colon cancer presented with gradual eruption of erythematous vesiculobullous lesions on the scalp, upper extremities, and both feet for 2 weeks. No mucosal involvement was found. The diagnosis of bullous pemphigoid was confirmed with typical histological findings and positive DIF. The DIF analysis showed a linear staining pattern with immunoglobulin G/complement C3 along the dermoepidermal junction as shown in Figure 2. Topical treatment of betamethasone dipropionate 0.05% ointment and oral prednisolone 10 mg per day were given to control his skin lesions. No recurrence of colon cancer had been found. His medications included metformin, pioglitazone, sitagliptin, rosuvastatin, and baby aspirin. Sitagliptin was started for 65 months before the diagnosis of BP and was continued for 15 months after the diagnosis. Until August 2018, sitagliptin was discontinued, and oral pioglitazone was titrated up to 30 mg per day due to increasingly reported cases of DPP4i-associated BP. His skin lesions went into remission without any oral steroid treatment within 2 weeks after DPP4i discontinuation. The clinical pictures before and after DPP4i withdrawal in this patient are depicted in Figure 3.

However, the patient had relapsed BP again at 4 months later, and oral prednisolone 10 mg per day was needed to restart to control skin lesions. Later on, the skin lesions are relapsing and remitting 1 to 2 times per year without

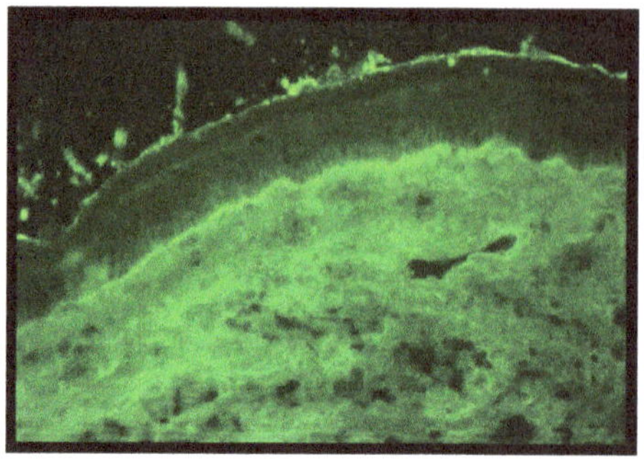

FIGURE 2: Direct immunofluorescence (DIF) analysis of skin biopsy from the patient no.4 showed a linear staining pattern with immunoglobulin G/complement C3 along the dermoepidermal junction.

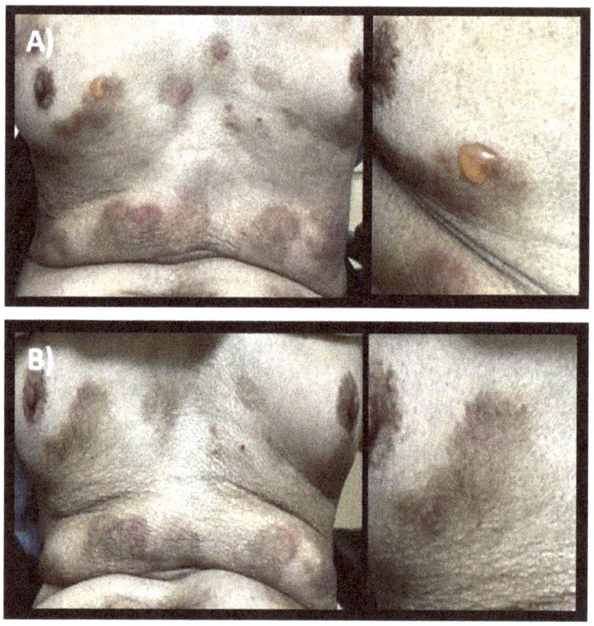

FIGURE 3: (a) Disseminated bullous pemphigoid and a close up image of bullae on the chest wall in Case no.4 before sitagliptin withdrawal and (b) improvements of skin lesions in this patient after 2 weeks of sitagliptin discontinuation.

requiring hospitalization. Current, his glycemic control is stable with metformin and pioglitazone, and BP could be controlled with only topical steroid ointment.

4.5. Case 5. A 72-year-old man with underlying T2DM, Graves' disease, and Parkinson's disease presented with acute eruption of erythematous tense bullous lesions at the left leg after 20 months of starting vildagliptin. No mucosal involvement was found. The diagnosis of bullous pemphigoid was suspected based on typical histological examination. No direct immunofluorescence (DIF) method or serological tests were performed to further confirm the diagnosis. His medications included metformin, vildagliptin, simvastatin, Tapazole, sertraline, and levodopa/benserazide. Vildagliptin was added to metformin at 20 months earlier to better glycemic control. Topical treatment of desoximetasone 0.25% ointment and oral prednisolone 20 mg per day were given to control his skin lesions. After the BP diagnosis, vildagliptin was continued for 2 months before stopping due to the potential association of DPP4i and BP. After discontinuation, his skin lesions still progressed gradually to the trunk and upper extremities. However, oral prednisolone was tapered to 10 mg per day. Unfortunately, his Parkinson's disease progressed, and he became bed ridden. Finally, he passed away from sudden cardiac arrest at home 6 months after the diagnosis of BP. In summary, the clinical course of BP did improve after stopping vildagliptin. Underlying neurological disease and long-duration exposure of DPP4i had been postulated as potential implicating factors.

5. Discussion

This is the first case series from Southeast Asian patients to describe the clinical features and outcomes of DPP4i-associated BP. Based on our present series from a single center institute, the incidence of DPP4i-associated BP is rare with only 1.4 cases per 1,000 DPP4i-treated patients but slightly higher than a previous report of Japanese patients (0.9 cases per 1,000 DPP4i-treated patients) [9]. The occurrence of BP is known to be common in very elderly patients (70s-80s) with neurological diseases such as Alzheimer's disease, stroke, and Parkinson's disease. As shown in our series, some patients in our series already had some underlying conditions or were taking another potential culprit drug, which had been reported in the development of BP. Previous studies showed that the increased risk of BP has been observed in patients older than 70 years, female patients, patients with T2DM, patients having dementia, and other well-known precipitating drugs such as spironolactone [1]. However, T2DM patients taking metformin or second-generation sulphonylurea had lower BP risks when compared with DPP4i [10, 11]. Clinicians prefer prescribing DPP4i as a part of antidiabetic medications in elderly T2DM patients who are prone to hypoglycemia due to its safety profiles. Therefore, DPP4i probably increases the risk of BP but does not independently induce the disease on its own. Moreover, the latency period from an introduction of DPP4i could be several years, and the clinical course after DPP4i discontinuation varied.

DPP4 (also known as CD26) is a ubiquitous cell surface glycoprotein expressed throughout the body including the skin, and its inhibition may lead to modification of the immune response [15]. Some animal studies showed that DPP4i induces infiltration of eosinophil into the skin and also change in the antigenic properties of the epidermal basement membrane [16]. Moreover, the global effects of DPP4 inhibition might affect other subtypes of DPP (DPP8 and DPP9). However, the exact pathogenesis of DPP4i-associated BP remains unknown. A recent study from Japan suggested that HLA-DQB1 * 03 : 01 could be a potential biomarker for the genetic susceptibility toward noninflammatory DPP4i-associated BP among the Japanese population [17]. Further studies are required to verify this finding in other ethnicities.

Since the first anecdotal case report of DPP4i-BP cases in 2011 [18], increasing publications from various countries confirmed that DPP4i had been implicated in the onset of BP with higher odds ratios than previously known major BP-induced drugs such as furosemide, spironolactone, and captopril. Interestingly, vildagliptin had been repeatedly reported as the most increased risk of developing BP. Our present series also corroborated this observation as 3 from 5 cases had been treated with vildagliptin even though sitagliptin was the most common used DPP4i during study period. The mechanism of vildagliptin in the pathogenesis of this rare adverse event is unknown, but the molecule of this medication and relatively lesser DPP4 selectivity of vildagliptin had been proposed as a potential mechanism [7]. Earlier reports suggested that this condition tended to develop within 12 months after the introduction of DPP4i, and BP control could be achieved in the majority of cases after drug withdrawal [7, 8]. However, it should be emphasized that BP usually has a remitting-relapsing clinical course, and most previous reports had a short follow-up duration. As demonstrated in our Case no. 4, the complete remission after DPP4i withdrawal could sustain only for 4 months, and then, low-dose oral prednisolone needed to be restarted. Another possible hypothesis is that the prolonged use of DPP4i after the onset of BP in our cases might lead to a refractory disease course as suggested in a recent review [19]. Moreover, the majority of elderly T2DM patients received polypharmacy, some of which had shown an association with BP [20]. DPP4i-associated BP could be the result of interaction of DPP4i with those medications rather than by DPP4i solely as a trigger drug. Further accumulated cases are required to understand the complete clinical course of this rare side effect.

Advanced age is associated with the onset of both BP and underlying comorbidities, so clinicians should be aware of increased mortality risk in patients with BP [21]. As revealed in our case series, 3 out of 5 cases passed away within months after the diagnosis of BP. In Case no. 1, the association between malignancy and BP remained controversial, especially in Asian patients [22]. The latest population-based study from Taiwan did not demonstrate malignancy as a risk factor for BP [23]. In light of these uncertainties, DPP4i should be stopped immediately if the patient develops BP, and the clinical course after DPP4i discontinuation should be observed closely. It also should be noted that a prodromal phase of chronic eczema or urticarial eruptions could develop before blisters appear [24]. Early consultation with dermatologists in DPP4i-treated elderly T2DM patients should be done for further investigations.

Several limitations of our study should be acknowledged. First, this is a retrospective study conducted in a tertiary diabetes center, which composed of mainly elderly T2DM patients with multiple comorbidities. Second, only one case had the serological tests for anti-BP180 and anti-BP230. Detailed studies of autoantibodies and HLA genotype should be further investigated. Third, we were not able to evaluate the BP severity score in this retrospective study [25]. Further multicenter case-control studies or prospective study should be conducted to clarify the clinical outcomes of this rare adverse effect.

In conclusion, our case series is the first study in Southeast Asia to illustrate the clinical features and outcomes of DPP4i-assoicated BP. The latency period from an introduction of DPP-4i could be several years. Clinicians prescribing DPP4i should be aware of this association and consider stopping this medication before a refractory disease course ensues.

Acknowledgments

The authors wish to thank the staff of the Diabetes and Thyroid Center, Theptarin Hospital, for all their supports, Dr. Tinapa Himathongkam for language editing, and Dr. Weeranut Phothong, Department of Dermatology, Faculty of Medicine, Siriraj Hopsital, Mahidol University, for suggestions and guidance.

References

[1] B. E. Katherine, W. H. Chad, L. M. Christine et al., "Incidence and mortality rates of bullous pemphigoid in olmsted county, Minnesota, over 6 decades," *Journal of The American Academy of Dermatology*, vol. 71, no. 1, pp. 92–99, 2014.

[2] S. A. Giovanni, D. Ilaria, N. Besmir, M. Chiara, M. Edoardo, and M. Matteo, "Bullous pemphigoid and dipeptidyl peptidase-4 inhibitors: a meta-analysis of randomized controlled trials," *Endocrine*, vol. 69, no. 3, pp. 504–507, 2020.

[3] J. Béné, G. Moulis, I. Bennani et al., "Bullous pemphigoid and dipeptidyl peptidase IV inhibitors: a case-noncase study in the French Pharmacovigilance Database," *British Journal of Dermatology*, vol. 175, no. 2, pp. 296–301, 2016.

[4] M. Benzaquen, L. Borradori, P. Berbis et al., "Dipeptidyl peptidase IV inhibitors, a risk factor for bullous pemphigoid: retrospective multicenter case-control study from France and Switzerland," *Journal of The American Academy of Dermatology*, vol. 78, no. 6, pp. 1090–1096, 2018.

[5] A. Reolid, E. Muñoz-Aceituno, P. Rodríguez-Jiménez et al., "Bullous pemphigoid associated with dipeptidyl peptidase-4 inhibitors. A case series and analysis of cases reported in the Spanish pharmacovigilance database," *International Journal of Dermatology*, vol. 59, no. 2, pp. 197–206, 2019.

[6] H. Horikawa, Y. Kurihara, T. Funakoshi et al., "Unique clinical and serological features of bullous pemphigoid associated with dipeptidyl peptidase-4 inhibitors," *British Journal of Dermatology*, vol. 178, no. 6, pp. 1462-1463, 2018.

[7] O. Varpuluoma, A.-K. Försti, J. Jokelainen et al., "Vildagliptin significantly increases the risk of bullous pemphigoid: a Finnish nationwide registry study," *Journal of Investigative Dermatology*, vol. 138, no. 7, pp. 1659–1661, 2018.

[8] K. Kridin and R. Bergman, "Association of bullous pemphigoid with dipeptidyl-peptidase 4 inhibitors in patients with diabetes," *JAMA Dermatology*, vol. 154, no. 10, pp. 1152–1158, 2018.

[9] Y. Kawaguchi, R. Shimauchi, N. Nishibori et al., "Dipeptidyl peptidase-4 inhibitors-associated bullous pemphigoid: a retrospective study of 168 pemphigoid and 9,304 diabetes mellitus patients," *Journal of Diabetes Investigation*, vol. 10, no. 2, pp. 392–398, 2019.

[10] S. G. Lee, H. J. Lee, M. S. Yoon, and D. H. Kim, "Association of dipeptidyl peptidase 4 inhibitor use with risk of bullous pemphigoid in patients with diabetes," *JAMA Dermatology*, vol. 155, no. 2, pp. 172–177, 2019.

[11] C. T. Hung, J. S. Liu, C. Y. Cheng et al., "Increased risk of bullous pemphigoid in dipeptidyl peptidase 4 inhibitors: a nationwide, population-based, cohort study in Taiwan," *The Journal of Dermatology*, vol. 47, no. 3, pp. 245–250, 2020.

[12] C. A. Naranjo, U. Busto, E. M. Sellers et al., "A method for estimating the probability of adverse drug reactions," *Clinical Pharmacology and Therapeutics*, vol. 30, no. 2, pp. 239–245, 1981.

[13] K. Chanprapaph, V. Ounsakul, D. Pruettivorawongse, and K. Thadanipon, "Anti-BP180 and anti-BP230 enzyme linked immunosorbent assays for diagnosis and disease activity tracking of bullous pemphigoid: a prospective cohort study," *Asian Pacific Journal of Allergy and Immunology*, 2019.

[14] D. F. Murrell, B. S. Daniel, P. Joly et al., "Definitions and outcome measures for bullous pemphigoid: recommendations by an international panel of experts," *Journal of The American Academy of Dermatology*, vol. 66, no. 3, pp. 479–485, 2012.

[15] K. Ohnuma, N. H. Dang, and C. Morimoto, "Revisiting an old acquaintance: CD26 and its molecular mechanisms in T cell function," *Trends in Immunology*, vol. 29, no. 6, pp. 295–301, 2008.

[16] U. Forssmann, C. Stoetzer, M. Stephan et al., "Inhibition of CD26/dipeptidyl peptidase IV enhances CCL11/eotaxin-mediated recruitment of eosinophils in vivo," *The Journal of Immunology*, vol. 181, no. 2, pp. 1120–1127, 2008.

[17] H. Ujiie, K. Muramatsu, T. Mushiroda et al., "HLA-DQB1 $*$ 03 : 01 as a biomarker for genetic susceptibility to bullous pemphigoid induced by DPP-4 inhibitors," *Journal of Investigative Dermatology*, vol. 138, no. 5, pp. 1201–1204, 2018.

[18] E. Pasmatzi, A. Monastirli, J. Habeos, S. Georgiou, and D. Tsambaos, "Dipeptidyl peptidase-4 inhibitors cause bullous pemphigoid in diabetic patients: report of two cases," *Diabetes Care*, vol. 34, no. 8, p. e133, 2011.

[19] W. Nishie, "Dipeptidyl peptidase IV inhibitor-associated bullous pemphigoid: a recently recognized autoimmune blistering disease with unique clinical, immunological and genetic characteristics," *Immunological Medicine*, vol. 42, no. 1, pp. 22–28, 2019.

[20] A. Lloyd-Lavery, C. C. Chi, F. Wojnarowska, and K. Taghipour, "The associations between bullous pemphigoid and drug use: a UK case-control study," *JAMA Dermatology*, vol. 149, no. 1, pp. 5–62, 2013.

[21] S. C. S. Cai, J. C. Allen, Y. L. Lim, S. H. Chua, S. H. Tan, and M. B. Y. Tang, "Mortality of bullous pemphigoid in Singapore: risk factors and causes of death in 359 patients seen at the National Skin Centre," *British Journal of Dermatology*, vol. 170, no. 6, pp. 1319–1326, 2014.

[22] R. J. Lucariello, S. E. Villablanca, J. M. Mascaró, and M. Reichel, "Association between bullous pemphigoid and malignancy: a meta-analysis," *Australasian Journal of Dermatology*, vol. 59, no. 4, pp. 253–260, 2018.

[23] C. T. Chen, H. Y. Hu, Y. T. Chang, C. P. Li, and C. Y. Wu, "Cancer is not a risk factor for bullous pemphigoid: 10-year population-based cohort study," *British Journal of Dermatology*, vol. 180, no. 3, pp. 553–558, 2019.

[24] C. V. Bakker, J. B. Terra, H. H. Pas, and M. F. Jonkman, "Bullous pemphigoid as pruritus in the elderly," *JAMA Dermatology*, vol. 149, no. 8, pp. 950–953, 2013.

[25] B. S. Daniel, M. Hertl, V. P. Werth, R. Eming, and D. F. Murrell, "Severity score indexes for blistering diseases," *Clinics in Dermatology*, vol. 30, no. 1, pp. 108–113, 2012.

Denosumab-Induced Hypocalcemia after Billroth II Gastric Bypass Surgery

Abigail M. Schmucker[1] **Dina E. Green,**[2] **and Philip M. Montemuro**[2]

[1]*Sidney Kimmel Medical College, Thomas Jefferson University, 1025 Walnut Street, Philadelphia, PA 19107, USA*
[2]*Lankenau Medical Center, 100 East Lancaster Avenue, Wynnewood, PA 19096, USA*

Correspondence should be addressed to Abigail M. Schmucker; abigail.m.schmucker@gmail.com

Academic Editor: Takeshi Usui

Hypocalcemia is a known risk following bariatric surgery and can contribute to the development of osteoporosis. Osteoporosis is commonly treated with denosumab, though denosumab can exacerbate underlying abnormalities in calcium homeostasis. We present the case of a 59-year-old female with severe hypocalcemia who had been treated with denosumab for osteoporosis three months before and had Billroth II gastric bypass surgery 15 years before, for bariatric purposes. Intravenous calcium supplementation was used to correct the initial electrolyte abnormality, and the patient was able to maintain appropriate calcium levels on high doses of oral calcium before discharge. Denosumab-induced hypocalcemia has been previously reported in patients with predisposing conditions including chronic kidney disease, primary sclerosing cholangitis, Crohn's disease, and a history of sleeve gastrectomy for marginal gastric ulcers. A few cases of hypocalcemia have been reported in patients with a history of bariatric surgery secondary to vitamin D deficiency, but this report is unique in demonstrating denosumab-induced hypocalcemia after bariatric surgery with normal vitamin D levels, suggesting a primary malabsorption of calcium. The risk of severe hypocalcemia should be considered before initiating denosumab to treat osteoporosis in patients with a history of bariatric surgery. If denosumab is initiated, serum calcium levels should be closely monitored, and patients should be educated about the importance of adherence to calcium supplementation.

1. Introduction

With rising rates of obesity globally, bariatric surgery for weight loss has become an increasingly safe and effective option for managing excess weight and associated metabolic and mechanical complications [1, 2]. While bariatric surgical procedures continue to be modified to maximize weight loss while minimizing morbidity and mortality, they are not without risk [1]. Suboptimal preoperative nutrition, anatomical changes, and postoperative dietary constraints can lead to significant micronutrient and vitamin deficiencies after bariatric surgery, including hypocalcemia [2].

The combination of these nutritional deficiencies with mechanical and hormonal changes resulting from bariatric surgery can also contribute to the development of osteoporosis [3]. Antiresorptive therapies such as bisphosphonates and denosumab are first-line treatments for osteoporosis, yet they also pose a risk of hypocalcemia in predisposed patients, ranging from minor and asymptomatic to life-threatening conditions [4, 5]. Hypocalcemia is a known risk of both bariatric surgical procedures and antiresorptive osteoporosis therapies [2, 4, 6], but the hypocalcemia risk of these two factors combined and the optimal treatment of those with osteoporosis secondary to a history of bariatric surgery have received little attention in the literature.

In this report, we present the case of a 59-year-old female who developed severe hypocalcemia three months after treatment with denosumab for osteoporosis and fifteen years after Billroth II gastric bypass surgery. This case was prepared in accordance with the CARE guidelines for case reports (see Appendix 1 in Supplementary Materials for CARE checklist).

2. Case Presentation

A 59-year-old postmenopausal woman with a past medical history of Billroth II gastric bypass surgery 15 years before for bariatric purposes, Barrett esophagus, pericarditis secondary to suspected rheumatologic disease status treated with a pericardial window 3 years before, rheumatoid arthritis with negative rheumatoid factor, paroxysmal atrial fibrillation, amiodarone-induced hypothyroidism, and osteoporosis treated with denosumab 3 months before was referred to the emergency department by her endocrinologist after outpatient labs revealed profound hypocalcemia, hypophosphatemia, and hypomagnesemia. The patient had recently returned from vacation, where she experienced 2-3 episodes of diarrhea. She reported compliance to her medications, which included 50,000 IU ergocalciferol daily and 630 mg calcium citrate 2-3 times daily, apart from taking a decreased dose of calcium for the last 4 days of her vacation since she was running low on pills. She noted fatigue and intermittent tingling in her hands, feet, and perioral region for 2-3 days prior to admission. She denied weight loss, fever, muscle cramping, seizures, loss of consciousness, or lightheadedness.

On presentation, the patient was afebrile with a temperature of 98.2oF, blood pressure of 136/74 mmHg, heart rate of 71 beats/min, and respiratory rate of 15 breaths/min. Her oxygen saturation was 100% on room air. Physical examination revealed a well-appearing woman with a body mass index (BMI) of 30 kg/m^2 in no acute distress. Neck was supple with no thyromegaly. There were no abnormalities on cardiac or pulmonary exam. Abdomen was soft, nontender, and nondistended with normal bowel sounds. Patient had a positive Chvostek's sign. No muscle twitches or spasms were appreciated. Strength, sensation, reflexes, and cranial nerves were intact. The patient had no signs of confusion or psychosis.

Blood tests from the emergency department revealed a calcium of 5.8 mg/dL, phosphorus of <1 mg/dL, and magnesium of 1.7 mg/dL. Albumin was 3.8 g/dL, so the corrected calcium was 6.0 mg/dL. Ionized calcium was 0.8 mg/dL. Parathyroid hormone was 136 ng/L. 25-Hydroxy vitamin D was normal at 46 ng/mL, and 1-25-hydroxy vitamin D was normal at 30 pg/mL. Urinalysis was within normal limits, and urine calcium was <2 mg/dL. Creatinine was 0.61 mg/dL, and blood urea nitrogen was 11 mg/dL. TSH was normal at 0.78 μU/mL. An electrocardiogram performed in the emergency department showed normal sinus rhythm with a corrected QT interval of 493 ms.

In the emergency department, the patient was given 2 g of IV magnesium sulfate, 30 mmol of IV sodium phosphate, and 1 g of IV calcium gluconate. During her 4-day hospital stay, the patient continued to receive IV calcium, as well as oral calcitriol, phosphate, and magnesium. When she was able to consistently maintain serum calcium of at least 8.0 mg/dL on oral calcium citrate supplementation, she was discharged with a calcium level of 8.0 mg/dL, magnesium of 1.9 mg/dL, and phosphorus of 2.3 mg/dL. She was instructed to take calcium citrate of 1260 mg 4 times daily, calcitriol of 0.25 mcg 2 times daily, phosphorus of 250 mg 3 times daily, and magnesium oxide of 400 mg 2 times daily and to be followed up closely with her endocrinologist. Since discharge, the patient has been able to maintain adequate calcium levels on a low dose of calcium supplementation, and she is interested in considering further doses of denosumab.

3. Discussion

The risk of hypocalcemia following denosumab use for osteoporosis has been demonstrated in multiple case reports and case series for patients with chronic kidney disease [7–10] and in individual case reports for patients with primary sclerosing cholangitis [11], Crohn's disease [8, 12, 13], and a history of sleeve gastrectomy for marginal gastric ulcers [12]. A few cases of hypocalcemia with denosumab have been reported in patients with a history of bariatric surgery, but each of these was likely secondary to vitamin D deficiency [14, 15]. In our case, normal active and storage forms of vitamin D, low phosphate, and normal kidney function tests suggested that the hypocalcemia was not due to renal failure or vitamin D deficiency. With these etiologies excluded, the most likely cause of hypocalcemia was primary calcium malabsorption from the bariatric Billroth II procedure 15 years before, exacerbated by denosumab use 3 months before and insufficient calcium supplementation during the week prior to admission.

Billroth II gastrectomy is a form of gastric bypass surgery often used for refractory peptic ulcer disease and gastric adenocarcinoma, but it can also be used for weight loss since it reduces the volume of the stomach, causing early satiety [16]. Due to a combination of anatomical changes, postoperative dietary changes, and suboptimal preoperative nutrition, many patients develop micronutrient deficiencies after bariatric surgery [2], and Billroth II procedure has been shown to cause calcium and vitamin D absorption disturbances [17]. Because of the risk of hypocalcemia following bariatric surgery, calcium supplementation and vitamin D supplementation are recommended to prevent postoperative hypocalcemia [14].

Even with adequate supplementation, the malabsorption resulting from bariatric surgery, combined with mechanical and hormonal factors related to weight loss, predisposes patients to osteoporosis after bariatric surgery [3]. Denosumab, a common first-line treatment for osteoporosis, is a monoclonal antibody approved for prevention of skeletal-related events in postmenopausal women at risk for osteoporosis (as Prolia®) and is given as a subcutaneous injection every six months [4, 18]. Denosumab functions by inhibiting osteoclast-mediated bone resorption by binding to the receptor activator of nuclear factor kappa B ligand (RANKL), thus preventing RANKL from binding to its receptor. As a result, less skeletal calcium is released into the circulation [19]. Denosumab is known to exacerbate existing hypocalcemia, so correction of preexisting hypocalcemia is suggested prior to administration. Additionally, monitoring of calcium, phosphorus, and magnesium is recommended, and supplementation with at least 1000 mg daily of calcium and 400 IU of vitamin D is recommended, particularly during the first 14 days after administration [20].

Our patient experienced profound hypocalcemia 15 years after bariatric surgery and 3 months after denosumab administration. Prior to this episode, the patient was on a longstanding dose of 50,000 IU ergocalciferol daily, as well as 630 mg calcium citrate 2-3 times daily, which is well within the recommendations of the Prolia® insert [20]. She was closely monitored by her rheumatologist and endocrinologist during the interval immediately after denosumab administration, and she never experienced profound hypocalcemia during this time. Considering our patient had two separate indications for calcium and vitamin D supplementation, perhaps she needed higher doses of oral supplements, or she was particularly susceptible to a few days of a decreased calcium dose while on vacation.

One previous study sought to identify risks for denosumab-induced hypocalcemia and found no significant associations between clinical parameters and development of hypocalcemia [5]. Notably, however, previous gastrointestinal surgeries were not included among the clinical parameters they assessed. The study concluded that high baseline bone turnover, as evidenced by increased serum bone turnover markers, was associated with denosumab-induced hypocalcemia [5]. Given that our patient likely had a decreased ability to absorb calcium via the gastrointestinal tract, it seems reasonable to hypothesize that she had high baseline bone turnover.

Strengths of this case include the fact that the patient was a reliable historian with a well-documented surgical and medical history within the electronic medical record. Additionally, her established outpatient endocrinologist followed her in the hospital, allowing for continuity of care and effective outpatient follow-up. A weakness of the case is that there is no way to parse out the relative contribution to hypocalcemia of each potential factor—denosumab use, chronic absorption issues from prior bariatric surgery, and missed calcium supplementation and diarrhea in the days leading up to admission. Additionally, given the timing of the patient's bariatric surgery relative to the current episode, we do not have access to the degree of her weight loss after the surgery; however, based on the history from the patient and a current BMI of 30, we do not suspect that malabsorptive issues were a result of an overly aggressive bariatric surgery. Further research is needed to determine the risk of denosumab-induced hypocalcemia for various bariatric surgical techniques, as well as to determine a safe and cost-effective way to select patients for extended calcium monitoring after denosumab administration.

This case demonstrates that the risk of profound hypocalcemia should be weighed when considering initiation of denosumab in a patient with a history of bariatric surgery. While bariatric surgery has been shown to decrease bone mineral density, a 2012 study in the British Medical Journal showed that bariatric surgery does not have a significant effect on fracture risk, at least over the short term [21]. So, perhaps, treatment of osteoporosis secondary to bariatric surgery can be less aggressive than treatment of primary osteoporosis. For those patients with a bariatric surgery history who are started on denosumab for osteoporosis, monitoring of calcium, phosphorus, and magnesium should be extended beyond the 14-day interval recommended in the Prolia® insert, and higher doses of calcium, phosphorus, magnesium, and vitamin D should be considered than those recommended for general denosumab use. Finally, patients should be educated about the importance of long-term adherence to supplementation, as well as what symptoms should prompt them to visit the emergency department.

Acknowledgments

This work was supported in part by Thomas Jefferson University and Philadelphia University Open Access Fund.

References

[1] H.-U. Spiegel and S. Skawran, "From longitudinal gastric resection to sleeve gastrectomy-revival of a previously established surgical procedure," *Journal of Gastrointestinal Surgery*, vol. 15, no. 1, pp. 219–228, 2011.

[2] M. Shah, A. Sharma, R. A. Wermers, K. A. Kennel, T. A. Kellogg, and M. S. Mundi, "Hypocalcemia after bariatric surgery: prevalence and associated risk factors," *Obesity Surgery*, vol. 27, no. 11, pp. 2905–2911, 2017.

[3] A. Jammah, "Endocrine and metabolic complications after bariatric surgery," *Saudi Journal of Gastroenterology*, vol. 21, no. 5, pp. 269–277, 2015.

[4] K. N. Tu, J. D. Lie, C. K. V. Wan et al., "Osteoporosis: a review of treatment options," *A Peer-Reviewed Journal for Formulary Management*, vol. 43, no. 2, pp. 92–104, 2018.

[5] K. Ishikawa, T. Nagai, K. Sakamoto et al., "High bone turnover elevates the risk of denosumab-induced hypocalcemia in women with postmenopausal osteoporosis," *Therapeutics and Clinical Risk Management*, vol. 12, pp. 1831–1840, 2016.

[6] W.-X. Qi, F. Lin, A.-N. He, L.-N. Tang, Z. Shen, and Y. Yao, "Incidence and risk of denosumab-related hypocalcemia in cancer patients: a systematic review and pooled analysis of randomized controlled studies," *Current Medical Research and Opinion*, vol. 29, no. 9, pp. 1067–1073, 2013.

[7] R. Cernes, Z. Barnea, A. Biro, G. Zandman-Goddard, and Z. Katzir, "Severe hypocalcemia following a single denosumab injection," *Israel Medical Association Journal*, vol. 19, no. 11, pp. 719–721, 2017.

[8] J. Strickling and M. J. Wilkowski, "Severe, symptomatic hypocalcemia due to denosumab administration: treatment and clinical course," *Case Reports in Nephrology and Dialysis*, vol. 9, no. 1, pp. 33–41, 2019.

[9] R. D. Bhanot, J. Kaur, and Z. Bhat, "Severe hypocalcemia and dramatic increase in parathyroid hormone after denosumab in a dialysis patient: a case report and review of the literature," *Case Reports in Nephrology*, vol. 2019, pp. 1–4, 2019.

[10] R. Jalleh, G. Basu, R. Le Leu, and S. Jesudason, "Denosumab-induced severe hypocalcaemia in chronic kidney disease," *Case Reports in Nephrology*, vol. 2018, pp. 1–7, 2018.

[11] Y. Yasuda, S. Iwama, and H. Arima, "Severe hypocalcemia following denosumab treatment in a patient with secondary osteoporosis associated with primary sclerosing cholangitis," *Endocrine Journal*, vol. 66, no. 3, pp. 271–275, 2019.

[12] R. Kalayanamitra, I. Yaghnam, R. Patel, A. Groff, and R. Jain, "The calcium culprit: a case of denosumab-induced hypocalcemia," *Cureus*, vol. 11, 2019.
[13] V. Chandurkar and E. B. Marliss, "Multiple factors in recurrent symptomatic hypocalcemia following denosumab in a patient receiving home parenteral nutrition," *Journal of Parenteral and Enteral Nutrition*, vol. 40, no. 5, pp. 734–738, 2016.
[14] I. Miñambres, A. Chico, and A. Pérez, "Severe hypocalcemia due to vitamin D deficiency after extended roux-en-Y gastric bypass," *Journal of Obesity*, vol. 2011, pp. 1–3, 2011.
[15] V. Baptista Lopes, D. Robbrecht, S. van Thiel, and C. van Guldener, "[Symptomatic hypocalcaemia on denosumab use]," *Ned Tijdschr Geneeskd*, vol. 157, no. 29, p. A6159, 2013.
[16] E. P. Weledji, "Overview of gastric bypass surgery," *International Journal of Surgery Open*, vol. 5, pp. 11–19, 2016.
[17] M. Fukuda, H. Shibata, K. Hatakeyama et al., "Difference in calcium metabolism following billroth-I and billroth-II procedures for gastric and duodenal ulcers," *The Japanese Journal of Surgery*, vol. 9, no. 4, pp. 295–303, 1979.
[18] M. Muqeet Adnan, J. Morton, S. Hashmi, S. Abdul Mujeeb, W. Kern, and B. J. Cowley, "Anti-GBM of pregnancy: acute renal failure resolved after spontaneous abortion, plasma exchange, hemodialysis, and steroids," *Case Reports in Nephrology*, vol. 2014, pp. 1–4, 2014.
[19] L. K. Laskowski, D. S. Goldfarb, M. A. Howland, K. Kavcsak, D. M. Lugassy, and S. W. Smith, "A RANKL wrinkle: denosumab-induced hypocalcemia," *Journal of Medical Toxicology*, vol. 12, no. 3, pp. 305–308, 2016.
[20] Amgen, *Prolia Highlights of Prescribing Information*, Amgen, Thousand Oaks, CA, USA, 2010.
[21] L. Angrisani, A. Santonicola, P. Iovino, G. Formisano, H. Buchwald, and N. Scopinaro, "Bariatric surgery worldwide 2013," *Obesity Surgery*, vol. 25, no. 10, pp. 1822–1832, 2015.

Successful Treatment of Tumor-Induced Osteomalacia by Multidisciplinary Therapy with Radiation to Intracranial Fibromyxoid Tumor

Mariangela Massaccesi,[1] Francesco Micciché,[1] Mario Rigante,[2] Gianluigi Petrone,[3] Elisabetta Lepre,[4] Maria Antonietta Gambacorta,[1,4] and Vincenzo Valentini[1,4]

[1]*Fondazione Policlinico Universitario "A. Gemelli" IRCCS, Unità Operativa Complessa di Radioterapia, Dipartimento di Diagnostica per Immagini, Radioterapia Oncologica ed Ematologia, Roma, Italy*
[2]*Fondazione Policlinico Universitario "A. Gemelli" IRCCS, Unità Operativa Complessa di Otorinolaringoiatria, Dipartimento di scienze dell'invecchiamento, Neurologiche, Ortopediche e della testa-collo, Roma, Italy*
[3]*Fondazione Policlinico Universitario "A. Gemelli" IRCCS, Unità Operativa Complessa di Anatomia Patologica, Dipartimento di scienze della salute della donna, del bambino e di sanità pubblica, Roma, Italy*
[4]*Università Cattolica del Sacro Cuore Facoltà di Medicina e Chirurgia, Roma, Italy*

Correspondence should be addressed to Mariangela Massaccesi; mariangela.massaccesi@policlinicogemelli.it

Academic Editor: Osamu Isozaki

Background. Tumor-induced osteomalacia (TIO) is a rare paraneoplastic syndrome caused by protein fibroblast-growth-factor-23 (FGF-23) secreting tumors. Complete tumor resection is the current standard of care for TIO; however, some patients may develop tumor recurrence. Due to the rarity of this paraneoplastic syndrome, the role of radiotherapy is unclear. This case is worth reporting because it adds to our knowledge some insights about the potential role of radiotherapy in this rare condition. *Case Presentation.* After multidisciplinary consultation, in July 2015, postoperative adjuvant radiotherapy was offered to a 52-year-old man with a multiple recurrent ossifying fibromyxoid tumor in the right frontal sinus causing TIO. The patient had a history of multiple bone fractures and pain since more than 20 years. The tumor had been removed in 2003 for the first time. Subsequent endoscopic resections of the tumor had been performed for recurrences of TIO in May 2012, October 2013, and July 2015. Starting from October 2015, external beam radiotherapy was delivered with a volumetric modulated arc technique to the tumor bed with a daily dose of 2 Gy up to a total dose of 60 Gy. After five years from treatment, the patient is free from local tumor relapse, TIO progression, and radiation-induced side effects. *Conclusions.* Radiotherapy may provide long-term TIO remission and tumor control, thus being a treatment option in cases where surgery is unfeasible or unsuccessful.

1. Introduction

Tumor-induced osteomalacia (TIO) or oncogenic osteomalacia is a rare paraneoplastic syndrome resulting from excessive production of the protein fibroblast growth factor-23 (FGF-23). FGF-23 act as a phosphaturic hormone and also favors inactivation of 1, 25 dihydroxyvitamin D, thus leading to compensatory hyperparathyroidism. Patients typically present with symptoms of gradually progressive weakness, bone pain, and pathological fractures. Benign mesenchymal or mixed connective tissue tumor is the most common histological feature of neoplasms associated with TIO. Complete tumor resection is the current standard of care for TIO [1]. However, some patients may develop tumor recurrence and benefit from a second excision [2]. Radiotherapy has been rarely used in case of inoperable tumors or incomplete resections [3–9]. We report the case of a patient who had a multiple recurrent ossifying fibromyxoid tumor in the left frontal sinus causing TIO.

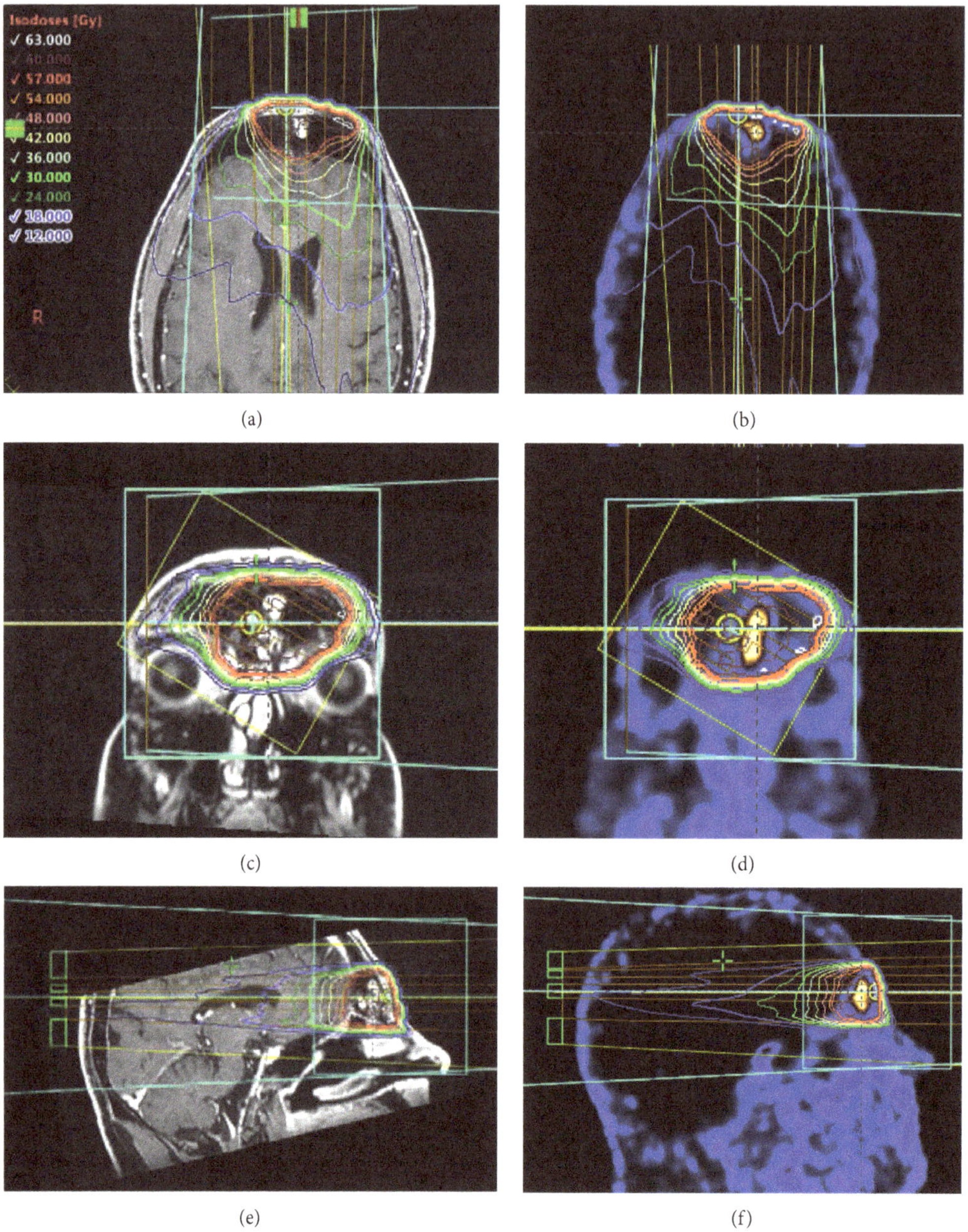

FIGURE 1: Dose distribution of postoperative VMAT for a multiple recurrent ossifying fibromyxoid tumor of the left frontal sinus causing TIO. Isodose lines are shown on axial (a, b), coronal (c, d), and sagittal (e, f) planes of coregistered preoperative MR (a, c, and e), ^{68}Ga-DOTATATE PET, and simulation CT images (b, d, and f). The red line represents the 95% isodose.

2. Case Presentation

The patient was a 52-year-old man with no family history of cancer and no significant comorbidity except hypercholesterolemia and arterial hypertension.

The patient had a history of bone pain, weakness, and multiple pathological fractures for more than 20 years. In 2003, osteomalacia was diagnosed by bone biopsy at the level of the right knee. In the same period, the patient underwent also surgical removal of a small lesion on the left frontal sinus that was diagnosed as an ossifying fibromyxoid tumor. After surgery, the patient experienced a period of symptom improvement, but again, over the following years, bone pain progressively worsened, and many nontraumatic bone fractures occurred in the right femur, ribs, right tibia, right fibula, and metatarsal bones despite therapy with vitamin D3 and calcium. In 2012, the diagnostic hypothesis of osteomalacia of oncogenic origin finally arose, and the patient underwent targeted investigations.

A total body computed tomography (CT) scan documented the presence of dense tissue in the left frontal sinus. At that level, a magnetic resonance (MR) examination showed a lobulated lesion measuring 2 cm, which was hypointense in the T1 sequences and hyperintense in the T2 sequences and had intense contrast enhancement. The lesion highly expressed somatostatin receptors on a ^{68}Ga-

TABLE 1: Dose received by organs at risk.

Organ at risk	Maximum dose (Gy)	Mean dose (Gy)
Left eye	41.7	5.6
Right eye	26.8	6.0
Left lens	5.9	3.3
Right lens	5.5	3.6
Optic chiasm	5.8	3.1
Left optic nerve	14.7	6.2
Right optic nerve	16.8	6.9
Brain	62.0	7.4

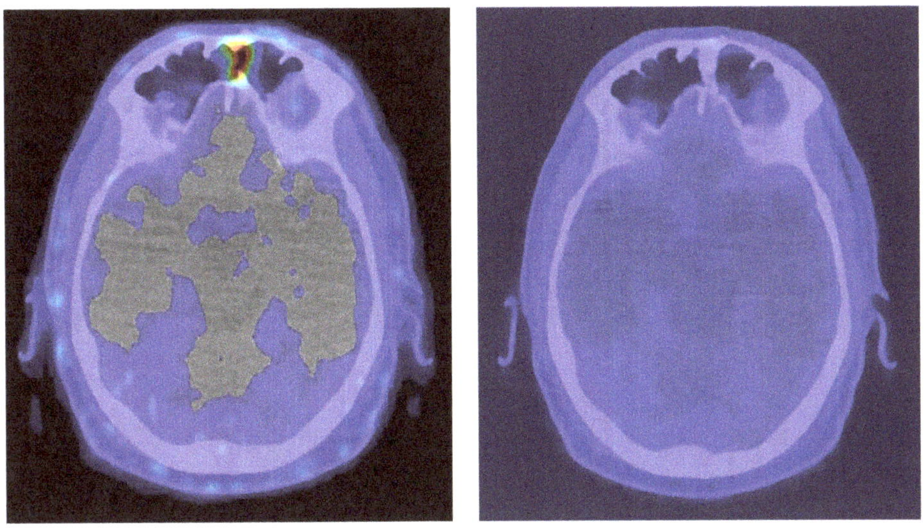

(a) (b)

FIGURE 2: ^{68}Ga-DOTATATE PET-CT images showing complete response of the recurrent ossifying fibromyxoid tumor in the left frontal sinus after surgery and adjuvant radiotherapy. ^{68}Ga-DOTATATE PET-CT images before treatment (a) and after treatment (b).

DOTATATE positron emission tomography (PET) scan. Blood tests documented low levels of phosphate and high levels of FGF-23.

In May 2012, the lesion of the left frontal sinus was removed through an endoscopic approach. Histological examination documented an ossifying fibromyxoid tumor that was framed as a recurrence of the lesion that had been removed in 2003. After a brief period of clinical and laboratory remission, TIO symptoms reappeared and gradually worsened. In April 2013, a ^{68}Ga-DOTATATE PET scan showed a small lesion in the left frontal sinus with hyperexpression of somatostatin receptors. Six months later, a MR scan confirmed the presence of a contrast-enhancing lesion measuring 1.5 cm in the medial wall of the left frontal sinus, without signs of bone or orbital infiltration. In October 2013, the patient underwent an endoscopic frontal senectomy to remove the recurrence of the ossifying fibromyxoid tumor. Again, after less than two years of clinical remission, TIO symptoms worsened. In March 2015, an MR scan confirmed the presence of a small recurrence of the tumor, without signs of bone or orbital infiltration. A fourth surgical intervention was performed in July 2015 through a combined endoscopic and open approach to completely remove the lesion. A postoperative contrast-enhanced computed tomography was performed four weeks later, and it did not show any suspect sign of disease persistence. In August 2015, the case was discussed in a multidisciplinary tumor board and adjuvant radiation therapy was proposed to reduce the risk of further tumor recurrence. This multidisciplinary decision was shared with the patient who gave his consent to the treatment. Starting from October 2015, external beam radiotherapy was delivered with a volumetric modulated arc technique (VMAT) to the tumor bed with a daily dose of 2 Gy up to a total dose of 60 Gy. The patient was treated in the supine position with a thermoplastic facemask. The tumor bed was identified on coregistered preoperative MR, ^{68}Ga-DOTATATE PET, and planning CT simulation images. The clinical target volume (CTV) included the tumor bed plus 1 cm margin along the frontal sinus walls. The planning target volume (PTV) included the CTV plus 3 mm margin. The organs at risk (OARs) were the optic chiasm, right and left cochlea, right and left lens, right and left eyeballs, and right and left optic nerves. Details of the radiation treatment are shown in Figure 1 and Table 1. Orthogonal planar kilo-voltage images were used daily before treatment as image guidance. Radiotherapy was completed without any treatment-related side effects.

Figure 2 shows the complete disappearance of the recurrent ossifying fibromyxoid tumor in the left frontal sinus after surgery and adjuvant radiotherapy.

Table 2: Details of all published cases of radiotherapy use for TIO.

Reference	Case	Age	Sex	Histopathology	Lesion site	Previous surgery	Radiotherapy indication	Radiotherapy treatment modality	EBRT, total dose (Gy)	EBRT, fraction dose (Gy)	EBRT technique	Follow-up time (months)	Local tumor control	Status osteomalacia
Uramoto, 2009	1	48	M	Malignant PMTMCT	Tongue	Yes, 1 time	Unresectable recurrence of the lesion	EBRT	66	Not specified	Not specified	24	Unknown	Cured
Tarasova, 2013	2	67	F	Unknown	Intracranial	No	Surgery refusal	EBRT	60	Not specified	SRT	12	Unknown	Cured
Hautmann, 2014	3	45	M	PMTMCT	Distal tibia	Yes, 1 time	Postoperative, partial resection	EBRT	45	1.8	Not specified	34	Complete remission	Cured
Basu, 2016	4	53	F	Benign giant-cell tumor	Base of the skull	Yes, multiple	Unresectable recurrence of the lesion	PPRT (peptide receptor radiotherapy)	-	-	-	3	Partial response	Cured
	5	46	M	Hemangiopericytoma	Left petrous tumor	Yes, 1 time	Postoperative, partial resection	EBRT	Not specified	Not specified	Not specified	96	Complete remission	Cured
Shah, 2019	6	53	F	PMTMCT	Base of the skull	Yes, multiple	Postoperative, partial resection	PPRT (peptide receptor radiotherapy)	-	-	-	13	Stable disease	Cured
	7	60	M	PMTMCT	Left ethmoid sinus	Yes, multiple	Postoperative, partial resection	EBRT	54	1.8	IMRT	36	Unknown	Cured
Present case	8	52	M	Ossifying fibromyxoid tumor	Frontal sinus	Yes, multiple	Postoperative, complete resection	EBRT	60	2	VMAT	55	Complete remission	Cured

PMTMCT, phosphaturic mesenchymal tumor mixed connective tissue type; EBRT, external beam radiotherapy; PPRT, peptide receptor radiotherapy; SRT, stereotactic radiotherapy; IMRT, intensity-modulated radiotherapy, VMAT, volumetric modulated arc therapy.

After 60 months from treatment, the patient is free from both tumor recurrence and TIO.

3. Discussion

The role of radiotherapy in the multidisciplinary treatment of TIO is far to be defined due to the rarity of this condition. This report described the case of a patient with TIO caused by a multiple recurrent ossifying fibromyxoid tumor, who was cured by surgery and postoperative radiotherapy. To our knowledge, only eight cases of radiotherapy treatment for TIO have been reported so far [3, 4, 6, 7, 9]. Table 2 reports characteristics of all published cases. Five patients were male, and three were female. Patients' age ranged between 43 and 67 years. The cause of oncogenic osteomalacia was a phosphaturic mesenchymal tumor in most cases, and most tumors were in the head region. All patients but one had tumor recurrence after surgery, that was multiple in four cases. In patients with tumor recurrence after previous surgery, radiotherapy was used alone (two patients) or after either partial (four cases) or complete (present case) tumor reresection. A patient who refused surgery for an intracranial lesion underwent radiotherapy as the sole treatment modality.

External beam radiotherapy was used in six cases. Peptide receptor radiotherapy (PPRT) was used in the other two cases. External beam radiation treatment was poorly detailed in published reports. When specified, the total radiation dose ranged between 45 and 66 Gy, and treatment was delivered with conventional fractionation. All patients who underwent radiotherapy had complete remission of TIO. Particularly, three patients who had more than three years of follow-up experienced long-term tumor control and TIO remission.

In conclusion, external beam radiotherapy might provide long-term tumor control and TIO remission, thus being a possible option whenever surgery is unfeasible or unsuccessful.

References

[1] P. Florenzano, I. R. Hartley, M. Jimenez, K. Roszko, R. I. Gafni, and M. T. Collins, "Tumor-induced osteomalacia," *Calcified Tissue International*, vol. 108, no. 1, pp. 128–142, 2021.

[2] Z.-j. Sun, J. Jin, G.-x. Qiu, P. Gao, and Y. Liu, "Surgical treatment of tumor-induced osteomalacia: a retrospective review of 40 cases with extremity tumors," *BMC Musculoskeletal Disorders*, vol. 16, no. 1, p. 43, 2015.

[3] R. Shah, A. R. Lila, R. S. Jadhav et al., "Tumor induced osteomalacia in head and neck region: single center experience and systematic review," *Endocrine Connections*, vol. 8, pp. 1330–1353, 2019.

[4] N. Uramoto, M. Furukawa, and T. Yoshizaki, "Malignant phosphaturic mesenchymal tumor, mixed connective tissue variant of the tongue," *Auris, Nasus, Larynx*, vol. 36, pp. 104-105, 2009.

[5] F. A. Sandhu and R. L. Martuza, "Craniofacial hemangiopericytoma associated with oncogenic osteomalacia: case report," *Journal of Neuro-Oncology*, vol. 46, pp. 241–247, 2000.

[6] V. D. Tarasova, A. G. Trepp-Carrasco, R. Thompson et al., "Successful treatment of tumor-induced osteomalacia due to an intracranial tumor by fractionated stereotactic radiotherapy," *The Journal of Clinical Endocrinology and Metabolism*, vol. 98, pp. 4267–4272, 2013.

[7] A. H. Hautmann, J. Schroeder, P. Wild et al., "Tumor-induced osteomalacia: increased level of FGF-23 in a patient with a phosphaturic mesenchymal tumor at the tibia expressing periostin," *Case Reports in Endocrinology*, vol. 2014, Article ID 729387, 2014.

[8] P. J. Catalano, M. Brandwein, D. K. Shah, M. L. Urken, W. Lawson, and H. F Biller, "Sinonasal hemangiopericytomas: a clinicopathologic and immunohistochemical study of seven cases," *Head and Neck*, vol. 18, pp. 42–53, 1996.

[9] S. Basu and P. Fargose, "177Lu-DOTATATE PRRT in recurrent skull-base phosphaturic mesenchymal tumor causing osteomalacia: a potential application of PRRT beyond neuroendocrine tumors," *Journal of Nuclear Medicine Technology*, vol. 44, no. 4, pp. 248–250, 2016.

40

ARMC5 Primary Bilateral Macronodular Adrenal Hyperplasia Associated with a Meningioma: A Family Report

M. J. Ferreira,[1,2,3] **J. Pedro**,[1,2,3] **D. Salazar**,[1,2,3] **C. Costa**,[4,5] **J. Aragão Rodrigues**,[5] **M. M. Costa**,[6] **A. Grangeia**,[2,7] **J. L. Castedo**,[1] **and D. Carvalho**[1,2,3]

[1]*Department of Endocrinology, Diabetes and Metabolism of Centro Hospitalar Universitário de São João, Porto, Portugal*
[2]*Faculty of Medicine of the Universidade do Porto, Porto, Portugal*
[3]*Instituto de Investigação e Inovação em Saúde, Universidade do Porto, Porto, Portugal*
[4]*Portuguese Institute of Oncology, Porto, Portugal*
[5]*Department of Pathology of Centro Hospitalar Universitário de São João, Porto, Portugal*
[6]*Department of Endocrinology, Diabetes and Metabolism of Hospital Garcia de Orta, Porto, Portugal*
[7]*Department of Genetics of Centro Hospitalar Universitário de São João, Porto, Portugal*

Correspondence should be addressed to M. J. Ferreira; mj.ferreira0@gmail.com

Academic Editor: Osamu Isozaki

Primary bilateral adrenal macronodular hyperplasia is characterized by functioning adrenal macronodules and variable cortisol secretion. Familial clustering suggests a genetic cause that has been confirmed with the identification of some genetic mutations, including inactivating germline mutations, in *armadillo repeat containing 5 (ARMC5)* gene. The identification of the pathogenic variant enables the physician to identify and treat these patients earlier and more effectively. It has also been noticed that patients with germline causative variants show a different clinical spectrum, presenting specific clinical characteristics, as the association with the presence of meningiomas.

1. Introduction

Primary bilateral macronodular adrenal hyperplasia (PBMAH) is a rare cause of Cushing's syndrome, presenting multiple benign nodules in both adrenal cortexes [1]. In contrast to micronodular adrenal hyperplasia, adrenal nodules observed in patients with PBMAH are typically larger than 1 cm and detectable by abdominal imaging [2]. PBMAH may lead to overt Cushing's syndrome and long-term consequences of cortisol excess are frequent despite appropriate treatment. This might be due to diagnostic delay, as mild clinical presentation is often observed [2–4]. PBMAH is most frequently diagnosed in patients between 40 and 70 years of age and frequently in the course of investigation of an adrenal incidentaloma [2]. Because of its clinical variability, the prevalence of this disease is not well-established, but is thought to represent less than 2% of all endogenous cases of Cushing's syndrome [1, 5].

The pathophysiological process that leads to PBMAH has not been fully clarified [6–8]. Steroidogenesis has been shown to be relatively inefficient in PBMAH, which explains the indolent natural history of the disease, and the late manifestation of clinical hypercortisolism, present only after severe and irregular enlargement of the adrenal glands [2].

Although previously considered an ACTH-independent Cushing syndrome, it now appears that cortisol secretion by the adrenals is regulated by corticotropin, which is locally produced by a subpopulation of steroidogenic cells in the hyperplastic adrenals [7, 9]. The abnormal expression of ACTH by these cells seems to represent a secondary pathophysiological process that is common to diverse molecular defects and is seen in both sporadic and familial cases [7]. In most patients with PBMAH, there are also aberrant receptors that regulate steroidogenesis by mimicking the cellular events that are triggered normally by the ACTH receptor [10]. As so, the secretion of cortisol often involves stimulation of ectopic membrane receptors that shows hyperactivity or paradoxical stimulation to glucose-dependent insulinotropic peptide, beta-adrenergic receptors, serotonin, glucagon, and probably angiotensin; as well as eutopic receptors such as those for vasopressin, LH/human chorionic gonadotropin, or serotonin [11–13].

Germline and somatic mutations were also reported to be involved in the mechanism causing PBMAH. Genes associated with PBMAH include ARMC5 (*armadillo repeatcontaining 5*), PDE11A (*Phosphodiesterase 11A*), APC (*Adenomatous polyposis coli*), and FH (*Fumarate hydratase*) [6]. ARMC5 mutations were found to be the most frequently mutated gene in PBMAH. Different studies show prevalences of ARMC5 mutations ranging from 19.6% to 55%, mostly sporadic cases [3, 4, 14]. ARMC5 likely functions as a tumor suppressor gene, and somatic mutations have been detected in addition to the germline mutations in patients with PBMAH, supporting the "two-hit" model for ARMC5 as a tumor suppressor gene [3, 15, 16]. The occurrence of intracranial meningiomas has also been associated with PBMAH, suggesting a possible role of ARMC5 for the development of other neoplasia [17].

2. Case Presentation

A 64-year-old man, referred to endocrinology due to bilateral adrenal incidentalomas on a CT scan, measuring 4 × 4.3 cm on the left and 4.3 × 4.2 cm on the right side, with characteristics of adenoma/hyperplasia (Figure 1). He had assumed type 2 diabetes mellitus, hypertension, and dyslipidemia for about 4 years and had suffered an acute myocardial infarction 3 years before. He was being treated with four different antihypertensive medications (bisoprolol, spironolactone, olmesartan, and amlodipine), as well as gliclazide and simvastatin. Physical examination revealed thin and dry skin, obesity with centripetal fat distribution, multiple ecchymosis, and facial erythrosis.

He had a 41-year-old son diagnosed with schizophrenia and an apparently healthy 37-year-old daughter. No known familial relevant diseases.

His laboratory workup revealed hypercortisolism: failure to suppress on the 1 mg overnight dexamethasone suppression test-cortisol 27.6 μg/dL-and on the low-dose dexamethasone suppression test (0.5 mg every 6 h for 48 h) end of the test-cortisol 24 μg/dL-associated to morning ACTH < 1 ng/L.

He underwent stimulation tests with Tetracosactide, LHRH (luteinizing hormone-releasing hormone), TRH (thyrotropin-releasing hormone), vasopressin, metoclopramide, glucagon, and upright posture test, which were overall negative, with the exception of partial response to the upright posture test (cortisol variation of 42.5%).

It was then decided to proceed bilateral adrenalectomy. However, due to surgical complications, only right adrenalectomy was performed. On gross examination, a right adrenalectomy specimen was surrounded by fat with 94,6 g with 8,5 × 4,3 × 2 cm adrenal gland in size was removed. The adrenal gland was compact and yellow, with nodular appearance on section. On histological examination, the adrenal tissue had architectural disorganization associated with ill-defined multinodular hyperplasia of the cortical fasciculata layer. These aspects were consistent with adrenal nodular hyperplasia (Figures 2–5).

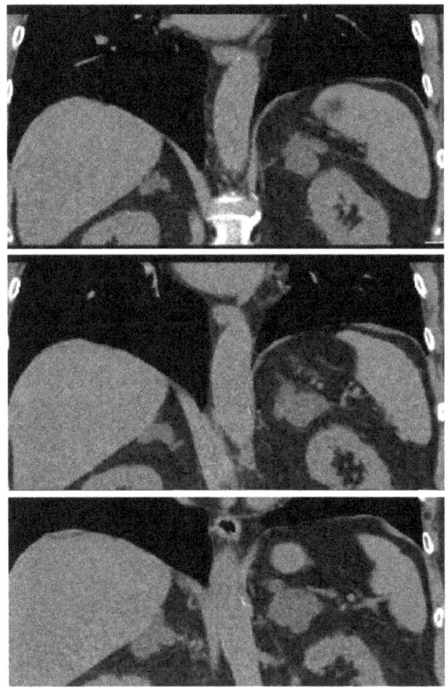

Figure 1: Adrenal CT scan of the index patient.

The patient now remains free of hypercortisolism, with normal blood pressure and glucose control, with no need of medication.

A molecular study in DNA extracted from peripheral blood leucocyte and in the adrenal gland revealed the presence in heterozygosity of the pathogenic mutation c.1379T < C in the ARMC5 gene, which encodes the protein variant p(Leu460Pro). Due to this finding, the patient underwent a cerebral CT scan, which showed a meningioma in the posterior left temporal convexity (Figure 6).

Genetic testing was also performed on the daughter and son, which revealed the same pathogenic mutation. They were also tested for hypercortisolism and underwent adrenal and cerebral CT scan (Figure 7).

His son had no physical signs of hypercortisolism. His blood tests did not reveal any finding suggesting hypercortisolism: 1 mg overnight dexamethasone suppression test–cortisol 0.8 μg/dL, morning ACTH 18.6 ng/L. His adrenal and cerebral CT scans showed no abnormalities. His daughter had a history of easy bruising, but no other signs suggestive of hypercortisolism. As with her brother, her blood tests did not reveal hypercortisolism: 1 mg overnight dexamethasone suppression test–cortisol 1.0 μg/dL and morning ACTH 19.1 ng/L; and her cerebral CT scan was normal. Her adrenal CT scan, however, showed enlargement of the left adrenal gland, with aspects suggestive of nodular hyperplasia, with a more evident and nodular area of 14 mm in diameter.

Both of them are currently under annual active surveillance, with yearly evaluation for hypercortisolism.

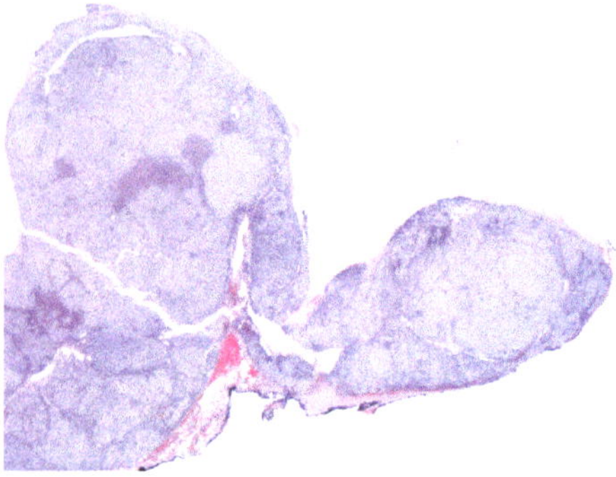

Figure 2: (H&E, original magnification x2.5)-Histologically, there is evidence of adrenal cortex thickening, with architectural disorganization and multinodular appearance.

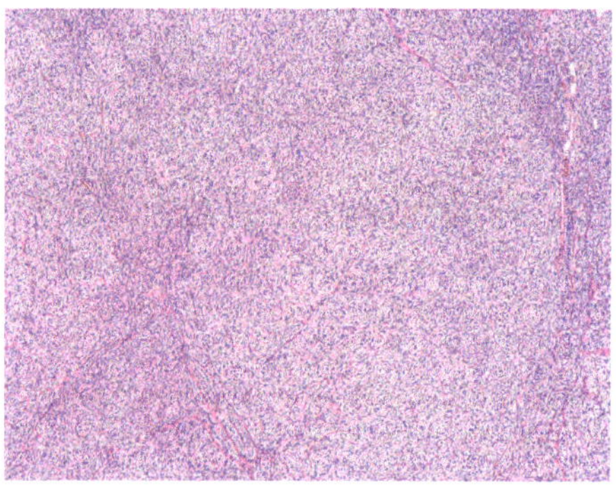

Figure 3: (H&E, original magnification x4 and x10)-There is ill-defined multinodular hyperplasia of the cortical fasciculata layer of the adrenal tissue.

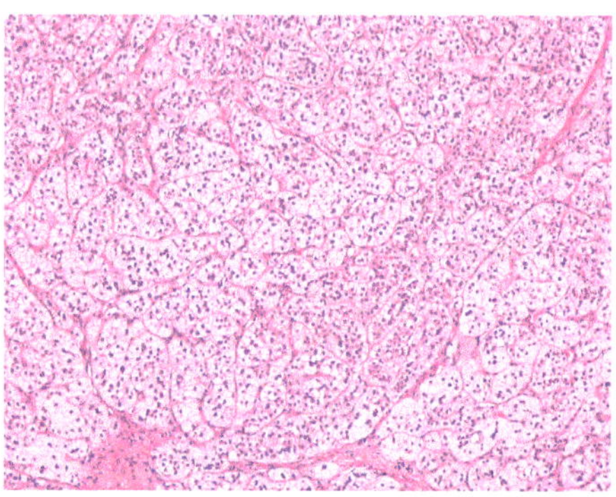

Figure 4: H&E, original magnification x4 and x10)-There is ill-defined multinodular hyperplasia of the cortical fasciculata layer of the adrenal tissue.

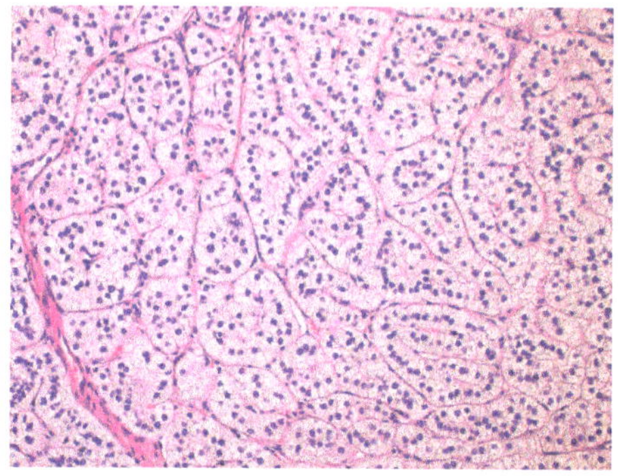

Figure 5: (H&E, original magnification x20)-The hyperplastic cortical fasciculata layer is characterized by a large number of cord organized cells with well-defined membranes, clear and vacuolated cytoplasm and, small nuclei.

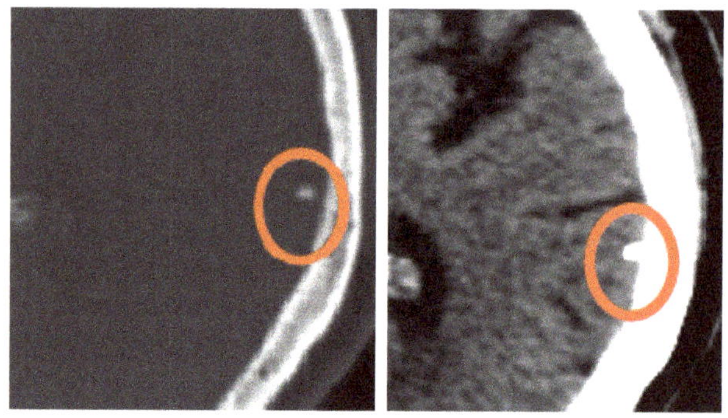

Figure 6: Cerebral CT scan of the index patient.

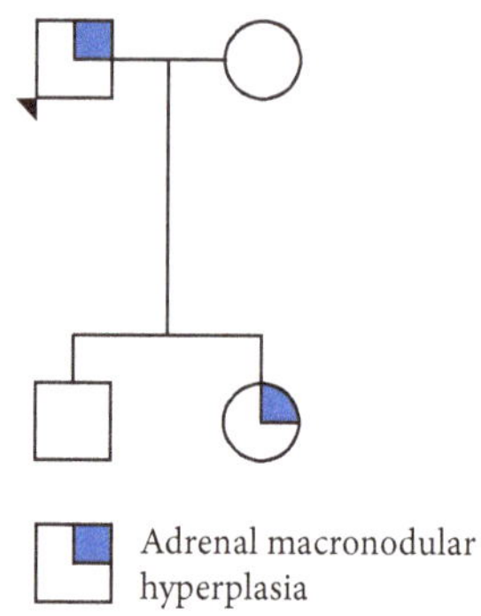

Figure 7: Family tree: 1. Proband, 2. affected daughter, 3. healthy son. Circles: females; squares: males.

3. Discussion

PBMAH is a heterogeneous and complex disorder with varying degrees of hypercortisolism (from subclinical to overt Cushing's syndrome), variable size and number of nodules, and expression of illegitimate membrane receptors. The frequency of such illegitimate receptors in PBMAH is high, varying from 77% to 87% [2, 18]. This illegitimate receptors are G protein-coupled receptors stimulating adenylyl cyclase, inducing cortisol secretion [19]. PBMAH is also associated with paracrine intraadrenal ACTH secretion. This ectopic ACTH is secreted by adrenocortical cells, located in the subcapsular region and in hyperplasic nodules which express both proconvertase 1, the ACTH-precursor cleavage enzyme, and the usual enzymatic resources of cells capable of steroidogenesis. This condition is slightly more prevalent in women, but the reason is not clear [19].

ARMC5 gene mutations has been identified in a large number of patients and familial cases with PBMAH [3, 6–8, 17]. ARMC5 is a cytosolic protein with no enzymatic activity, containing 7 armadillo domains and one BTB domain towards its C-terminus, which allows its dimerization or trimerization [20]. More proteins are known to contain armadillo domains, including the well-known beta-catenin. Armadillo-containing proteins are involved in many different functions, including T-cell, neural tube, and adrenal cortex development as well as tumor suppression. ARMC5 inactivation leads to decreased steroidogenesis. Despite the reduced cortisol secretion capacity of each cell, progressive hypercortisolism results from the increased number of adrenocortical cells, explaining the slow and progressive development of Cushing syndrome [3]. The ARMC5 antiapototic effect is responsible for the growth of bilateral masses [2, 8, 16]. The presence or absence of ARMC5 mutations may be associated with diverse phenotypes [16]. Patients with ARMC5 mutation tend to present a more severe presentation, with younger age at diagnosis, larger adrenal nodules and a higher prevalence of clinical CS [2, 16]. These patients also seem to show a higher abnormal cortisol response during the upright posture test, which was also seen in our index patient [2]. In addition, ARMC5-mutated patients have hypertension more often than wild-type patients [16, 21]. In fact, ARMC5 mutations are also responsible for some cases of primary hyperaldosteronism, mainly in Afro-American patients [21]. Intracranial meningiomas have also been described in patients harboring (p.Ala110fs ∗ 9) ARMC5 mutation with PBMAH, while others lacking these mutations do not develop this condition [7, 16, 17, 21]. Our patient also had a meningioma, despite having a different mutation than described (c.1379T < C, p.Leu460Pro). It seems that some degree of genotype-phenotype correlation is present [16].

Bilateral adrenalectomy has been considered the treatment of choice for PBMAH, but it leads to permanent adrenal insufficiency, requiring lifelong glucocorticoid and mineralocorticoid replacement and impaired quality of life [22]. Unilateral adrenalectomy has recently been proposed as an alternative in selected patients, with some advocating for the removal of the larger gland, especially in older patients [23]. Recently the use of mifepristone has also been proposed [24].

No specific follow-up protocol has been proposed to mutation carriers without Cushing syndrome diagnosis. In our center, we perform a yearly biochemical evaluation.

4. Conclusion

All patients with PBMAH or suspected of having the disease should be tested, and once a germline mutation is identified, first degree patients should also undergo genetic testing and counseling [7]. Considering the insidious nature of this disease and the known deleterious effects of hypercortisolism, this will allow physicians to timely identify and treat this patients.

Our findings correlate with the literature available, and they support the idea of a new "syndrome" which may include the association between PBMAH and meningioma. More studies are needed to confirm this hypothesis.

References

[1] A. De Venanzi, G. A. Alencar, I. Bourdeau, M. C. B. V. Ragoso, and A. Lacroix, "Primary bilateral macronodular adrenal hyperplasia," *Current Opinion in Endocrinology & Diabetes and Obesity*, vol. 21, no. 3, pp. 177–184, 2014.

[2] S. Espiard, L. Drougat, R. Libé et al., "ARMC5Mutations in a large cohort of primary macronodular adrenal hyperplasia: clinical and functional consequences," *The Journal of Clinical Endocrinology & Metabolism*, vol. 100, no. 6, pp. E926–E935, 2015.

[3] G. Assié, R. Libé, S. Espiard et al., "ARMC5Mutations in macronodular adrenal hyperplasia with cushing's syndrome," *New England Journal of Medicine*, vol. 369, no. 22, p. 2105, 2013.

[4] N. M. Albiger, D. Regazzo, B. Rubin et al., "A multicenter experience on the prevalence of ARMC5 mutations in patients with primary bilateral macronodular adrenal hyperplasia: from genetic characterization to clinical phenotype," *Endocrine*, vol. 55, no. 3, p. 959, 2017.

[5] H.-P. Hsiao, L. S. Kirschner, I. Bourdeau et al., "Clinical and genetic heterogeneity, overlap with other tumor syndromes, and atypical glucocorticoid hormone secretion in adrenocorticotropin-independent macronodular adrenal hyperplasia compared with other adrenocortical tumors," *The Journal of Clinical Endocrinology & Metabolism*, vol. 94, no. 8, p. 2930, 2009.

[6] L. Yu, J. Zhang, X. Guo, X. Chen, Z. He, and Q. He, "ARMC5 mutations in familial and sporadic primary bilateral macronodular adrenal hyperplasia," *PLoS One*, vol. 13, no. 1, p. 16, 2018.

[7] G. A. Alencar, A. M. Lerario, M. Y. Nishi et al., "ARMC5-Mutations are a frequent cause of primary macronodular adrenal hyperplasia," *The Journal of Clinical Endocrinology & Metabolism*, vol. 99, no. 8, pp. E1501–E1509, 2014.

[8] T. Rego, F. Fonseca, S. Espiard, K. Perlemoine, J. Bertherat, and A. Agapito, "ARMC5 mutation in a Portuguese family with primary bilateral macronodular adrenal hyperplasia (PBMAH)," *Endocrinol Diabetes Metab Case Reports*, vol. 99, 2017.

[9] E. Louiset, C. Duparc, J. Young et al., "Intraadrenal corticotropin in bilateral macronodular adrenal hyperplasia," *New England Journal of Medicine*, vol. 369, no. 22, pp. 2115–2125, 2013.

[10] N. E. Ghorayeb, I. Bourdeau, and A. Lacroix, "Multiple aberrant hormone receptors in Cushing's syndrome," *European Journal of Endocrinology*, vol. 173, no. 4, pp. M45–M60, 2015.

[11] X. Bertagna, L. Groussin, J.-P. Luton, and J. Bertherat, "Aberrant receptor-mediated cushing's syndrome," *Hormone Research in Paediatrics*, vol. 59, no. 1, pp. 99–103, 2003.

[12] Y. Reznik, V. Allali-Zerah, J. A. Chayvialle et al., "Food-dependent cushing's syndrome mediated by aberrant adrenal sensitivity to gastric inhibitory polypeptide," *New England Journal of Medicine*, vol. 327, no. 14, p. 981, 1992.

[13] A. Lacroix, E. Bolté, J. Tremblay et al., "Gastric inhibitory polypeptide-dependent cortisol hypersecretion-a new cause of cushing's syndrome," *New England Journal of Medicine*, vol. 327, no. 14, p. 974, 1992.

[14] F. R. Faucz, M. Zilbermint, M. B. Lodish et al., "Macronodular adrenal hyperplasia due to mutations in an armadillo repeat containing 5 (ARMC5) Gene: a clinical and genetic investigation," *The Journal of Clinical Endocrinology & Metabolism*, vol. 99, no. 6, 2014.

[15] L. Drougat, S. Espiard, and J. Bertherat, "Genetics of primary bilateral macronodular adrenal hyperplasia: a model for early diagnosis of Cushing's syndrome?" *European Journal of Endocrinology*, vol. 173, no. 4, pp. M121–M131, 2015.

[16] Q. Liu, D. Tong, J. Xu et al., "A novel germline ARMC5 mutation in a patient with bilateral macronodular adrenal hyperplasia: a case report," *BMC Medical Genetics*, vol. 19, no. 1, pp. 1–5, 2018.

[17] U. Elbelt, A. Trovato, M. Kloth et al., "Molecular and clinical evidence for anARMC5Tumor syndrome: concurrent inactivating germline and somatic mutations are associated with both primary macronodular adrenal hyperplasia and meningioma," *The Journal of Clinical Endocrinology & Metabolism*, vol. 100, no. 1, p. E119, 2015.

[18] J. Hofland, L. J. Hofland, P. M. van Koetsveld et al., "ACTH-independent macronodular adrenocortical hyperplasia reveals prevalent aberrant in vivo and in vitro responses to hormonal stimuli and coupling of arginine-vasopressin type 1a receptor to 11β-hydroxylase," *Orphanet Journal of Rare Diseases*, vol. 8, no. 1, p. 142, 2013.

[19] F. Bonnet-Serrano and J. Bertherat, "Genetics of tumors of the adrenal cortex," *Endocrine-Related Cancer*, vol. 25, no. 3, p. R131, 2018.

[20] Y. Hu, L. Lao, J. Mao et al., "Armc5 deletion causes developmental defects and compromises T-cell immune responses," *Nature Communications*, vol. 8, no. 1, 2017.

[21] M. Zilbermint, P. Xekouki, F. R. Faucz et al., "Primary aldosteronism and ARMC5 variants," *The Journal of Clinical Endocrinology & Metabolism*, vol. 100, 2015.

[22] M. T. Hawn, D. Cook, C. Deveney, and B. C. Sheppard, "Quality of life after laparoscopic bilateral adrenalectomy for Cushing's disease," *Surgery*, vol. 132, no. 6, p. 1064, 2002.

[23] G. Di Dalmazi and M. Reincke, "Adrenal surgery for cushing's syndrome," *Endocrinology and Metabolism Clinics of North America*, vol. 47, no. 2, p. 385, 2018.

[24] P. Cohan, H. E. East, S.-J. Galati et al., "Mifepristone treatment in four cases of primary bilateral macronodular adrenal hyperplasia (BMAH)," *The Journal of Clinical Endocrinology & Metabolism*, vol. 104, no. 12, p. 6279, 2019.

41

PES Syndrome Presenting as Severe Hyponatremia in an Asymptomatic Septuagenarian

Rahul Pansare and Sangeetha Nanthabalan

Department of Internal Medicine, St. Mary Mercy Hospital, Livonia, MI 48154, USA

Correspondence should be addressed to Sangeetha Nanthabalan; sangeetha.nanthabalan@stjoeshealth.org

Academic Editor: Lucy Mastrandrea

Background. Hyponatremia is commonly seen in hospitalized patients. In euvolemic individuals, syndrome of inappropriate antidiuretic hormone secretion (SIADH) is a common differential. However, before establishing a diagnosis of SIADH, it is imperative to evaluate for hypocortisolism and hypothyroidism. The finding of endocrine abnormalities determined to be of pituitary origin should prompt evaluation by brain MRI. Furthermore, primary empty sella (PES) is commonly seen as an incidental neuroradiological finding. However, PES in association with endocrine abnormalities is recognized as a separate entity called primary empty sella syndrome (PESS). *Case Presentation.* We report the case of a 71-year-old male sans neurological symptoms who presented to us with severe hyponatremia in whom we used a stepwise approach which led us to the diagnosis of PESS. This methodical approach was crucial for timely correction of the endocrine abnormalities which in turn rectified hyponatremia. Intriguingly, the presence of an ectopic pituitary which is a very rare entity and the sudden manifestation of his underlying endocrine deficiencies in the 8th decade of life make this clinical scenario highly unusual. *Conclusion.* Clinicians should be aware that absence of an orderly approach to workup presumed SIADH or an assumption of PES (instead of PESS) could both lead to serious consequences in the face of missed endocrine deficiencies.

1. Background

Hyponatremia is a common electrolyte derangement observed in hospitalized patients. Severe hyponatremia (<120 mMol/L) has been reported to be a predictor of high mortality [1, 2]. Euvolemic hyponatremia requires evaluation for syndrome of inappropriate antidiuretic hormone (SIADH) but may also be the initial presentation of hypoadrenalism and/or hypothyroidism. We present a rare case of an older adult who presented with severe hyponatremia, subsequently diagnosed with panhypopituitarism. Although deficiencies involving multiple axes are common, panhypopituitarism is rare, described in 2% of primary empty sella (PES) cases [3]. This endocrine abnormality along with radiological evidence of PES led to a diagnosis of PES syndrome (PESS).

2. Case Presentation

A 71-year-old normotensive male, 149 cm in height (<1st percentile for height) and 56.3 kg in weight (BMI: 25), with an extensive smoking history, was referred to the hospital by his primary care physician (PCP) for severe hyponatremia (117 mMol/L). His past medical records showed normal sodium levels in multiple PCP visits in the previous two years. He denied any active complaints or neurological symptoms, and initial physical examination showed an euvolemic male with feminine features and short stature. Vital signs were significant for blood pressure of 131/70 mmHg. Laboratory values also revealed mild metabolic acidosis (HCO_3^-: 19) and normal potassium levels, BUN of 13.1 mg/dl, creatinine of 1.27 mg/dl, and GFR of 68 ml/min/1.73 m^2.

In the initial steps of evaluation of hyponatremia, low serum osmolality of 245 mOsm/kg but a normal urine osmolality of 309 mOsm/kg and inappropriately high urine sodium of 68 mEq/L were highly suggestive of SIADH. Due to his long-standing smoking history, we obtained a CT chest with contrast which conclusively ruled out lung malignancy as cause for ectopic SIADH.

Our suspicion for SIADH prompted us to further rule out thyroid and cortisol hormone deficiencies. Low morning serum cortisol levels (2 mcg/dl) followed by suboptimal cortisol response to cosyntropin stimulation test (injection of 1 mcg at 0 minutes, followed by cortisol measurements –8 mcg/dl at 30 minutes and 9 mcg/dl at 60 minutes) were noted. These findings coupled with a low morning serum adrenocorticotropic hormone (ACTH) level were suggestive of secondary hypocortisolism. Low free T4 with inappropriately normal TSH heralded the diagnosis of coexisting central hypothyroidism. Due to the finding of dual hormone deficiency, the diagnosis of panhypopituitarism was entertained.

LH, FSH, IGF, and testosterone levels were all low, indicating GH and gonadotropin deficiencies. Prolactin level was mildly elevated (Table 1). To complete the workup for panhypopituitarism, an MRI brain with contrast was obtained. It ruled out pituitary adenoma or stalk compression but revealed complete empty sella (complete absence of anterior/posterior pituitary glands and pituitary stalk) and an ectopic pituitary gland in the posterior hypothalamus (Figures 1(a) and 1(b)).

At that point, we approached the patient again to get in-depth history about any prior endocrine disorders. He did acknowledge that he had required growth hormone supplementation in his teenage years as a treatment for his short stature. However, he discontinued it in a few months when he noticed no improvement. Since his teens, he was lost to follow-up by endocrinology and thus had not received any hormone supplementation. Furthermore, his underlying endocrine problems had never manifested with such severe hyponatremia during his lifetime up until this encounter.

Levothyroxine and hydrocortisone supplementation was initiated with improvement in serum sodium to 130 mMol/l noted after three days. The patient was discharged to follow-up with PCP where labs after a week showed normal sodium levels. He continues to be healthy at subsequent PCP visits.

3. Discussion and Conclusion

Hyponatremia with the findings of euvolemia, decreased serum osmolality, normal to high urine osmolality (>100 mOsm/kg), paradoxical natriuresis (U_{Na} >40 mMol/L), and absence of adrenal and thyroid disorders characterizes SIADH [4]. However, a normal acid-base balance is considered part of the SIADH criteria but is often overlooked. Occasionally, SIADH may present as metabolic alkalosis [5]. However, the patient in our case had mild metabolic acidosis. We attributed this to type 4 renal tubular acidosis which is commonly seen in ACTH deficiency [6]. Thus, in retrospect, the metabolic acidosis also provided an important clue to an underlying endocrine pathology in our case.

Table 1: Endocrine profile.

Endocrine profile	Serum levels
Adrenocorticotropic hormone (ACTH)	12 pg/ml
Thyroid-stimulating hormone (TSH)	1.46 mcIU/ml
Free T4	0.47 ng/dl
Growth hormone (GH)	<0.1 ng/ml
IGF binding protein 3	0.6 mg/L
Luteinizing hormone (LH)	0.8 IU/ml
Follicle-stimulating hormone (FSH)	1.4 IU/ml
Testosterone	<10 ng/dL
Prolactin	19.4 ng/ml
Baseline serum cortisol	2 mcg/dl
After cosyntropin stimulation test at 30 mins	8 mcg/dl
After cosyntropin stimulation test at 60 mins	9 mcg/dl
Antidiuretic hormone (ADH)	<0.5 pg/ml

The correction of hyponatremia after hydrocortisone treatment is also congruent with "endocrine SIADH." In our patient, hyponatremia can be explained by both hypocortisolism as well as hypothyroidism. For hypocortisolism, the usual mechanism of action is related to the loss of inhibitory effect of cortisol and subsequent increase in CRH which is an ADH secretagogue [7]. For hypothyroidism, the resultant decline in cardiac output and subsequent compensation by increase in ADH levels and decrease in GFR have been proposed as possible mechanisms of action [8]. All these ultimately contribute to free water retention.

Intriguingly, our patient had low ADH levels suggesting increased tubular action or heightened sensitivity to available ADH. Low ADH levels bring to light a possible underlying hypothalamic deficiency. However, ADH levels were reported at a time when hyponatremia had already been corrected. Our patient refused further testing for hypothalamic hormones.

Our case had some common and uncommon features in terms of presenting symptoms. On the one hand, absence of symptoms and incidentally detected hyponatremia is not an uncommon presentation of chronic adrenal insufficiency in the elderly and should be considered as a differential for hyponatremia [7, 9, 10]. On the other hand, we came across only a few of the cases of PES syndrome with panhypopituitarism presenting as hyponatremia [11–14]. Interestingly, they had dramatic presentations such as mania, extrapontine myelinolysis, and adrenal crisis requiring ICU admission. This further reiterates the importance of timely diagnosis and initiation of appropriate treatment. Undiagnosed, uncorrected adrenal insufficiency could potentially result in significant morbidity and mortality, particularly during periods of stress [15].

The brain MRI findings in our patient were read as an "empty sella" which is extensively described as an incidental radiological finding [16] in 8–35% of cases. It is important to differentiate primary from secondary empty sella since management differs. Secondary causes include spontaneous necrosis in preexisting pituitary adenomas, infection, autoimmune causes, intracranial hypertension, brain surgery and/or radiotherapy, cerebral trauma, and pseudotumor

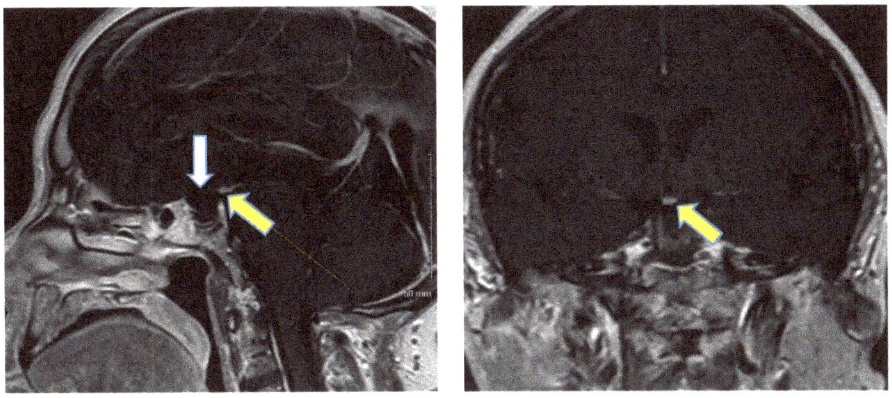

(a) (b)

FIGURE 1: MRI brain with contrast showing empty sella with complete absence of anterior and posterior pituitary glands/infundibulum and tissue representing an ectopic hypothalamic-pituitary gland. (a) Sagittal T1 section. (b) Coronal T1 section (white arrow shows the empty sella, and yellow arrows depict the ectopic pituitary gland).

cerebri [17]. No obvious secondary cause was observed in our patient, and thus, through diagnosis of exclusion, we arrived at PES. Unlike our case, PES is usually described in obese woman with hypertension, typically in the 4th and 5th decade. It is important to recognize that PES with concomitant underlying panhypopituitarism is a separate entity called "PES syndrome." It should also be borne in mind that such patients can have concomitant mild hyperprolactinemia [18] due to alterations in dopaminergic tone.

Lastly, an ectopic pituitary is a very rare condition but is a common cause of pediatric growth hormone deficiency, the likely diagnosis for this patient [19, 20]. The short stature and feminine facial features which were first noted during our patient's teenage years likely represent early evidence of hypopituitarism as a result of PES and ectopic posterior pituitary [21]. The patient's survival into old age without depending on hormonal supplementation and the sudden reappearance of endocrine deficiencies manifesting as hyponatremia remain an odd presentation.

The appropriate workup for hyponatremia in the case led to a diagnosis of panhypopituitarism enabling us to institute appropriate therapy. Even in asymptomatic individuals found to have PES, it is recommended that they should be evaluated further for underlying hypothalamic-pituitary axis deficiencies as highlighted by our patient's incidentally detected hyponatremia.

Abbreviations

SIADH: Syndrome of inappropriate antidiuretic hormone secretion
PES: Primary empty sella
PESS: Primary empty sella syndrome
PCP: Primary care physician
TSH: Thyroid-stimulating hormone
ACTH: Adrenocorticotropic hormone
ADH: Antidiuretic hormone
FSH: Follicle-stimulating hormone
LH: Luteinizing hormone
GH: Growth hormone
IGF: Insulin-like growth factor.

Consent

Written informed consent was obtained from the patient for publication of this case report and any accompanying images.

Authors' Contributions

RP wrote the abstract and case report. SN proofread the abstract and case report and suggested changes to improvise. Both authors worked on the drafts to finalize it.

References

[1] T. Krummel, E. Prinz, C. Borni-Duval et al., "Prognosis of patients with severe hyponatremia is related not only to hyponatraemia but also to comorbidities and to medical management: results of an observational retrospective study," *BMC Nephrology*, vol. 17, p. 159, 2016.

[2] S. Mohan, A. Parikh, and J. Radhakrishnan, "Prevalence of hyponatremia and association with mortality: results from NHANES," *The American Journal of Medicine*, vol. 126, no. 12, pp. 1127–1137, 2013.

[3] A. Giustina, G. Aimaretti, M. Bondanelli et al., "Primary empty sella: why and when to investigate hypothalamic-pituitary function," *Journal of Endocrinological Investigation*, vol. 33, no. 5, pp. 343–346, 2010.

[4] G. Liamis, H. J. Milionis, and M. Elisaf, "Endocrine disorders: causes of hyponatremia not to neglect," *Annals of Medicine*, vol. 43, no. 3, pp. 179–187, 2011.

[5] Y. Izumi, Y. Nakayama, T. Onoue, H. Inoue, and M. Mukoyama, "Renal tubular acidosis complicated with hyponatremia due to cortisol insufficiency," *Oxford Medical Case Reports*, vol. 2015, no. 11, pp. 360–363, 2015.

[6] G. D. W. Musch, R. Penninckx, and A. Soupart, "Low plasma bicarbonate level in hyponatremia related to adrenocorticotropin deficiency," *The Journal of Clinical Endocrinology & Metabolism*, vol. 88, no. 11, pp. 5255–5257, 2003.

[7] N. Jessani, W. Jehangir, D. Behman, A. Yousif, and I. J. Spiler, "Secondary adrenal insufficiency: an overlooked cause of

hyponatremia," *Journal of Clinical Medicine Research*, vol. 7, no. 4, pp. 286–288, 2015.

[8] T. Nagata, S. Nakajima, A. Fujiya, H. Sobajima, and M. Yamaguchi, "Prevalence of hypothyroidism in patients with hyponatremia: a retrospective cross-sectional study," *PLoS One*, vol. 13, no. 10, Article ID e0205687, 2018.

[9] S. Diederich, N. Franzen, V. Bähr, and W. Oelkers, "Severe hyponatremia due to hypopituitarism with adrenal insufficiency: report on 28 cases," *European Journal of Endocrinology*, vol. 148, no. 6, pp. 609–617, 2003.

[10] T. Winchester Behr, "Hyponatremia in older people as a sign of adrenal insufficiency: a case-control study," *Internal Medicine Journal*, vol. 42, no. 3, pp. 306–310, 2012.

[11] I. 1 Aijazi, A. S. Abdullah, and S. H. Adam Mukhtar, "Primary empty sella syndrome presenting with severe hyponatremia and minimal salt wasting," *Journal of Ayub Medical College Abbottabad*, vol. 28, no. 3, pp. 605–608, 2016.

[12] V. A. Gupta, "Karnik N2, itolikar M1, vekariya K3.extrapontine myelinolysis in a case of pan-hypopituitarism due to empty sella syndrome," *JAPI: Journal of the Association of Physicians of India*, vol. 63, no. 10, pp. 86-87, 2015.

[13] C. H. Yang, Y. C. Lin, P. H. Chou, H. C. Chen, and C. H. Chan, "A case report of late onset mania caused by hyponatremia in a patient with empty sella syndrome," *Medicine (Baltimore)*, vol. 95, no. 6, e26, 29 pages, 2016.

[14] S. Okuno, M. Inaba, Y. Nishizawa, T. Miki, Y. Inoue, and H. Morii, "A case of hyponatremia in panhypopituitarism caused by the primary empty sella syndrome," *Endocrinologia Japonica*, vol. 34, no. 2, pp. 299–307, 1987.

[15] T. Asano, A. Aoki, M. Sasaki et al., "Hyponatremia is the valuable manifestation for initiating diagnosis of hypopituitarism in elderly," *Endocrine Journal*, vol. 59, no. 11, pp. 1015–1020, 2012.

[16] S. Chiloiro, A. Giampietro, A. Bianchi et al., "Diagnosis of endocrine disease: primary empty sella: a comprehensive review," *European Journal of Endocrinology*, vol. 177, no. 6, pp. R275–R285, 2017.

[17] M. K. Auer, M. R. Stieg, A. Crispin, C. Sievers, G. K. Stalla, and A. Kopczak, "Primary empty sella syndrome and the prevalence of hormonal dysregulation," *Deutsches Ärzteblatt International*, vol. 115, no. 7, pp. 99–105, 2018.

[18] H. Gharib, H. M. Frey, E. R. Laws, R. V. Randall, and B. W. Scheithauer, "Coexistent primary empty sella syndrome and hyperprolactinemia," *Archives of Internal Medicine*, vol. 143, no. 7, pp. 1383–1386, 1983.

[19] N. Mahomed and T. Motshudi, "The ectopic posterior pituitary gland," *South African Journal of Surgery*, vol. 51, no. 4, p. 148, 2013.

[20] S. Kurtoğlu, A. Özdemir, and N. Hatipoğlu, "Neonatal hypopituitarism: approaches to diagnosis and treatment," *Journal of Clinical Research in Pediatric Endocrinology*, vol. 11, no. 1, pp. 4–12, 2019.

[21] C. Bar, C. Zadro, Gwenaelle Diene et al., "Pituitary stalk interruption syndrome from infancy to adulthood: clinical, hormonal, and radiological assessment according to the initial presentation," *PLoS One*, vol. 10, no. 11, Article ID e0142354, 2015.

42

Autosomal Dominant Hypophosphatemic Rickets Presenting in a Phenotypically Normal Adult Female

Hala Mualla,[1] Su Ah Bae,[2] and Abid Yaqub[1]

[1]*Division of Endocrinology, Diabetes and Metabolism, University of Cincinnati, 231 Albert Sabin Way, Cincinnati, OH 45267-0542, USA*
[2]*Cotton O'Neil Diabetes & Endocrinology Clinic, 3520 SW 6th Ave, Topeka, KS 6660, USA*

Correspondence should be addressed to Abid Yaqub; yaqubad@ucmail.uc.edu

Academic Editor: Toshihiro Kita

We describe a presentation of Autosomal Dominant Hypophosphatemic Rickets (ADHR) in a 22-year-old female with normal pubertal growth and development and a negative family history in first-degree relatives. The patient presented with a 2-year history of upper and lower extremity proximal muscle pain and weakness and bilateral femoral neck and pubic bone insufficiency fractures. She had a normal serum calcium but a low phosphate as well as 25-hydroxyvitamin D (25(OH)D) levels leading initially to a diagnosis of osteomalacia. Urine phosphate reabsorption was low confirming a phosphate wasting disorder. She had an elevated Fibroblast Growth Factor 23 (FGF23) level. After Tumor-Induced Osteomalacia was ruled out by extensive imaging, she was sent for genetic testing for hereditary rickets which showed a previously reported missense variant in *FGF23*. Subsequently, she found out that her father's maternal aunt and grandfather had 'bone disorder' and were wheelchair-bound in adulthood. After replenishment of vitamin D, treatment with calcitriol and phosphate leads to complete resolution of patient's symptoms and laboratory abnormalities.

1. Introduction

Hypophosphatemic rickets (HR) is a rare genetic disorder characterized by renal phosphate wasting. It is usually transmitted by X-linked inheritance. Autosomal dominant (ADHR) inheritance is relatively uncommon. Here, we report a case of ADHR presenting in 22-year-old female with normal pubertal growth and skeletal phenotype and a negative family history in first-degree relatives. We review the pathophysiology, diagnosis, and treatment of ADHR with emphasis on the clinical presentation in the late-onset form.

2. Case Report

A 22-year-old female was referred to our endocrine clinic with 2-year history of gradually progressive proximal muscle pain and weakness involving both upper and lower extremities. Her pediatrician had treated her with prednisone for a period of two months without any improvement. MRI of pelvis and thighs completed before her referral had shown linear hypointense foci in both proximal medial femoral necks and the right ischium consistent with insufficiency fractures. She had a normal childhood development and pubertal growth and at presentation had a height of 154cm and a body weight of 57.1kg. There was no reported family history of rickets, osteomalacia, or any other metabolic bone disease. Her menstrual history was unremarkable.

Past medical history was significant for a diagnosis of carnitine palmitoyl transferase 2 (CPT2) deficiency at the age of 14 which was diagnosed in the context of a work-up for diffuse muscle pain and weakness. At that time, she was evaluated in the Neurology clinic and was found to have low serum carnitine levels, elevated serum alanine, normal lactate, and low pyruvate levels. C16, C18:2, C18:1, and C18 levels were elevated suggesting carnitine palmitoyltransferase II deficiency. However, genetic testing was negative for the S113L variant. Results of other biochemical testing at that time were not available in her medical records. Her symptoms had reportedly completely resolved a few months after she was started on oral carnitine replacement therapy.

Physical exam did not show any apparent kyphosis or scoliosis of spine, vertebral tenderness, or hyperextensibility of joints. There were no lower extremity deformities. She had proximal muscle weakness with 4/5 strength in upper and 3/5 in the lower extremities. There was tenderness in the thighs. Her neurological exam was otherwise normal. She had a waddling gait.

Laboratory work-up revealed the following results: calcium, 9.1 (ref: 8.6-10.2 mg/dl); phosphate level, 2.0 (ref: 2.5-4.5 mg/dl); alkaline phosphatase, 243 (ref: 39-136 Units/L); bone specific alkaline phosphatase, 119.6 (ref: 0-21.3 mg/dl); 25-hydroxy vitamin D, 8.2 (ref: 30-100 ng/ml); and PTH, 145 (ref: 22-84 pg/ml). A bone density scan showed an abnormally low bone density matched for age, gender, and ethnicity with the lowest Z score of -3.3 at the left femoral neck. Vertebral fracture assessment score was within normal limits.

A 24-hour urine collection revealed low calcium of 27.6 (ref: 100-300.0 mg/24 hr) and inappropriately normal urine phosphate excretion of 445 mg/dL (ref: 400.0-1300.0 mg/24 hr). Fractional excretion of phosphate was inappropriately normal at 19% (ref: 15–20%). Renal tubular reabsorption of phosphate (TmP/GFR) was low at 0.50 (ref: 3.18-6.41 for 16- to 25-year-old females). These results suggested renal phosphate wasting as a potential etiology for osteomalacia and we considered Tumor-Induced Osteomalacia (TIO) and Hereditary Hypophosphatemic Rickets (HRR) as diagnostic possibilities. However, in the absence of any family history of rickets and her normal childhood growth and stature, rickets appeared to be less likely and subsequent work-up was directed at ruling out TIO. An Octreotide scan with SPECT imaging came back negative and was followed by F-18 FDG PET/CT scan, which too failed to reveal any tumor. However, an FGF-23 level was found to be elevated at 580 (ref: 44-215 RU/mL). The assay used is a second-generation C-terminal assay that measures both the intact FGF-23 and its C-terminal fragments. At this stage, following the negative localization studies for TIO, the patient was counseled on genetic testing to look for the possibility of hereditary hypophosphatemic rickets. She consented for the genetic testing which revealed a heterozygous known pathogenic missense variant in FGF23: c.527 G>A p. Arg176Gln (R176Q) consistent with a diagnosis of "Autosomal Dominant Hypophosphatemic Rickets".

Genetic screens for variants in *PHEX* (X-linked Hypophosphatemic Rickets) and *DMP-1* (Autosomal Recessive Hypophosphatemic Rickets 1) were negative. These results were therefore consistent with a diagnosis of Autosomal Dominant Hypophosphatemic Rickets (ADHR) caused by a mutant FGF23. When we informed the patient about the genetic diagnosis, she did some further research regarding her family history and found out that her father's maternal aunt and grandfather had 'bone disorder' and were wheelchair-bound in early adulthood but her mother remained in good health and had no symptoms

She was started on Ergocalciferol 50,000 IU weekly and was encouraged to increase her dietary calcium to 1000 mg daily. She was also prescribed Potassium-Sodium-Phosphate 250 mg (8 mmol) 4 times a day. She continued to have pain and discomfort in her inner thighs. She was prescribed Diclofenac and Flexeril for pain. MRI of the pelvis

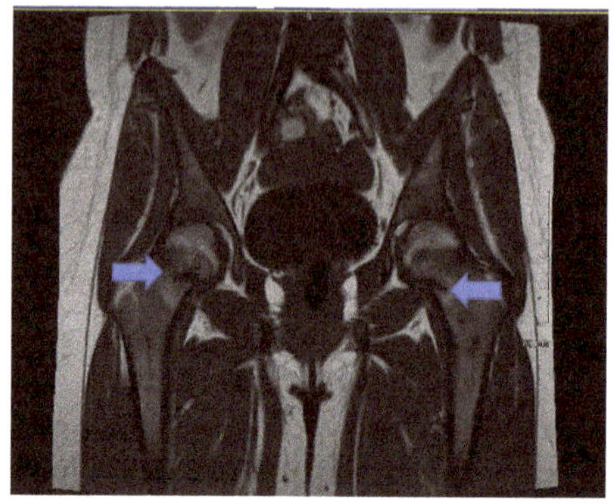

FIGURE 1: *MRI Pelvis showing bilateral stress insufficiency fractures of the hip, femoral neck.* On the right, the transcervical low signal line extends to the superior lateral cortex and is associated with marrow edema, suggestive of a nondisplaced transcervical fracture.

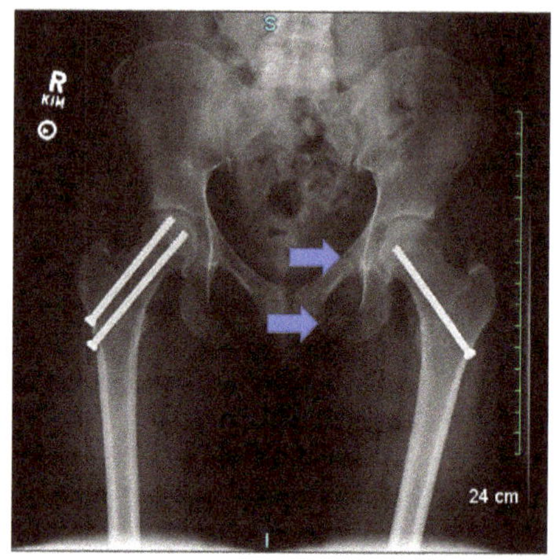

FIGURE 2: *X-ray of the hips and femurs.* New insufficiency fractures (arrows) were noted. There was interval placement of stabilizing screws for the previous right and left femoral neck insufficiency fractures.

was repeated to follow up on the insufficiency fractures and showed persistent bilateral femoral stress insufficiency fractures (Figure 1). She was referred to orthopedic surgery and underwent pinning of bilateral femoral necks. She had significant improvement in pain and discomfort in the right thigh and groin region but still had some discomfort in the left upper thigh.

Her 25(OH)D levels normalized to 46.2 ng/ml as did her serum phosphate level (2.7 mg/dL) with oral replacement therapy.

Due to persistent pain in her left groin, she was prescribed narcotic analgesics and underwent a steroid injection of the psoas muscle by orthopedics with no relief. A repeat X-ray of pelvis showed new insufficiency fractures of the left superior and inferior rami (Figure 2).

The patient had difficulty adhering to the regimen of potassium-sodium-phosphate 250 mg (8 mmol) four times daily. Therefore, she was started on calcitriol 0.25 mcg once a day. The dose of calcitriol was gradually increased up to 2 mcg per day. The patient reported significant improvement in her pain after the introduction of calcitriol to her regimen.

Although she missed a few follow-up appointments in the endocrine clinic, she was eventually seen a year later and reported feeling significantly better on the same treatment regimen of calcitriol 2 mcg daily, potassium-sodium-phosphate 250 mg (8 mmol) twice daily, vitamin D3 2000 units daily, and 600 mg of calcium supplement daily. She had complete resolution of her pain and was not on any pain medications. Her physical exam showed normal strength in the upper and lower extremities and no tenderness. Laboratory work-up at that time showed complete resolution of the previous abnormalities: serum phosphate level was 3.3 (ref: 2.5- 4.5 mg/dl); calcium, 9.4 (ref: 8.6-10.2 mg/dl); alkaline phosphatase, 88 (ref: 39-136 units/l); and 25(OH)D, 44.6 (ref: 30-100 ng/ml). A repeat X-ray of pelvis showed resolution of the previous left superior and inferior pubic rami fractures.

The patient subsequently enrolled in a clinical trial of iron supplementation for patients with ADHR at another institution. Correspondence received from that institution showed a hemoglobin 10.1 (ref: 12-15.5 g/dl), hematocrit 31 (ref: 39.4-44.5%), MCV 78 (80-96 fL), platelets 313, 000 (ref: 150,000-400,000/ml), WBC 8.400 (ref: 4,000-11,000 ml), Total Iron Binding Capacity (TIBC) 378 (ref: 240-450 mcg/dl), ferritin 6.4 (ref: 12-300 ng/ml), and percent iron saturation 3% (ref: 25-35%). These results are consistent with iron deficiency anemia. The patient has not followed up with our endocrine clinic since then and we have not been able to reach her despite multiple attempts to obtain any update on her condition following iron supplementation trial.

3. Discussion

Hypophosphatemic rickets (HR) is a rare genetic disorder that is characterized by renal phosphate wasting. X-linked inheritance, accounting for about 80% of cases, is the most common form of transmission, with the remaining 20% caused by autosomal dominant (ADHR) and autosomal recessive inheritance [1].

ADHR is caused by missense variants in the *FGF23* encoding Fibroblast Growth Factor 23 (FGF23). These variants disrupt amino acid sequences 176–179 (RXXR), altering the RXXR furin protease recognition site, which protects the mutant FGF23 molecule from proteolysis but does not alter biological activity, leading to increased levels of intact FGF23 molecules, which in turns leads to phosphate wasting at the level of the proximal tubules [2–5].

More than 80% of the filtered load of the phosphate in the kidney is reabsorbed the proximal tubule through the sodium dependent phosphate cotransporters (NPT2a and NPT2c) present on the apical surface of proximal renal tubular cells [6]. FGF23 induces phosphate wasting by reducing expression of the sodium-phosphate cotransporters (NPT2a and NPT2c) on the apical surface of proximal renal tubule cells. FGF23 also suppresses transcription of *CYP27B1*, which encodes the vitamin D 1α-hydroxylase, and increases transcription of CYP24A1 which encodes the 24-hydroxylase, resulting in decreased circulating levels of 1,25 (OH)2D which can further exacerbate hypophosphatemia [4, 7–10].

In contrast to X-linked Hypophosphatemic Rickets (XLH), which is the most frequent inherited form of hypophosphatemia [6, 11], characterized by complete penetrance affecting males and females equally, the age at presentation in ADHR can vary between childhood and adulthood due to incomplete penetrance.

In 1997, Econs and McEnery [12] described a large kindred of hypophosphatemic rickets with an inheritance pattern consistent with autosomal dominant transmission. The kindred had 23 affected members and had two subgroups of phenotypes based upon the age of presentation: one group presented in childhood between the ages of 1 and 3 with the typical Ricketic lower extremity bowing and all manifested phosphate wasting, whereas the second group presented with renal phosphate wasting after puberty, between the ages of 14 and 45. The later-onset subjects showed diffuse or localized bone aches, weakness, and insufficiency fractures but did not have the short stature or the typical Ricketic lower extremity deformities or short stature. Their clinical presentation is similar to that for Tumor-Induced Osteomalacia (TIO). In the above-described case series of ADHR, all 9 patients with delayed-onset disease were female and it has been proposed that the postpubertal increases in sex steroid levels may play a role in the delayed-onset or penetrance. Additionally, two patients in the childhood-onset group had spontaneous resolution of their phosphate wasting disorder after puberty. In some instances, the onset of clinically evident disease correlated with a physiological stress such as pregnancy in some of the females in the adult-onset group [12] and a similar case report has also been reported [13].

Following iron supplementation, there was resolution of hypophosphatemia and the need for continued calcitriol and phosphate supplementation, reported in a young girl with ADHR [14]. The girl presented at the age of 26 months with poor growth and severe rickets. She was also found to have iron deficiency without anemia. She required treatment with phosphate supplements and calcitriol twice a day with documented radiological improvement. She relapsed when treatment was stopped around the age of five. She responded to resumption of calcitriol and phosphate supplementation. Around the age of 8, she received high dose iron supplementation, which resulted in significant reduction in both calcitriol and phosphate doses. Around the age of 9, she was able to come off calcitriol and phosphate completely.

It has been proposed that the low iron stores, induced by pregnancy or any other stressors, may lead to disease manifestation or exacerbation later in life. It has been shown that FGF23 expression inversely correlates with iron stores in patients with ADHR as well as in controls. In patients with ADHR, the mutant intact FGF-23 is resistant to cleavage and this leads to exacerbation of disease at times of iron deficiency when there is increased expression of FGF-23. This is not the case in controls, where, despite increase FGF23 expression in the context of iron deficiency, the cleavage process remains active preventing a rise in intact FGF-23 levels [15–17].

Treatment of ADHR involves correction of the abnormalities caused by elevated FGF 23, including low 1,25(OH)2D and serum phosphate, by administration of calcitriol and phosphate. There is limited data on treatment of ADHR as compared to the more common form which is X-linked form of hereditary rickets. The aim of treatment is directed at resolution of symptoms and not just the correction of hypophosphatemia [18].

Our patient, like other reported adult-onset cases, did not have any growth retardation, lower extremity deformity, or any other dental or skeletal abnormality during her childhood or adolescence. Her only reported episode of muscle aches and weakness was in her early adolescence when she was diagnosed with CPTII deficiency biochemically, but with negative genetic testing. We do not have access to her biochemical work-up done at that time. Therefore, it is plausible that she might have had a presentation of ADHR at that time that may have resolved spontaneously. Moreover, iron studies were not checked in our patient prior to her referral or during the work-up at our clinic as the role of iron deficiency and supplementation in management of patients with ADHR was not clearly established at that time. An early diagnosis and management of iron deficiency in our patient would likely have facilitated her management. Our patient did not have full knowledge of her family history, but it appears from her description that ADHR may have had skipped one generation on her paternal side. ADHR has been associated with variable expressivity and penetrance as compared to XLH.

This case highlights the importance of suspecting the diagnosis of hypophosphatemic rickets even in adult patients presenting with musculoskeletal pain, weakness, and hypophosphatemia, renal phosphate wasting, and elevated FGF-23 levels. An in-depth family history is invaluable as it can prevent extensive diagnostic work-up to look for a cause of TIO.

Treatment with calcitriol and phosphate can be remarkably effective in reducing symptoms of pain and weakness as shown in our patient. However, treatment related adverse events can occur necessitating long-term monitoring. Nephrocalcinosis, related to intermittent hypercalcemia and hypercalciuria resulting from high calcitriol dose, and secondary hyperparathyroidism, related to intermittent hypocalcemia on phosphate treatment, have been described. This warrants the need to carefully monitor serum and urinary calcium along with careful adjustment of calcitriol and phosphate dosing to avoid such complications [19, 20]. As shown in the above discussion, treatment of ADHR with iron replacement has been shown to be helpful in some patients leading to complete resolution of pain and biochemical abnormalities without any further need for the conventional treatment with phosphate replacement and calcitriol. It is unclear if our patient was able to get off ADHR treatment regimen upon iron supplementation eventually as she was lost to follow up in our clinic.

Female patients with ADHR or with family history of ADHR need to be followed closely when planning for pregnancy due to possibility of flare-up or worsening of the clinical course. It is unclear if prophylactic iron can be effective in preventing pregnancy-related flare-up of ADHR in such patients.

Another potential future option for patients with ADHR is Burosumab which is a human monoclonal antibody that targets and binds excess Fibroblast Growth Factor 23 (FGF-23) and has been tested in clinical trials in children with X-linked Hypophosphatemic Rickets with success and recently approved by FDA in 2018 for that purpose. Phase 2 trials of Burosumab in children with X-linked hypophosphatemia revealed that it improved renal tubular phosphate reabsorption, serum phosphorus levels, linear growth, and physical function and reduced the pain and the severity of rickets. [21]. However, at present, Burosumab is only approved for children with XLH. Further studies are needed to ascertain if it can be effective in ADHR.

In summary, our case describes a patient with adult-onset ADHR in the absence of any skeletal deformities and highlights the importance of considering this diagnosis in the work-up of patients presenting with musculoskeletal pain, weakness and hypophosphatemia.

Disclosure

The abstract of this case report was presented as a poster at the 98th Annual Meeting of The Endocrine Society in March 2016, Boston, MA.

References

[1] V. Pavone, G. Testa, S. Gioitta Iachino, F. R. Evola, S. Avondo, and G. Sessa, "Hypophosphatemic rickets: etiology, clinical features and treatment," *European Journal of Orthopaedic Surgery and Traumatology*, vol. 25, no. 2, pp. 221–226, 2015.

[2] K. E. White, W. E. Evans, J. L. H. O'Riordan et al., "Autosomal dominant hypophosphataemic rickets is associated with mutations in FGF23," *Nature Genetics*, vol. 26, no. 3, pp. 345–348, 2000.

[3] T. Shimada, T. Muto, I. Urakawa et al., "Mutant FGF-23 responsible for autosomal dominant hypophosphatemic rickets is resistant to proteolytic cleavage and causes hypophosphatemia in vivo," *Endocrinology*, vol. 143, no. 8, pp. 3179–3182, 2002.

[4] K. E. White, K. B. Jonsson, G. Carn, G. Hampson, T. D. Spector, M. Mannstadt et al., "The autosomal dominant hypophosphatemic rickets (ADHR) gene is a secreted polypeptide overexpressed by tumors that cause phosphate wasting," *The Journal of Clinical Endocrinology & Metabolism*, vol. 86, no. 2, pp. 497–500, 2001.

[5] K. E. White, G. Carn, B. Lorenz-Depiereux, A. Benet-Pages, T. M. Strom, and M. J. Econs, "Autosomal-dominant hypophosphatemic rickets (ADHR) mutations stabilize FGF-23," *Kidney International*, vol. 60, no. 6, pp. 2079–2086, 2001.

[6] M. Christov and H. Jüppner, "Phosphate homeostasis disorders," *Best Practice & Research Clinical Endocrinology & Metabolism*, vol. 32, no. 5, pp. 685–706, 2018.

[7] H. S. Tenenhouse and L. Beck, "Renal Na^+-phosphate cotransporter gene expression in X-linked *Hyp* and *Gy* mice," *Kidney International*, vol. 49, no. 4, pp. 1027–1032, 1996.

[8] F. Perwad, M. Y. Zhang, H. S. Tenenhouse, and A. A. Portale, "Fibroblast growth factor 23 impairs phosphorus and vitamin D metabolism in vivo and suppresses 25-hydroxyvitamin D-1α-hydroxylase expression in vitro," *American Journal of Physiology-Renal Physiology*, vol. 293, no. 5, pp. F1577–F1583, 2007.

[9] T. Shimada, H. Hasegawa, Y. Yamazaki et al., "FGF-23 is a potent regulator of vitamin D metabolism and phosphate homeostasis," *Journal of Bone and Mineral Research*, vol. 19, no. 3, pp. 429–435, 2004.

[10] J. M. Pettifor and K. Thandrayen, "Hypophosphatemic rickets: unraveling the role of FGF23," *Calcified Tissue International*, vol. 91, no. 5, pp. 297–306, 2012.

[11] E. A. Imel and M. J. Econs, "Approach to the hypophosphatemic patient," *The Journal of Clinical Endocrinology & Metabolism*, vol. 97, no. 3, pp. 696–706, 2012.

[12] M. J. Econs and P. T. McEnery, "Autosomal dominant hypophosphatemic rickets/osteomalacia: clinical characterization of a novel renal phosphate-wasting disorder," *The Journal of Clinical Endocrinology & Metabolism*, vol. 82, no. 2, pp. 674–681, 1997.

[13] S. Tournis, T. Koromila, N. Chatzistamatas et al., "Hip fracture leading to the diagnosis of autosomal dominant hypophosphatemic rickets. A case report," *Journal of Musculoskeletal and Neuronal Interactions*, vol. 13, no. 3, pp. 391–393, 2013.

[14] K. Kapelari, J. Köhle, D. Kotzot, and W. Högler, "Iron supplementation associated with loss of phenotype in autosomal dominant hypophosphatemic rickets," *The Journal of Clinical Endocrinology & Metabolism*, vol. 100, no. 9, pp. 3388–3392, 2015.

[15] B. K. Goldsweig and T. O. Carpenter, "Hypophosphatemic rickets: lessons from disrupted FGF23 control of phosphorus homeostasis," *Current Osteoporosis Reports*, vol. 13, no. 2, pp. 88–97, 2015.

[16] E. G. Farrow, X. Yu, L. J. Summers, S. I. Davis, J. C. Fleet, M. R. Allen et al., "Iron deficiency drives an autosomal dominant hypophosphatemic rickets (ADHR) phenotype in fibroblast growth factor-23 (Fgf23) knock-in mice," *Proceedings of the National Academy of Sciences of the United States of America*, vol. 108, no. 46, pp. E1146–E1155, 2011.

[17] E. A. Imel, M. Peacock, A. K. Gray, L. R. Padgett, S. L. Hui, and M. J. Econs, "Iron modifies plasma FGF23 differently in autosomal dominant hypophosphatemic rickets and healthy humans," *The Journal of Clinical Endocrinology & Metabolism*, vol. 96, no. 11, pp. 3541–3549, 2011.

[18] A. Linglart, M. Biosse-Duplan, K. Briot et al., "Therapeutic management of hypophosphatemic rickets from infancy to adulthood," *Endocrine Connections*, vol. 3, no. 1, pp. R13–R30, 2014.

[19] M. Tieder, J. Blonder, S. Strauss et al., "Hyperoxaluria is not a cause of nephrocalcinosis in phosphate-treated patients with hereditary hypophosphatemic rickets," *Nephron*, vol. 64, no. 4, pp. 526–531, 1993.

[20] T. O. Carpenter, M. A. Mitnick, A. Ellison, C. Smith, and K. L. Insogna, "Nocturnal hyperparathyroidism: a frequent feature of X-linked hypophosphatemia.," *The Journal of Clinical Endocrinology & Metabolism*, vol. 78, no. 6, pp. 1378–1383, 1994.

[21] T. O. Carpenter, M. P. Whyte, E. A. Imel, A. M. Boot, W. Hogler, A. Linglart et al., "Burosumab therapy in children with X-linked hypophosphatemia," *The New England Journal of Medicine*, vol. 378, no. 21, pp. 1987–1998, 2018.

43

Diabetic Ketoacidosis Revealing a Severe Hypertriglyceridemia and Acute Pancreatitis in Type 1 Diabetes Mellitus

Fatima Zahra Zaher, Imane Boubagura, Sana Rafi, Ghizlane Elmghari, and Nawal Elansari

Department of Endocrinology, Diabetes, Metabolic Diseases and Nutrition, Mohammed VI University Hospital, Marrakech, Morocco

Correspondence should be addressed to Fatima Zahra Zaher; drzaherfz@gmail.com

Academic Editor: John Broom

Diabetic ketoacidosis (DKA) is a life-threatening acute metabolic complication occurring in patients with diabetes, especially in patients with type 1 diabetes (T1D), due to an insulin deficiency. Moderate hypertriglyceridemia is commonly observed in DKA but severe hypertriglyceridemia with a triglyceride level exceeding 10g/L is very rarely reported. We report a case of a 14-year-old boy who had type 1 diabetes for 4 years treated with insulin therapy, also having adrenal insufficiency treated with hydrocortisone who presented with ketoacidosis and excruciating abdominal pain. Investigations revealed hypertriglyceridemia at 64g/L, lipasemia at 1000 U/L, and stage E pancreatitis on abdominal CT. The patient was treated with intravenous insulin, rehydration, and fenofibrate with good clinical and biological evolution. Severe hypertriglyceridemia causing pancreatitis in type 1 diabetes mellitus is a rare but very serious complication of DKA in children.

1. Introduction

Diabetes ketoacidosis (DKA) is the association of hyperglycemia with serum glucose ≥200 mg/dL or 11 mmol/L, the presence of ketonemia or ketonuria and acidosis with serum bicarbonate <15 mEq/L, or venous pH < 7.3 [1]. DKA represents a common complication of T1D due to an absolute insulin deficiency; it can be the mode of revelation of type 1 diabetes in 25% of cases [2], as it can complicate the evolution of a known T1D. Severe hypertriglyceridemia is an uncommon T1D complication which is also due to insulin deficiency and which can trigger acute pancreatitis. The triad of DKA, severe hypertriglyceridemia, and acute pancreatitis have been rarely described in children, especially in those with new onset T1D. We report only the tenth observation of this triad in a child known to be diabetic for 4 years with poor glycemic control.

2. Case Report

We report a case of a 14-year-old boy with type 1 diabetes from the age of 9 years treated with insulin 4 injections per day and followed up one year ago for adrenal insufficiency treated with hydrocortisone 25mg per day. His maternal uncle had a type 2 diabetes and his sister has been diagnosed with corticoid-induced diabetes; no family history of dislipidemia was reported. This child presented to the emergency room with severe abdominal pain and vomiting and he was found to have DKA, with an elevated lipase of 1000 U/L, and his abdominal ultrasound was suggestive of acute pancreatitis associated with moderate peritoneal effusion. His abdominal computed tomography (CT) showed pancreatitis grade E with antropyloric parietal thickening extended to the 2nd part of the duodenum associated with peritoneal effusion and a moderate hepatomegaly; the imaging did not show any other anomaly causing acute pancreatitis (Figures 1, 2 and 3). His plasma triglyceride (TG) level at admission was very high 64 g/L, and C- reactive protein was elevated at 358 mg/L, and other biochemical values were at the normal range. Fluid resuscitation and insulin therapy have been started and, on arrival to the pediatric intensive care unit, he was treated with the continuous insulin infusion, fenofibrate 160mg per day, antibiotic (third-generation cephalosporins 2g per day), and hydrocortisone 50mg four times per day intravenously. The

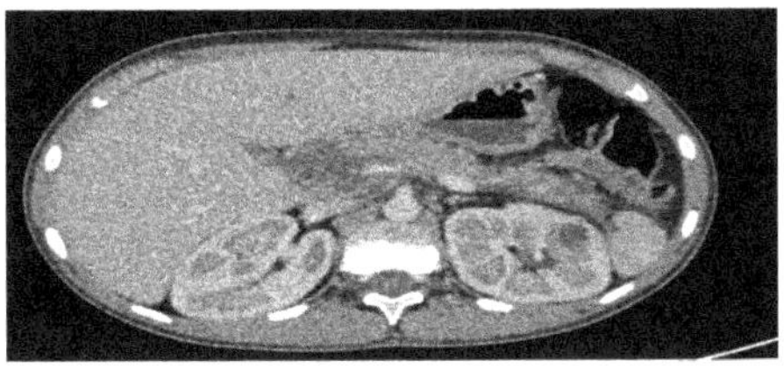

FIGURE 1: Abdominal CT showing a stage E pancreatitis.

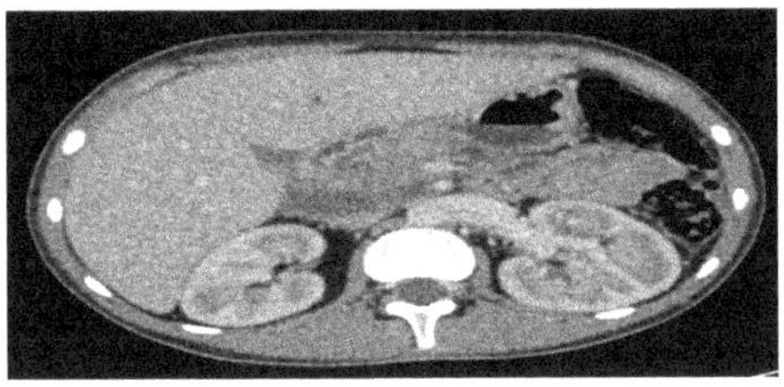

FIGURE 2: Abdominal CT showing a stage E pancreatitis.

TABLE 1: Evolution of biological parameters.

DAYS	TG (g/l)	LIPASE (U/l)	CRP (mg/l)
1st day	64	1000	358
2nd day	20	410	350
3rd day	12	285	169
4th day	4.31	-	76
5th day	3.37	159	20
6th day	4.20	-	5.38
7th day	3.32	65	5.25

indication of plasmapheresis was not retained in the light of the reduction in triglyceride levels.

He was transferred to our department one week after stabilization. History revealed steatorrhea 15 days before admission and a glycemic imbalance with hemoglobin A1c level of 11.5% (2 months before his admission). Our patient had a Glasgow score of 15/15, pulse rate 80/min, respiratory rate 16/min, and blood pressure 90/61mmHg. Anthropometric measurements showed weight of 44 kg, height 155 cm, body mass index 18.3 kg/m2, and a capillary glycemia of 3.38 g/L with presence of urine ketone; there was no eruptive or tuberous xanthoma or xanthelasma at the skin.

The therapeutic management was continued by correction of diabetic ketosis, fenofibrates, and the use of unsaturated oils: omega 3.6.9. The evolution was favorable: clinical improvement marked by disappearance of pain and a biological improvement (Table 1).

At the follow-up, the monitoring was favorable, the level of triglycerides gradually decreases until normalization, and the last rate is 1.56 g/L.

3. Discussion

Diabetic ketoacidosis (DKA) is associated with an increase in triglycerides (TG) level, which is observed in approximately 30-50% of cases [3]; however severe hypertriglyceridemia

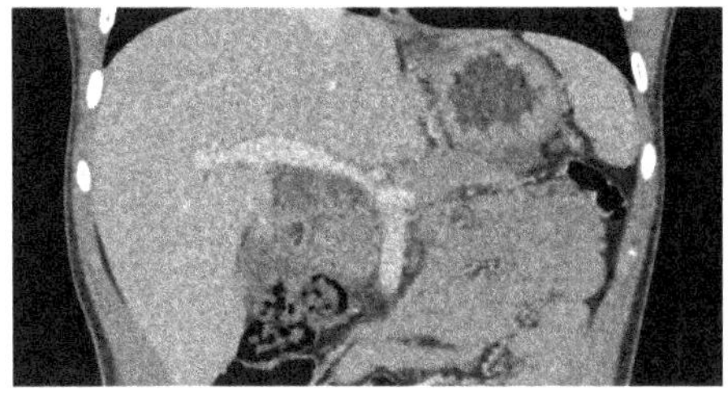

FIGURE 3: Abdominal CT showing a stage E pancreatitis.

(HTG), defined by a triglyceride level above 2000 mg/dL [4], is a rare complication of ketoacidosis which increases the risk of acute pancreatitis.

In many case reports, severe HTG is observed during DKA associated with newly diagnosed T1D [5, 6] or attributed to poor diabetes control [7] with severe insulin deficiency. In our case, the fact that his HbA1c was 11.5% signifies insulin deficiency for months, even if he did not report discontinuing his insulin therapy.

The mechanism of hypertriglyceridemia in DKA involves insulin deficiency which activate lipolysis in adipose tissue and increase the release of free fatty acid, which accelerate formation of very low-density lipoprotein by the liver [5]. Insulin deficiency is also associated with decreased activity of lipoprotein lipase (LPL), the enzyme responsible for TG metabolism, which reduces the clearance of VLDL and chylomicrons from the plasma, causing hypertriglyceridemia [8, 9].

However, in severe hypertriglyceridemia, the pathogenesis cannot be only explained by insulin deficiency, but may be aggravated by a coexisting genetic predisposition to hypertriglyceridemia, especially mutations in the gene coding for LPL which is located in chromosome 8 [10]. In the literature, more than 100 mutations of that gene with autosomal recessive inheritance were reported [11]. Young patients with homozygous mutation present with severe hypertriglyceridemia with abdominal pain, recurrent episodes of acute pancreatitis, and xanthomas [12] and those symptoms occur during the first year of life in approximately 25% of cases. However, in patients with a heterozygous mutation with normal health condition otherwise, blood lipid level is slightly increased or normal and disease symptoms occur during periods of insulin deficiency, stressful situation, or pregnancy [9, 11, 13].

Although severe hypertriglyceridemia is a rare condition, it may have devastating consequences such as lipidemia retinalis or acute pancreatitis [7]. Acute pancreatitis secondary to hypertriglyceridemia was reported in only 4% of DKA episodes in adults [14], and only nine cases are reported in children [5]. A triglyceride level more than 10g/L is associated with a risk of 5% for the development of acute pancreatitis; this risk is increased to 10%–20% when the triglyceride level is more than 20g/L [14]; DKA itself can cause pancreatic injury with false elevation of amylase and lipase. In our patient, the initial TG level was 64g/L. The mechanisms of this acute pancreatitis are composed of intrapancreatic release of free fatty acids resulting in cell injury, edema, and ischemia, as well as pancreatic ischemia caused directly by capillary hyperviscosity due to hyperchylomicronemia [15].

Management of DKA with HTG includes continuous insulin administration and intravenous fluid and according to diabetic ketoacidosis guidelines because the major mechanism of hypertriglyceridemia is insulin deficiency. However, some patients may require plasmapheresis, especially those with organ failure, which is the case of the patient reported by Lutfi who had extremely high TG level (163 g/L) with renal insufficiency, who failed with conservative treatment, but was successfully treated by plasmapheresis [16]. Heparin was also reported as a treatment for hypertriglyceridemia in adult with DKA, associated with fluid and insulin administration [17]. The use of lipid-lowering agents, such as fibrates, can be useful in most conditions accompanied by HTG but not beneficial in patients with lipoprotein lipase deficiency [18]. Omega oils are essential fatty acid naturally present in fish, algae, and other seafood; their use as a TG-lowering drug in the management of severe HTG is recommended by both the National Lipid Association [19] and the American Heart Association [20]. The EVOLVE study found a statistically significant reduction in serum TG in patients with severe HTG treated with omega 3 oil 2 g daily in comparison with those treated with olive oil 2 g daily, with a greater treatment effect in patients with very high baseline TG concentrations [21]. The proposed mechanisms to explain these finding include decreased VLDL synthesis by altering transcription factors such as sterol regulatory element-binding proteins involved in triglyceride synthesis and increased triglyceride clearance from the serum by increased lipoprotein lipase activity [22]. In our case, TG level was reduced from 64g/l to 3.37 g/L in 5 days, under insulin, fluid administration, fibrates, and omega oils.

The weakness of our case was that we could not perform appropriate genetic testing in our patient as well as his first-degree relatives. The genetic testing would have had an impact on the management of our patient since the majority of TG-lowering drugs, other than omega oils, decrease the plasma TG levels by the stimulation LPL activity, which makes them less effective in the case of a severely dysfunctional LPL protein. Surendran et al. have shown that a molecular diagnosis is effective in patients with severe HTG, and, by diagnosing the underlying genetic defect, different therapeutic strategies can be proposed [23]. For example, in the case of a genetic defect in GPIHBP1, where LPL itself is unaffected, Surendran et al. successfully used heparin infusion to facilitate activating LPL in the absence of GPIHBP1. On the other hand, in the case of patients with genetic LPL gene deficiency, LPL gene therapy has been used successfully. However, in the case of APOC2 or LMF1 deficiency, no clear treatment options are currently available, beyond strict dietary restrictions [23].

4. Conclusion

In patients with diabetic ketoacidosis and acute pancreatitis, clinicians should be aware of the possibility of associated hypertriglyceridemia caused by the severe insulin deficiency, recognition of this triad has important implications in the management of the patient as insulin requirements, and recovery period can be changed.

References

[1] J. I. Wolfsdorf, "The International Society of Pediatric and Adolescent Diabetes guidelines for management of diabetic ketoacidosis: do the guidelines need to be modified?" *Pediatric Diabetes*, vol. 15, no. 4, pp. 277–286, 2014.

[2] A. Rewers, G. Klingensmith, C. Davis et al., "Presence of diabetic ketoacidosis at diagnosis of diabetes mellitus in youth: The search for diabetes in youth study," *Pediatrics*, vol. 121, no. 5, pp. e1258–e1266, 2008.

[3] P. R. Blackett, J. H. Holcombe, P. Alaupovic, and J. D. Fesmire, "Plasma lipids and apolipoproteins in a 13-year-old boy with diabetic ketoacidosis and extreme hyperlipidemia," *The American Journal of the Medical Sciences*, vol. 291, no. 5, pp. 342–346, 1986.

[4] M. Fulop and H. Eder, "Severe hypertriglyceridemia in diabetic ketosis," *The American Journal of the Medical Sciences*, vol. 300, no. 6, pp. 361–365, 1990.

[5] P. K. Sharma, M. Kumar, and D. K. Yadav, "Severe hypertriglyceridemia causing pancreatitis in a child with new-onset type-i diabetes mellitus presenting with diabetic ketoacidosis," *Indian Journal of Critical Care Medicine*, vol. 21, no. 3, pp. 176–178, 2017.

[6] P. M. Wolfgram and M. J. MacDonald, "Severe hypertriglyceridemia causing acute pancreatitis in a child with new onset type I diabetes mellitus presenting in ketoacidosis," *Journal of Pediatric Intensive Care*, vol. 2, no. 2, pp. 77–80, 2013.

[7] T. Saengkaew, T. Sahakitrungruang, S. Wacharasindhu, and V. Supornsilchai, "DKA with Severe Hypertriglyceridemia and Cerebral Edema in an Adolescent Boy: A Case Study and Review of the Literature," *Case Reports in Endocrinology*, vol. 2016, Article ID 7515721, 4 pages, 2016.

[8] A. Radhakutty, J. Shen, A. J. Hooper et al., "Quantification and genotyping of lipoprotein lipase in patients with diabetic lipaemia," *Diabetic Medicine*, vol. 31, no. 12, pp. 1702–1707, 2014.

[9] J. Nocoń-Bohusz, B. Wikiera, A. Basiak, R. Śmigiel, and A. Noczyńska, "LPL gene mutation as the cause of severe hypertriglyceridemia in the course of ketoacidosis in a patient with newly diagnosed type 1 diabetes mellitus," *Pediatric Endocrinology, Diabetes and Metabolism*, vol. 21, no. 2, pp. 89–92, 2015.

[10] M. Fulop and H. A. Eder, "Plasma triglycerides and cholesterol in diabetic ketosis," *JAMA Internal Medicine*, vol. 149, no. 9, pp. 1997–2002, 1989.

[11] A. G. McLean, C. J. Petersons, A. J. Hooper, J. R. Burnett, M. G. Burt, and M. P. Doogue, "Extreme diabetic lipaemia associated with a novel lipoprotein lipase gene mutation," *Clinica Chimica Acta*, vol. 406, no. 1-2, pp. 167–169, 2009.

[12] C. Karagianni, S. Stabouli, K. Roumeliotou et al., "Severe hypertriglyceridaemia in diabetic ketoacidosis: Clinical and genetic study," *Diabetic Medicine*, vol. 21, no. 4, pp. 380–382, 2004.

[13] J. Rip, M. C. Nierman, N. J. Wareham et al., "Serum lipoprotein lipase concentration and risk for future coronary artery disease: The EPIC-Norfolk prospective population study," *Arteriosclerosis, Thrombosis, and Vascular Biology*, vol. 26, no. 3, pp. 637–642, 2006.

[14] S. Nair, D. Yadav, and C. S. Pitchumoni, "Association of diabetic ketoacidosis and acute pancreatitis: observations in 100 consec-

utive episodes of DKA," *American Journal of Gastroenterology*, vol. 95, no. 10, pp. 2795–2800, 2000.

[15] W. Tsuang, U. Navaneethan, L. Ruiz, J. B. Palascak, and A. Gelrud, "Hypertriglyceridemic pancreatitis: presentation and management," *American Journal of Gastroenterology*, vol. 104, no. 4, pp. 984–991, 2009.

[16] R. Lutfi, J. Huang, and H. R. Wong, "Plasmapheresis to treat hypertriglyceridemia in a child with diabetic ketoacidosis and pancreatitis," *Pediatrics*, vol. 129, no. 1, pp. e195–e198, 2012.

[17] R. P. Cole, "Heparin treatment for severe hypertriglyceridemia in diabetic ketoacidosis," *JAMA Internal Medicine*, vol. 169, no. 15, pp. 1439–1441, 2009.

[18] A. R. Rahalkar, F. Giffen, B. Har et al., "Novel LPL mutations associated with lipoprotein lipase deficiency: Two case reports and a literature review," *Canadian Journal of Physiology and Pharmacology*, vol. 87, no. 3, pp. 151–160, 2009.

[19] T. A. Jacobson, M. K. Ito, K. C. Maki et al., "National Lipid Association recommendations for patient-centered management of dyslipidemia: Part 1 - Executive summary," *Journal of Clinical Lipidology*, vol. 8, no. 5, pp. 473–488, 2014.

[20] M. Miller, N. J. Stone, C. Ballantyne et al., "Triglycerides and cardiovascular disease: a scientific statement from the American Heart Association," *Circulation*, vol. 123, no. 20, pp. 2292–2333, 2011.

[21] E. S. G. Stroes, A. V. Susekov, T. W. A. de Bruin, M. Kvarnström, H. Yang, and M. H. Davidson, "Omega-3 carboxylic acids in patients with severe hypertriglyceridemia: EVOLVE II, a randomized, placebo-controlled trial," *Journal of Clinical Lipidology*, vol. 12, no. 2, pp. 321–330, 2018.

[22] W. S. Harris, M. Miller, A. P. Tighe, M. H. Davidson, and E. J. Schaefer, "Omega-3 fatty acids and coronary heart disease risk: clinical and mechanistic perspectives," *Atherosclerosis*, vol. 197, no. 1, pp. 12–24, 2008.

[23] R. P. Surendran, M. E. Visser, S. Heemelaar et al., "Mutations in LPL, APOC2, APOA5, GPIHBP1 and LMF1 in patients with severe hypertriglyceridaemia," *Journal of Internal Medicine*, vol. 272, no. 2, pp. 185–196, 2012.

44

Persistent vs Recurrent Cushing's Disease Diagnosed Four Weeks Postpartum

Leena Shah ,[1] Emily V. Nosova ,[1] Joshua B. Bederson,[2] and Khadeen Christi Cheesman[1]

[1]*Division of Endocrinology, Diabetes, and Bone Disease, Department of Medicine, Icahn School of Medicine at Mount Sinai, New York, NY, USA*
[2]*Department of Neurosurgery, Icahn School of Medicine at Mount Sinai, New York, NY, USA*

Correspondence should be addressed to Leena Shah; leena.y.shah@gmail.com

Academic Editor: Wayne V. Moore

Background. Cushing's disease (CD) recurrence in pregnancy is thought to be associated with estradiol fluctuations during gestation. CD recurrence in the immediate postpartum period in a patient with a documented dormant disease during pregnancy has never been reported. *Case Report.* A 30-year-old woman with CD had improvement of her symptoms after transsphenoidal resection (TSA) of her pituitary lesion. She conceived unexpectedly 3 months postsurgery and had no symptoms or biochemical evidence of recurrence during pregnancy. After delivering a healthy boy, she developed CD 4 weeks postpartum and underwent a repeat TSA. Despite repeat TSA, she continued to have elevated cortisol levels that were not well controlled with medical management. She eventually had a bilateral adrenalectomy. *Discussion.* CD recurrence may be higher in the peripartum period, but the link between pregnancy and CD recurrence and/or persistence is not well studied. Potential mechanisms of CD recurrence in the postpartum period are discussed below. *Conclusion.* We describe the first report of recurrent CD that was quiescent during pregnancy and diagnosed in the immediate postpartum period. Understanding the risk and mechanisms of CD recurrence in pregnancy allows us to counsel these otherwise healthy, reproductive-age women in the context of additional family planning.

1. Introduction

Despite a relatively high prevalence of Cushing's syndrome (CS) in women of reproductive age, it is rare for pregnancy to occur in patients with active disease [1]. Hypercortisolism leads to infertility through impairment of the hypothalamic gonadal axis. Additionally, while Cushing's disease (CD) is the leading etiology of CS in nonpregnant adults, it is less common in pregnancy, accounting for only 30–40% of the CS cases in pregnant women [2]. It has been suggested that in CD there is hypersecretion of both cortisol and androgens, impairing fertility to a greater extent, while in CS of an adrenal origin, hypersecretion is almost exclusively of cortisol with minimal androgen production [3]. Regardless of the cause, active CS in pregnancy is associated with a higher maternal and fetal morbidity, hence, prompt diagnosis and treatment are essential.

Pregnancy is considered a physiological state of hypercortisolism, and the peripartum period is a common time for women to develop CD [3, 4]. A recent study reported that 27% of reproductive-age women with CD had onset associated with pregnancy [4]. The high rate of pregnancy-associated CD suggests that the stress of pregnancy and peripartum pituitary corticotroph hyperstimulation may promote or accelerate pituitary tumorigenesis [4–6]. During pregnancy, the circulating levels of corticotropin-releasing hormone (CRH) in the plasma increase exponentially as a result of CRH production by the placenta, decidua, and fetal membranes rather than by the hypothalamus. Unbound circulating placental CRH stimulates pituitary ACTH secretion and causes maternal plasma ACTH levels to rise [4]. A review of the literature reveals many studies of CD onset during the peripartum period, but CD recurrence in the peripartum period has only been

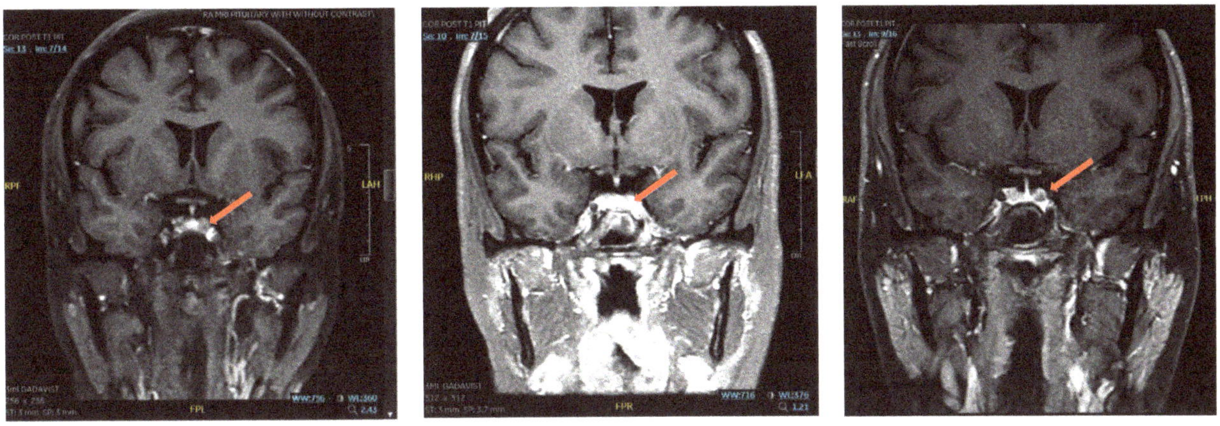

(a) (b) (c)

FIGURE 1: (a) Initial: MRI pituitary with and without contrast showing a coronal T1 postcontrast image immediately prior to our patient's pituitary surgery. The red arrow points to a 3 × 3 × 5 mm hypoenhancing focus representing a pituitary microadenoma. (b) Postsurgical: MRI pituitary with and without contrast showing a coronal T1 postcontrast image obtained three months after transsphenoidal pituitary surgery. The red arrow shows that a hypoenhancing focus is no longer seen and has been resected. (c) Postpartum: MRI pituitary with and without contrast showing a coronal T1 postcontrast image obtained four weeks postpartum. The red arrow points to a 3 mm relatively hypoenhancing lesion representing a recurrent pituitary adenoma.

reported a handful of times [7–10]. Of these, most cases recurred during pregnancy. CD recurrence in the immediate postpartum period has only been reported once [7]. Below, we report for the first time a case of CD recurrence that occurred 4 weeks postpartum, with a documented dormant disease throughout pregnancy.

2. Case Presentation

A 30-year-old woman initially presented with prediabetes, weight gain, dorsal hump, abdominal striae, depression, lower extremity weakness, and oligomenorrhea with a recent miscarriage 10 months ago. Diagnostic tests were consistent with CD. Results included the following: three elevated midnight salivary cortisols: 0.33, 1.38, and 1.10 μg/dL (<0.010–0.090); 1 mg dexamethasone suppression test (DST) with cortisol 14 μg/dL (<1.8); elevated 24 hr urine cortisol (UFC) measuring 825 μg/24 hr (6–42); ACTH 35 pg/mL (7.2–63.3). MRI of the pituitary gland revealed a left 4 mm focal lesion (Figure 1(a)). After transsphenoidal resection (TSA), day 1, 2, and 3 morning cortisol values were 18, 5, and 2 μg/dL, respectively. Pathology did not show a definitive pituitary neoplasm. She was rapidly titrated off hydrocortisone (HC) by six weeks postresection. Her symptoms steadily improved, including improved energy levels, improved mood, and resolution of striae. She resumed normal menses and conceived unexpectedly around 3 months post-TSA. Hormonal evaluation completed a few weeks prior to her pregnancy indicated no recurrence: morning ACTH level, 27.8 pg/mL; UFC, 5 μg/24 hr; midnight salivary cortisol, 0.085 and 0.014 μg/dL. Her postop MRI at that time did not show a definitive adenoma (Figure 1(b)). During pregnancy, she had a normal oral glucose tolerance test at 20 weeks and no other sequela of CD. Every 8 weeks, she had 24-hour urine cortisol measurements. Of these, the highest was 93 μg/24 hr at 17 weeks and none were in the range of CD (Table 1). Towards the end of her 2nd trimester, she started to complain of severe fatigue. Given her low 24 hr urine cortisol level of 15 μg/24 hr at 36 weeks gestation, she was started on HC. She underwent a cesarean section at 40 weeks gestation for oligohydramnios and she subsequently delivered a healthy baby boy weighing 7.6 pounds with APGAR scores at 1 and 5 minutes being 9 and 9. HC was discontinued immediately after delivery. Around four weeks postpartum she developed symptoms suggestive for CD. Diagnostic tests showed an elevated midnight salivary cortisol of 0.206 and 0.723 μg/dL, and 24-hour urine cortisol of 400 μg/24 hr. MRI pituitary illustrated a 3 mm adenoma in the left posterior region of the gland, which was thought to represent a recurrent tumor (Figure 1(c)). A discrete lesion was found and resected during repeat TSA. Pathology confirmed corticotroph adenoma with MIB-1 < 3%. On postoperative days 1, 2, and 3, the cortisol levels were 26, 10, and 2.8 μg/dL, respectively. She was tapered off HC within one month. Her symptoms improved only slightly and she continued to report weight gain, muscle weakness, and fatigue. Three months after repeat TSA, biochemical data showed 1 out of 2 midnight salivary cortisols elevated at 0.124 μg/dL and elevated urine cortisol of 76 μg/24 hr. MRI pituitary demonstrated a 3 × 5 mm left enhancement, concerning for residual or enlarged persistent tumor. Subsequent lab work continued to show a biochemical excess of cortisol, and the patient was started on metyrapone but reported no significant improvement of her symptoms and only mild improvement of excess cortisol. After a multidisciplinary discussion, the patient made the decision to pursue bilateral adrenalectomy, as she refused further medical management and opted against radiation given the risk of hypogonadism.

Table 1: 24-hour urine-free cortisol measurements collected approximately every 8 weeks throughout our patient's pregnancy.

Time in relation to pregnancy	4 months before conception and 2 months pre-TSA	2 weeks before conception and 7 weeks post-TSA	10 weeks	17 weeks	29 weeks	36 weeks	4 weeks postpartum
24-hour urine-free cortisol (μg/24 hr) nonpregnant reference range (LabCorp): 6–42 μg/24 hr	825.6	5	34	93	29	15	408

*Pregnancy reference ranges have not been well established. UFC levels are typically higher in pregnancy, up to twice the upper limit of normal. Our patient was therefore said to have low UFC levels at 36 weeks gestation.

3. Discussion

The symptoms and signs of Cushing's syndrome overlap with those seen in normal pregnancy, making diagnosis of Cushing's disease during pregnancy challenging [1]. Potential mechanisms of gestational hypercortisolemia include increased systemic cortisol resistance during pregnancy, decreased sensitivity of plasma ACTH to negative feedback causing an altered pituitary ACTH setpoint, and non-circadian secretion of placental CRH during pregnancy causing stimulation of the maternal HPA axis [5]. Consequently, both urinary excretion of cortisol and late-night salivary cortisol undergo a gradual increase during normal pregnancy, beginning at the 11th week of gestation [2]. Cushing's disease is suggested by 24-hour urinary-free cortisol levels greater than 3-fold of the upper limit of normal [2]. It has also been suggested that nocturnal salivary cortisol be used to diagnose Cushing's disease by using the following specific trimester thresholds: first trimester, 0.25 μg/dL; second trimester, 0.26 μg/dL; third trimester 0.33, μg/dL [11]. By these criteria, our patient had no signs or biochemical evidence of CD during pregnancy but developed CD 4 weeks postpartum.

A recent study by Tang et al. proposed that there may be a higher risk of developing CD in the peripartum period, but did not test for CD during pregnancy, and therefore was not able to definitively say exactly when CD onset occurred in relation to pregnancy [4]. Previous literature suggests that there may be a higher risk of ACTH-secreting pituitary adenomas following pregnancy as there is a significant surge of ACTH and cortisol hormones at the time of labor. This increased stimulation of the pituitary corticotrophs in the immediate postpartum period may promote tumorigenesis [6]. It has also been suggested that the hormonal milieu during pregnancy may cause accelerated growth of otherwise dormant or small slow-growing pituitary corticotroph adenomas [4, 5]. However, the underlying mechanisms of CD development in the postpartum period have yet to be clarified. We highlight the need for more research to investigate not only the development, but also the risk of CD recurrence in the postpartum period. Such research would be helpful for family planning.

4. Conclusion

Hypothalamic-pituitary-adrenal axis activation during pregnancy and the immediate postpartum period may result in higher rates of CD recurrence in the postpartum period, as seen in our patient. In general, more testing for CS in all reproductive-age females with symptoms suggesting CS, especially during and after childbirth, is necessary. Such testing can also help us determine when CD occurred in relation to pregnancy, so that we can further understand the link between pregnancy and CD occurrence, recurrence, and/or persistence. Learning about the potential mechanisms of CD development and recurrence in pregnancy will help us to counsel these reproductive-age women who desire pregnancy.

Abbreviations

CD: Cushing's disease
TSA: Transsphenoidal resection
DST: Dexamethasone suppression test
ACTH: Adrenocorticotropic hormone
MRI: Magnetic-resonance imaging
HC: Hydrocortisone
CTH: Corticotroph-releasing hormone
HPA: Hypothalamic-pituitary-adrenal.

Additional Points

Note. Peripartum refers to the period immediately before, during, or after pregnancy and postpartum refers to any period after pregnancy up until 1 year postdelivery.

Disclosure

This case report is a follow up to an abstract that was presented in ENDO 2020 Abstracts.

Acknowledgments

The authors thank Dr. Puneet Pawha for his help in reviewing MRI images and his suggestions.

References

[1] J. R. Lindsay and L. K. Nieman, "The hypothalamic-pituitary-adrenal axis in pregnancy: challenges in disease detection and

treatment," *Endocrine Reviews*, vol. 26, no. 6, pp. 775–799, 2005.
[2] W. Huang, M. E. Molitch, and M. E. Molitch, "Pituitary tumors in pregnancy," *Endocrinology and Metabolism Clinics of North America*, vol. 48, no. 3, pp. 569–581, 2019.
[3] M. C. Machado, M. C. B. V. Fragoso, M. D. Bronstein, and M. Delano, "Pregnancy in patients with cushing's syndrome," *Endocrinology and Metabolism Clinics of North America*, vol. 47, no. 2, pp. 441–449, 2018.
[4] K. Tang, L. Lu, M. Feng et al., "The incidence of pregnancy-associated Cushing's disease and its relation to pregnancy: a retrospective study," *Frontiers in Endocrinology*, vol. 11, p. 305, 2020.
[5] S. K. Palejwala, A. R. Conger, A. A. Eisenberg et al., "Pregnancy-associated Cushing's disease? an exploratory retrospective study," *Pituitary*, vol. 21, no. 6, pp. 584–592, 2018.
[6] G. Mastorakos and I. Ilias, "Maternal and fetal hypothalamic-pituitary-adrenal axes during pregnancy and postpartum," *Annals of the New York Academy of Sciences*, vol. 997, no. 1, pp. 136–149, 2003.
[7] G. F. Yaylali, F. Akin, E. Yerlikaya, S. Topsakal, and D. Herek, "Cushing's disease recurrence after pregnancy," *Endocrine Abstracts*, vol. 32, 2013.
[8] C. V. L. Fellipe, R. Muniz, L. Stefanello, N. M. Massucati, and L. Warszawski, "Cushing's disease recurrence during peripartum period: a case report," *Endocrine Abstracts*, vol. 70, 2020.
[9] P. Recinos, M. Abbassy, V. Kshettry et al., "Surgical management of recurrent Cushing's disease in pregnancy: a case report," *Surgical Neurology International*, vol. 6, no. 26, pp. S640–S645, 2015.
[10] A. Nakhleh, L. Saiegh, M. Reut, M. S. Ahmad, I. W. Pearl, and C. Shechner, "Cabergoline treatment for recurrent Cushing's disease during pregnancy," *Hormones*, vol. 15, no. 3, pp. 453–458, 2016.
[11] L. M. L. Lopes, R. P. V. Francisco, M. A. K. Galletta, and M. D. Bronstein, "Determination of nighttime salivary cortisol during pregnancy: comparison with values in non-pregnancy and cushing's disease," *Pituitary*, vol. 19, no. 1, pp. 30–38, 2015.

45

Diagnostic Challenges in Ovarian Hyperthecosis: Clinical Presentation with Subdiagnostic Testosterone Levels

Sanket Shah,[1] **Callie Torres**,[2] **and Naser Gharaibeh**[3]

[1]*Department of Internal Medicine, Medical College of Wisconsin, Milwaukee, WI 53226, USA*
[2]*Department of Pathology & Immunology, Washington University in St Louis, St Louis, MO 63110, USA*
[3]*Department of Endocrinology, Mercy Hospital, 100 Mercy Way, Joplin, MO 64804, USA*

Correspondence should be addressed to Sanket Shah; shah_sanket22@yahoo.com

Academic Editor: Osamu Isozaki

Symptoms of hyperandrogenism and virilization in postmenopausal women warrant workup for ovarian hyperthecosis. In this case series, we discuss two patients who presented with symptoms of hyperandrogenism and metabolic abnormalities including insulin resistance stemming from ovarian hyperthecosis. Imaging revealed normal ovaries in both patients. However, both patients had total serum testosterone levels below the lower diagnostic limit for ovarian hyperthecosis. Due to high clinical suspicion of ovarian hyperthecosis, both patients underwent bilateral oophorectomy without venous sampling for ovarian androgens. The diagnosis of ovarian hyperthecosis was confirmed on histological examination. Both women had improvement in their hyperandrogenic symptoms, testosterone levels, and biochemical features of insulin resistance after surgical intervention. This presentation of ovarian hyperthecosis with subdiagnostic total serum testosterone levels demonstrates the need for continued research into the pathophysiology of the disease, discussion of the diagnostic threshold of total serum testosterone, as well as the inclusion of ovarian hyperthecosis in the differential of postmenopausal women with hyperandrogenism and insulin resistance.

1. Introduction

Ovarian hyperthecosis refers to a process in which ovarian cells differentiate into clusters of luteinized thecal cells in the ovarian stroma producing excessive amounts of testosterone. This condition commonly presents in postmenopausal women with symptoms similar to that of polycystic ovarian syndrome [1]. The disorder can result in metabolic abnormalities such as insulin resistance which can then lead to hyperinsulinemia. Hyperinsulinemia can result in an increased risk for type 2 diabetes mellitus and cardiovascular disease [2]. Acne and hirsutism secondary to high testosterone levels are also commonly present [3]. In this article, we discuss two patients with symptomatic ovarian hyperthecosis and laboratory levels below the standard diagnostic criteria. The discussed cases highlight the importance of using clinical impression and metabolic symptomology to confirm the diagnosis of ovarian hyperthecosis, although testosterone levels may be below the usual diagnostic threshold for the disease [4].

2. Case Presentation

2.1. Case 1. A 60-year-old female with a history of dyslipidemia, hypertension, polycystic ovarian syndrome, and obstructive sleep apnea was referred to endocrinology for management of severe hirsutism, fatty liver disease, hyperlipidemia, and type 2 diabetes mellitus. She reported a longstanding history of hirsutism with frontal balding that progressed over five years and was being treated with spironolactone. She described her libido as normal and denied any clitoromegaly or acne. Compared to one year prior, laboratory results revealed mild elevations in ALT (increasing from 34 to 52) and AST (increasing from 34 to 43). Additionally, hemoglobin A1c (HbA1c) increased from 6.7% to 8.0%. Total serum testosterone levels were at 145 ng/dL.

The patient was started on metformin 2000 mg and subcutaneous semaglutide 0.5 mg to manage her diabetes. Due to her abnormal liver enzyme levels, she was screened for chronic hepatitis which was negative. Pelvic ultrasound revealed a 2.5 cm simple cyst within the right ovary and an incidental 9 mm calcification within the endometrial canal. Her gonadotropin levels were below normal for her post-menopausal state, and DHEA-S, 17-hydroxyprogesterone, and prolactin levels were normal. She was referred to an obstetrician-gynecologist due to suspicion of ovarian hyperthecosis. No adrenal/ovarian vein sampling was performed as it was not available at the facility.

After discussion with the patient and the gynecological team, it was decided that a complete hysterectomy was a reasonable option due to the high suspicion of ovarian hyperthecosis and the presence of rectocele and cystocele. Posthysterectomy, the pathology report was remarkable for atrophic endometrium and bilateral ovarian hyperthecosis as shown in Figure 1. Labs collected during the one-month posthysterectomy follow-up visit were significant, in which liver transaminase levels had returned to normal and HbA1c had improved to 6.3%. Additionally, total serum testosterone decreased to 7 ng/dL, and the patient noted that her hirsutism had mildly improved.

2.2. Case 2. A 58-year-old female with a history of hysterectomy in 1999 and hyperlipidemia was referred to endocrinology for management of type 2 diabetes mellitus and hirsutism. She noted excessive hair growth for the past three years which required her to shave and pluck her facial hair daily. She also complained of worsening acne, folliculitis, clitoromegaly, and occasional light vaginal bleeding. She described her libido as normal. She voiced concerns about a rising HbA1c increasing from normal to 8.2% over a six-month period. Additional laboratory tests showed a normal TSH at 3.38 uU/mL and elevated total serum testosterone of 135 ng/dL.

The patient was started on metformin 2000 mg for management of her diabetes. The patient's rapid progression of diabetes and recent development of hirsutism was worrisome for insulin resistance in the setting of an underlying etiology such as high testosterone levels. Pelvic ultrasound showed normal bilateral ovaries containing small cysts or follicles. Pelvic MRI demonstrated bilateral ovarian enlargement for the patient's age, which was more pronounced in the right ovary than the left ovary. Additional laboratory testing revealed normal prolactin, 17-hydroxyprogesterone, and androstenedione levels. However, the patient had subnormal age-specific LH and FSH levels. Based on the imaging and laboratory results, the patient was referred to the gynecological team. The patient then underwent bilateral oophorectomy due to a high suspicion of ovarian hyperthecosis.

The oophorectomy pathology report was significant for bilateral ovarian hyperthecosis as shown in Figure 2. Laboratory results collected one-month postoophorectomy demonstrated an improvement in HbA1c from 8.2% to 6.1% and testosterone from 135 ng/dL to 16 ng/dL. The patient denied significant improvement in hirsutism after the surgery and stated that she continued to have excess hair on the abdomen and bilateral upper extremities. However, she reported significant improvement in clitoromegaly.

3. Discussion

These cases emphasize the importance of including ovarian hyperthecosis in the differential diagnosis when a post-menopausal woman presents with hirsutism, symptoms of virilization, or symptoms of rapidly progressive insulin resistance (in the absence of clinical or biochemical abnormalities of other etiologies such as Cushing's syndrome or hypothyroidism). Current guidelines recommend that ovarian hyperthecosis is less likely if total serum testosterone levels are below 150 ng/dL [4]. As described in the cases, both patients had a total serum testosterone level below 150 ng/dL and were still diagnosed with ovarian hyperthecosis and had significant improvement in symptoms postoophorectomy. In patients with symptoms of severe hyperandrogenism, it is important to rule out androgen-secreting ovarian and adrenal tumors. In the cases discussed, adrenal tumors were lower on the differential due to normal adrenal androgen levels. A gonadotropin secreting pituitary adenoma was also unlikely given that the patients did not have any suggestive symptoms or laboratory findings consistent with adenoma. Congenital adrenal hyperplasia was additionally ruled out due to normal 17-hydroxyprogesterone levels. Exposure to synthetic androgens was also ruled out due to normal androstenedione levels and patient denial of exogenous hormone intake. Both patients had a significant improvement in their hemoglobin A1C as well as their total serum testosterone levels after oophorectomy as given in Table 1.

In the workup of patients presenting with elevated total serum testosterone levels and virilization, the first step is to identify the source of the excess androgen production. Pelvic ultrasound in women with hyperthecosis is recommended to rule out androgen-producing tumors and usually shows a bilateral increase in ovarian size and stroma [5]. If imaging is negative and a strong suspicion of ovarian hyperthecosis remains, the next step is to perform ovarian venous sampling. It is important to note, however, that ovarian venous sampling is an advanced procedure requiring technical expertise, and evidence for using it in clinical practice is not substantiated [6, 7]. Additionally, the procedure is not offered at all facilities.

Insulin resistance is a key component in identifying ovarian hyperthecosis [8]. It is important to measure sex hormone-binding globulin (SHBG) levels as low levels can serve as a predictive marker for insulin resistance when underlying hyperandrogenism is a suspected cause [9]. Once hyperthecosis is suspected, it is vital to address and manage the various complications caused by increased androgen levels. Patients should be counseled on weight control, lifestyle modifications, and started on metformin for better glycemic control if HbA1c is elevated [10]. The definitive treatment for patients with hyperthecosis is bilateral oophorectomy, and diagnosis of hyperthecosis is confirmed only by histological analysis. If patients are unable to tolerate surgery, treatment with a long-term gonadotropin-releasing hormone agonist is recommended to suppress the HPG axis. Currently, a surgical approach is preferred for the management of hyperthecosis over medical management [3, 11].

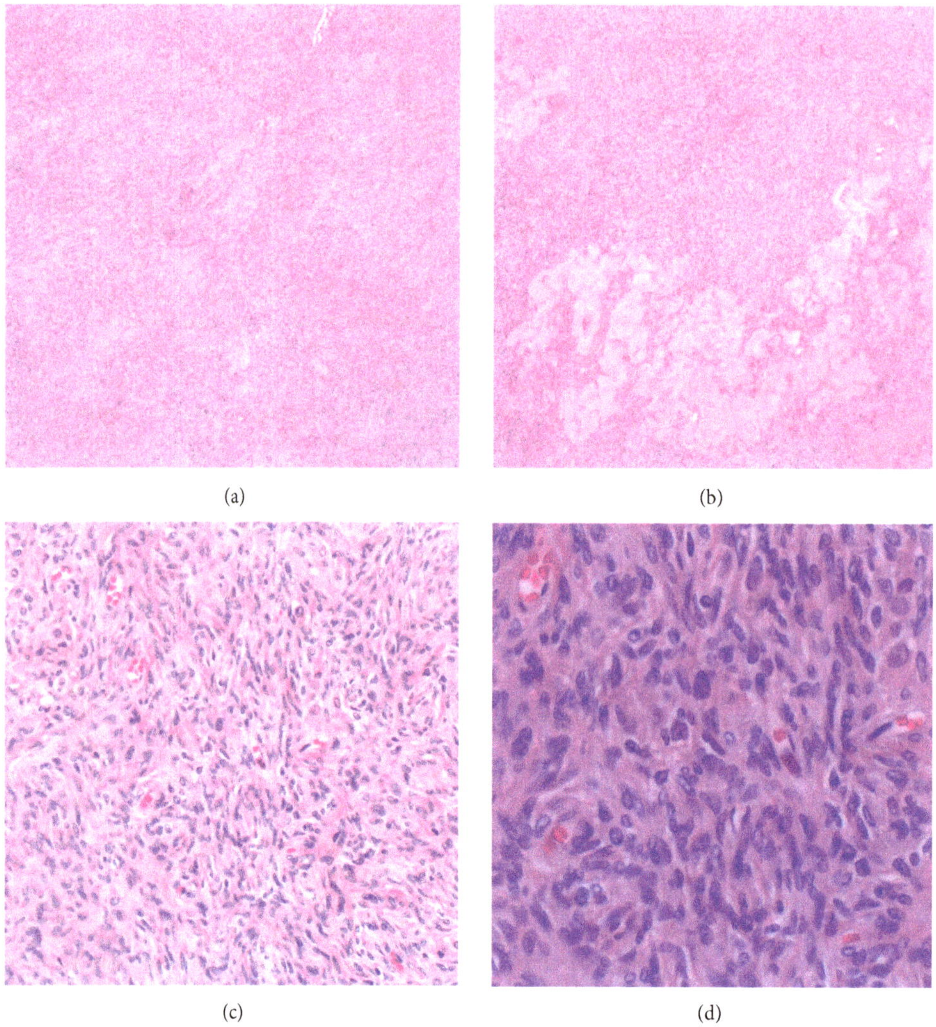

Figure 1: Microscopic images depict ovarian hyperthecosis with stromal hyperplasia and abundant spindled theca cells. Corpora albicantia (B) was also apparent throughout the specimen. Hematoxylin and eosin stain, original magnification: (a) 4x, (b) 4x, (c) 20x, and (d) 40x.

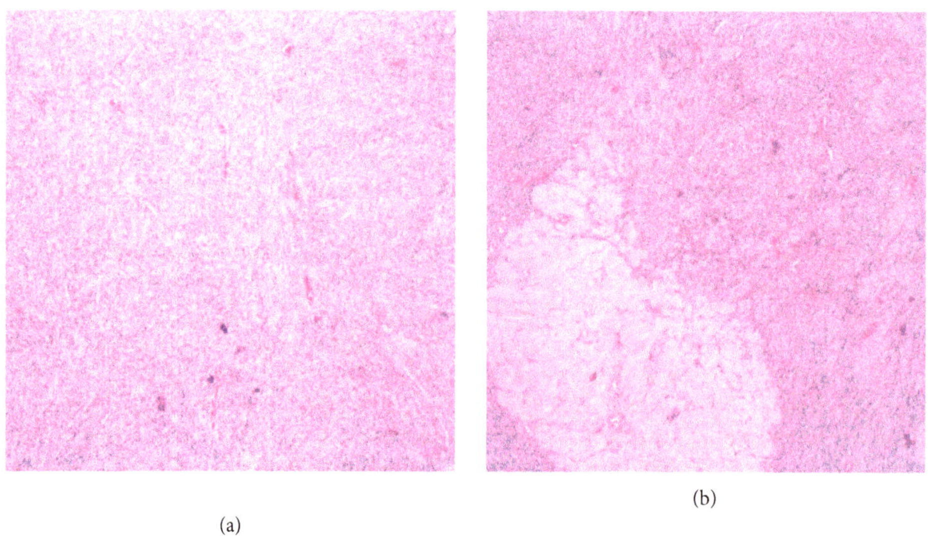

Figure 2: Continued.

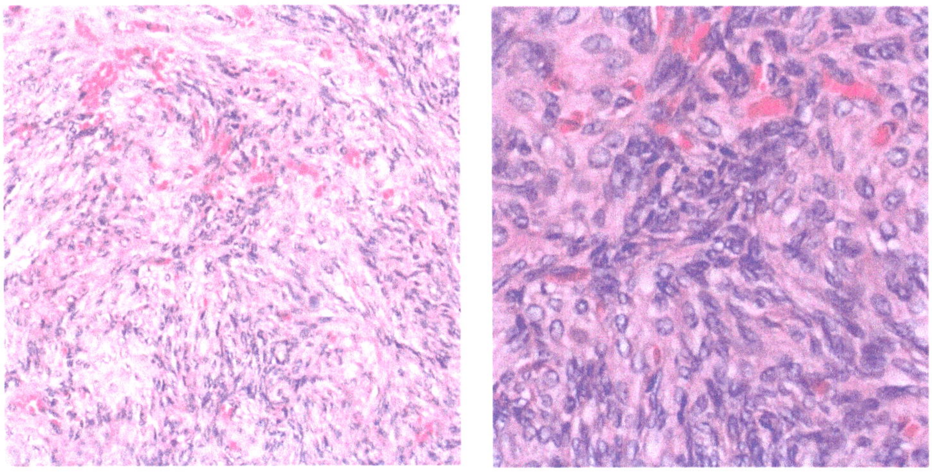

(c) (d)

FIGURE 2: Microscopic images depicting ovarian hyperthecosis with stromal hyperplasia and abundant spindled theca cells. Corpora albicantia (B) was also apparent throughout the specimen. Hematoxylin and eosin stain, original magnification: (a) 4x, (b) 4x, (c) 20x, and (d) 40x.

TABLE 1: Pre and postbilateral oophorectomy laboratory results for case 1 and case 2.

	Case 1: pre and postsurgery lab results		Case 2: pre and postsurgery lab results	
Labs	Presurgery	Postsurgery	Presurgery	Postsurgery
HbA1c (%)	8	6.3	8.2	6.1
Serum testosterone (ng/dL)	145	7	135	16
LH (IU/L)	15.9	N/A	21.2	49.9
FSH (IU/L)	20.9	24.4	31.5	74.1
DHEA-S (mcg/dL)	25		47	
17-Hydroxyprogesterone (ng/dL)	72		195	
Prolactin (ng/mL)	8.8		7.9	
Hb (g/dL)	14.0	12.7	14.7	14.8
Hct (%)	42.3	41.0	45.5	46.2

4. Conclusion

In postmenopausal patients presenting with symptoms of hyperandrogenism, it is important to evaluate for malignant androgen-producing ovarian or adrenal tumors, congenital adrenal hyperplasia, and Cushing's disease. While the testosterone levels in patients discussed were not markedly elevated, the clinical picture was suggestive of ovarian hyperthecosis. After reviewing the patient history, physical exam findings, imaging, and laboratory results, the diagnosis of hyperthecosis was at the top of the differential. Post-oophorectomy, both patients showed remarkable improvement in HbA1c and serum testosterone levels. Interestingly, the identification and diagnosis of ovarian hyperthecosis in the presented cases involved testosterone levels below the recommended diagnostic threshold. The discussed cases show that there is a need for continued research and a further discussion into the diagnostic guidelines to better understand the pathophysiology of this disease including the clinical presentation and biochemical findings.

References

[1] J. M. Goldman and L. J. Kapadia, "Virilization in a postmenopausal woman due to ovarian stromal hyperthecosis," *Postgraduate Medical Journal*, vol. 67, no. 785, pp. 304–306, 1991.

[2] J. H. Barth, M. Jenkins, and P. E. Belchetz, "Ovarian hyperthecosis, diabetes and hirsuties in post-menopausal women," *Clinical Endocrinology*, vol. 46, no. 2, pp. 123–128, 1997.

[3] S. H. Geist and J. A. Gaines, "Diffuse luteinization of the ovaries associated with the masculinization syndrome," *American Journal of Obstetrics and Gynecology*, vol. 43, no. 6, pp. 975–983, 1942.

[4] J. B. O'Driscoll, H. Mamtora, J. Higginson, A. Pollock, J. Kane, and D. C. Anderson, "A prospective study of the prevalence of clear-cut endocrine disorders and polycystic ovaries in 350 patients presenting with hirsutism or androgenic alopecia," *Clinical Endocrinology*, vol. 41, no. 2, pp. 231–236, 1994.

[5] A. Bühler-Christen, V. Tischler, P. A. Diener, and M. Brändle, "New onset alopecia and hirsutism in a postmenopausal women," *Gynecological Endocrinology*, vol. 25, p. 324, 2009.

[6] G. A. Kaltsas, J. J. Mukherjee, B. Kola et al., "Is ovarian and adrenal venous catheterization and sampling helpful in the investigation of hyperandrogenic women?" *Clinical Endocrinology*, vol. 59, no. 1, pp. 34–43, 2003.

[7] Y. Mamoojee, M. Ganguri, N. Taylor, and R. Quinton, "Clinical Case Seminar: postmenopausal androgen excess-challenges in diagnostic work-up and management of ovarian the cosis," *Clinical Endocrinology*, vol. 88, no. 1, pp. 13–20, 2018.

[8] M. Nagamani and C. A. Stuart, "Specific binding sites for insulin-like growth factor I in the ovarian stroma of women with polycystic ovarian disease and stromal hyperthecosis," *American Journal of Obstetrics and Gynecology*, vol. 163, no. 6, pp. 1992–1997, 1990.

[9] N. Kajaia, H. Binder, R. Dittrich et al., "Low sex hormone-binding globulin as a predictive marker for insulin resistance in women with hyperandrogenic syndrome," *European Journal of Endocrinology*, vol. 157, no. 4, pp. 499–507, 2007.

[10] S. T. Sharma, E. P. Wickham, and J. E. Nestler, "Changes in glucose tolerance with metformin treatment in polycystic ovary syndrome: a retrospective analysis," *Endocrine Practice*, vol. 13, no. 4, pp. 373–379, 2007.

[11] K. A. Steingold, H. L. Judd, R. K. Nieberg, J. K. H. Lu, and R. J. Chang, "Treatment of severe androgen excess due to ovarian hyperthecosis with a long-acting gonadotropin-releasing hormone agonist," *American Journal of Obstetrics and Gynecology*, vol. 154, no. 6, pp. 1241–1248, 1986.

Permissions

All chapters in this book were first published by Hindawi Publishing Corporation; hereby published with permission under the Creative Commons Attribution License or equivalent. Every chapter published in this book has been scrutinized by our experts. Their significance has been extensively debated. The topics covered herein carry significant findings which will fuel the growth of the discipline. They may even be implemented as practical applications or may be referred to as a beginning point for another development.

The contributors of this book come from diverse backgrounds, making this book a truly international effort. This book will bring forth new frontiers with its revolutionizing research information and detailed analysis of the nascent developments around the world.

We would like to thank all the contributing authors for lending their expertise to make the book truly unique. They have played a crucial role in the development of this book. Without their invaluable contributions this book wouldn't have been possible. They have made vital efforts to compile up to date information on the varied aspects of this subject to make this book a valuable addition to the collection of many professionals and students.

This book was conceptualized with the vision of imparting up-to-date information and advanced data in this field. To ensure the same, a matchless editorial board was set up. Every individual on the board went through rigorous rounds of assessment to prove their worth. After which they invested a large part of their time researching and compiling the most relevant data for our readers.

The editorial board has been involved in producing this book since its inception. They have spent rigorous hours researching and exploring the diverse topics which have resulted in the successful publishing of this book. They have passed on their knowledge of decades through this book. To expedite this challenging task, the publisher supported the team at every step. A small team of assistant editors was also appointed to further simplify the editing procedure and attain best results for the readers.

Apart from the editorial board, the designing team has also invested a significant amount of their time in understanding the subject and creating the most relevant covers. They scrutinized every image to scout for the most suitable representation of the subject and create an appropriate cover for the book.

The publishing team has been an ardent support to the editorial, designing and production team. Their endless efforts to recruit the best for this project, has resulted in the accomplishment of this book. They are a veteran in the field of academics and their pool of knowledge is as vast as their experience in printing. Their expertise and guidance has proved useful at every step. Their uncompromising quality standards have made this book an exceptional effort. Their encouragement from time to time has been an inspiration for everyone.

The publisher and the editorial board hope that this book will prove to be a valuable piece of knowledge for researchers, students, practitioners and scholars across the globe.

List of Contributors

David H. Jelley
Pediatric Department, University of Oklahoma School of Community Medicine, Tulsa, 4444 E 41st St., Tulsa, OK 74135, 918-619-4803, USA

Deborah Zayneb Mohamad Ali
Pediatric Department, University of Oklahoma School of Community Medicine, Tulsa, 4502 E 41st St, Tulsa, OK 74135, 918-660-3400, USA

Michelle Condren
University of Oklahoma College of Pharmacy, Pediatric Department, University of Oklahoma School of Community Medicine, Tulsa, 4502 E. 41st St, Tulsa, OK 74135, 918-660-3578, USA

Evance K. Godfrey Fatima Mussa, Parvina Kazahura, Aika Shoo, Helga Naburi and Karim P. Manji
Department of Paediatrics and Child Health, Muhimbili University of Health and Allied Sciences (MUHAS), Dar es Salaam, Tanzania

Elizabeth Jasola Omoniyi and Richard J. Robbins
From the Division of Endocrinology, Diabetes and Metabolism, Department of Medicine, Houston Methodist Hospital, Houston, TX, USA
Weill Cornell Medical College, New York, NY, USA

Yunyun Yang, Yang Ou, Yan Ren, Haoming Tian and Tao Chen
Department of Endocrinology and Metabolism, Adrenal Center, West China Hospital of Sichuan University, Chengdu, Sichuan 610041, China

Miguel Angel De los Santos-La Torre, Luis Rómulo Lu-de Lama, Eliana Manuela Chávez-Tejada, Oscar Antonio Espinoza-Robles, Paola Marianella Pinto-Ibárcena and Martha Rosario Calagua-Quispe
Department of Endocrinology and Metabolism, e Child's Health National Institute (Instituto Nacional de Salud del Niño), Lima, Peru

Carlos Manuel Del Águila-Villar and swaldo Nuñez-Almache
Department of Endocrinology and Metabolism, Child's Health National Institute (Instituto Nacional de Salud del Niño), Lima, Peru
Faculty Member of the Medical School, Universidad Nacional Federico Villareal, Lima, Peru

Ibrahim Alali and Younes Kabalan
Al-Assad University Hospital, Damascus University, Damascus, Syria

Reem Saad
Al-Mowassat University Hospital, Damascus University, Damascus, Syria

Ken Yajima
Division of Diabetes, Endocrinology and Metabolism, Department of Internal Medicine, Federation of National Public Service Personnel Mutual Aid Associations Tachikawa Hospital, 4-2-22 Nishikicho, Tachikawa, Tokyo 190-8531, Japan

Yushi Akise
Department of Urology, Federation of National Public Service Personnel Mutual Aid Associations Tachikawa Hospital, 4-2-22 Nishikicho, Tachikawa, Tokyo 190-8531, Japan

Jerrold Spapen
Department of Cardiology, Universitair Ziekenhuis Brussel, Brussels, Belgium

Stijn Lochy
Department of Cardiology, Universitair Ziekenhuis Brussel, Brussels, Belgium
Department of Intensive Care Medicine, Universitair Ziekenhuis Brussel, Brussels, Belgium

Jeroen de Filette
Department of Endocrinology, Universitair Ziekenhuis Brussel, Brussels, Belgium

Herbert Spapen
Development, Ageing and Pathology Research Group, Vrije Universiteit Brussel, Brussels, Belgium

Kiana Karimi
Student Research Committee, Hamadan University of Medical Sciences, Hamadan, Iran
Universal Scientific Education and Research Network (USERN), Tehran, Iran

Mohsen Nikzad
Department of Internal Medicine, School of Medicine, Hamadan University of Medical Sciences, Hamadan, Iran

Sohrab Kulivand
Department of Radiology, School of Medicine, Hamadan University of Medical Sciences, Hamadan, Iran

Shiva Borzouei
Department of Endocrinology, School of Medicine, Hamadan University of Medical Sciences, Hamadan, Iran

Kazuhito Oba, Yuko Chiba, Takeshi Kumakawa, Miho Akahoshi, Seiji Hashimoto, Aya Tachibana, Koichi Toyoshima, Remi Kodera, Kenji Toyoshima, Yoshiaki Tamura and Atsushi Araki
Departments of Diabetes, Metabolism, and Endocrinology, Tokyo Metropolitan Geriatric Hospital Tokyo, Tokyo, Japan

Yoko Matsuda
Department of Pathology, Tokyo Metropolitan Geriatric Hospital, Tokyo, Japan

Rie Aoyama
Department of Cardiology, Tokyo Metropolitan Geriatric Hospital and Institute of Gerontology, Tokyo, Japan

Takashi Nagata
Department of Urology, Tokyo Metropolitan Geriatric Hospital, Tokyo, Japan

Yuto Yamazaki and Hironobu Sasano
Department of Pathology, Tohoku University Graduate School of Medicine, Sendai, Japan

Wasita Warachit Parksook
Division of General Internal Medicine, Department of Medicine, Faculty of Medicine, Chulalongkorn University, and King Chulalongkorn Memorial Hospital, Thai Red Cross Society, Patumwan, Bangkok 10330, Thailand
Division of Endocrinology and Metabolism, Department of Medicine, and Hormonal and Metabolic Research Unit, Excellence Center in Diabetes, Hormone and Metabolism, Faculty of Medicine, Chulalongkorn University, and King Chulalongkorn Memorial Hospital, Thai Red Cross Society, Patumwan, Bangkok 10330, Thailand

Nitchakarn Laichuthai and Sarat Sunthornyothin
Division of Endocrinology and Metabolism, Department of Medicine, and Hormonal and Metabolic Research Unit, Excellence Center in Diabetes, Hormone and Metabolism, Faculty of Medicine, Chulalongkorn University, and King Chulalongkorn Memorial Hospital, Thai Red Cross Society, Patumwan, Bangkok 10330, Thailand

Chin Voon Tong
Department of Medicine, Malacca Hospital, 75400, Malaysia

Subashini Rajoo
Department of Medicine, Kuala Lumpur Hospital, 50586, Malaysia

Kundan Jana, Kalyana Janga, Sheldon Greenberg and Amit Gulati
Division of Nephrology and Hypertension, Maimonides Medical Center, Brooklyn, NY 11219, USA

Abdullah Al-Kandari, Hussain Sadeq and Rita Alfattal
Department of Pediatrics, Al-Amiri Hospital, General Pediatrics Unit, Kuwait city, Kuwait

Maryam AlRashid
Department of Pediatrics, Al-Amiri Hospital, Pediatric Endocrine Unit, Kuwait city, Kuwait

Mayra Alsaeid
Department of Pediatrics, Faculty of Medicine, Kuwait University, Kuwait city, Kuwait

Wafa Abdallah Fadle and Maryam Khamis Al-Badi
Department of Pediatric Endocrinology, National Diabetes and Endocrine Center, Royal Hospital, Muscat, Oman

Ali Al Reesi
Department of Internal Medicine, Sohar Hospital, Sohar, Oman

Saud Al-Shabibi
Department of Radiology, Royal Hospital, Muscat, Oman

Carlotta Giani, Teresa Ramone, Cristina Romei, Raffaele Ciampi, Alessia Tacito, Laura Valerio, Laura Agate, Simona Borsari, Filomena Cetani, Rossella Elisei and Michele Marinò
Endocrine Unit, Department of Clinical and Experimental Medicine, University Hospital of Pisa, 56124 Pisa, Italy

Clara Ugolini and Fulvio Basolo
Pathology Unit, Department of Surgical and Medical Pathology, University Hospital of Pisa, 56124 Pisa, Italy

Alessandro Franchi
Pathology Unit, Department of Translational Research and New Technologies in Medicine and Surgery, University Hospital of Pisa, 56124 Pisa, Italy

Angela Michelucci
Unit of Molecular Genetics, Department of Laboratory Medicine, University Hospital of Pisa, 56126 Pisa, Italy

Cesare Selli
Division of Urology, Department of Translational Research and New Technologies in Medicine and Surgery University Hospital of Pisa, 56124 Pisa, Italy

Gabriele Materazzi
Surgery Unit, Department of Surgical and Medical Pathology, University Hospital of Pisa, 56124 Pisa, Italy

Marco Ciacciarelli, Carmen Misurale, Eleonora D'Armiento, Alessandro Polidoro, Cristina Napoli, Alberto Lombardini, Umberto Ceratti, Ruben Manuel Luciano Colunga Biancatelli, Leonardo Calvosa, Romina Milanese, Sonia Ferri, Teresa Massaro, Andrea Lorusso and Luigi Iuliano
Department of Medico-Surgical Sciences and Biotechnologies, Internal Medicine Unit, ICOT Hospital, "Sapienza" University of Rome, Via Franco Faggiana 1668, Latina 04100, Italy

Gianluca Caruso, Veronica Sorrentino and Vincenzo Petrozza
Department of Medico-Surgical Sciences and Biotechnologies, Pathology Unit, ICOT Hospital, "Sapienza" University of Rome, Via Franco Faggiana 1668, Latina 04100, Italy

Marco Rengo, Piero Maceroni
Department of Radiological Sciences, Oncology and Pathology, ICOT Hospital, "Sapienza" University of Rome, Via Franco Faggiana 1668, Latina 04100, Italy

Mohd. Ashraf Ganie and Atul Sharma
Department of Endocrinology, Sher-I-Kasmir Institute of Medical Sciences, Srinagar, India

Bhanu Malhotra
Department of Endocrinology, PGIMER, Chandigarh 160012, India

Manpreet Saini
Baba Farid University, Faridkot, Punjab, India

Arshiya Dutta
MMC and Hospital, Solan, Himachal Pradesh, India

Kim Vaiphie
Department of Histopathology, PGIMER, Chandigarh 160012, India

Bakr Swaid and Ghassan Bachuwa
Department of Internal Medicine, Hurley Medical Center/Michigan State University, Flint, MI, USA

Frank Kalaba
Department of Combined Internal Medicine & Pediatrics Residency Program, Hurley Medical Center/ Michigan State University, Flint, MI, USA

Stephen E. Sullivan
Department of Neurosurgery and the Pituitary and Neuroendocrine Center, University of Michigan, Ann Arbor, MI, USA

Jessica Cao and Cindy Kim
Western University of Health Sciences, Community Memorial Hospital, Department of Internal Medicine, 147 N Brent St, Ventura, California 93003, USA

Thatcher Huynh, Amanda Frugoli, Heidi Henson and Vera Valdez
Community Memorial Hospital, Department of Graduate Medical Education, Department of Internal Medicine, 147 N Brent St, Ventura, California 93003, USA

Tricia Westhoff-Pankratz
Community Memorial Hospital, Department of Internal Medicine, Department of Endocrinology, 147 N Brent St, California 93003, USA

Fadi Nabhan and Katie Roll
Division of Endocrinology, Diabetes, and Metabolism, The Ohio State University and Arthur G. James Cancer Center, Columbus, OH 43235, USA

Elizabeth Kander, Vineeth Sukrithan, Ye Zhou, Ashima Goyal, Manisha Shah and Bhavana Konda
Division of Medical Oncology, Department of Internal Medicine, The Ohio State University Comprehensive Cancer Center, Columbus, OH, USA

Rulong Shen
Department of Pathology, The Ohio State University Wexner Medical Center, The Ohio State University, Columbus, OH, USA

Amit Agrawal
Department of Otolaryngology—Head and Neck Surgery, The Ohio State University James Cancer Hospital and Solove Research Institute, Columbus, OH, USA

Lucinda Barry, Ash Gargya and Anthony Marren
Royal Prince Alfred Hospital, Sydney, Australia

Selvan Pather
Chris O'Brien Lifehouse, Sydney, Australia

Daniel J. Olivieri
Warren Alpert Medical School of Brown University, Providence, RI, USA

Lauren J. Massingham and Jennifer L. Schwab
Division of Genetics, Hasbro Children's Hospital/ Warren Alpert Medical School of Brown University, 593 Eddy Street, Providence, RI 02903, USA

Jose Bernardo Quintos
Division of Pediatric Endocrinology and Diabetes, Hasbro Children's Hospital/Warren Alpert Medical School of Brown University, 593 Eddy Street, Providence, RI 02903, USA

Le Hoang Bao, Tran Viet Thang and Tran Quang Nam
Department of Endocrinology, University Medical Center, Ho Chi Minh City, Vietnam

Thieu-Thi Tra My
Department of Radiology, Hanoi Medical University, Ha Noi, Vietnam

Nguyen Minh Duc
Department of Radiology, Hanoi Medical University, Ha Noi, Vietnam
Department of Radiology, Pham Ngoc ach University of Medicine, Ho Chi Minh City, Vietnam
Department of Radiology, Children's Hospital 2, Ho Chi Minh City, Vietnam

Phan Cong Chien
Department of Radiology, University Medical Center, Ho Chi Minh City, Vietnam

Prathamesh Chandrapattan and Amitabh Jena
Department of Surgical Oncology, IMS & SUM Medical College and Hospital, Bhubaneswar, Odisha, India

Rashmi Patnayak and Sujata Naik
Department of Pathology, IMS and SUM Medical College and Hospital, Bhubaneswar, Odisha, India

Swayamsidha Mangaraj
Department of Endocrinology, IMS & SUM Medical College and Hospital, Bhubaneswar, Odisha, India

Saroj Panda
Department of Medical Oncology, IMS & SUM Medical College and Hospital, Bhubaneswar, Odisha, India

Christina N. DiMaria, Lorena I. Rasquin and Wikien A. Hung Pinto
Department of Internal Medicine, Einstein Medical Center, Philadelphia, PA, 19141, USA

Cyril Garcia, Mathilde Sollier, Sika Nassouri and Lyse Bordier
Hôpital d'Instruction des Armées BEGIN, Service d'endocrinologie, 69 avenue de Paris, Saint-Mande 94160, France

Marie Dusaud and Paul Chiron
Hôpital d'Instruction des Armées BEGIN, Service d'urologie, 69 avenue de Paris, Saint-Mande 94160, France

Lionel Groussin
Hôpital COCHIN, Service d'endocrinologie, 27 rue du Faubourg Saint Jacques, Paris 75014, France

Mathilde Sibony
Hôpital COCHIN, Service d'anatomopathologie, 27 rue du Faubourg Saint Jacques, Paris 75014, France

Claire Goursaud and Florence Roucher-Boulez
Hospices Civils de Lyon-Bron, Laboratoire de Biochimie et Biologie Moléculaire Grand Est, Lyon 69000, France

Jill D. Jacobson and Julia R. Broussard
Division of Endocrinology and Diabetes, Department of Pediatrics, Children's Mercy, University of Missouri-Kansas City School of Medicine, Kansas, MO 64111, USA

Courtney Marsh
Division of Reproductive Endocrinology and Infertility, Department of Obstetrics and Gynecology, University of Kansas School of Medicine, Kansas, KS 66160, USA

Brandon Newell
Division of Dermatology, Department of Pediatrics, Children's Mercy Hospital, University of Missouri-Kansas City School of Medicine, Kansas, MO 64111, USA

Rahul Gupta and Shakun Chaudhary
Department of Endocrinology, Post Graduate Institute of Medical Education and Research, Chandigarh, India

Pinaki Dutta
Department of Endocrinology, Post Graduate Institute of Medical Education and Research, Chandigarh, India
Department of Endocrinology, PGIMER, Chandigarh 160012, India

Urmimala Bhattacharjee, K. S. Lekshmon, Prashant Sharma and Aditya Jandial
Department of Clinical Hematology and Medical Oncology, Post Graduate Institute of Medical Education and Research, Chandigarh, India

R. El Qadiry, K. Danaoui, H. Nassih, A. Bourrahouat and I. Ait Sab
Pediatric B Department, Mother-Child Pole, Mohammed VI University Hospital, Marrakesh, Morocco

Ayesha Hassan and Apoorva Iyer
Department of Internal Medicine, West Virginia University Hospital, Morgantown, WV, USA

Jessica Perini
Department of Endocrinology and Metabolism, West Virginia University Hospital, Morgantown, WV, USA

Jia Wei Tan and Anant Shukla
Department of Internal Medicine, Yale New Haven Health, Bridgeport Hospital, Bridgeport, CT, USA

Sachin K. Majumdar
Department of Internal Medicine, Yale New Haven Health, Bridgeport Hospital, Bridgeport, CT, USA
Department of Endocrinology, Yale New Haven Health, Bridgeport Hospital, Bridgeport, CT, USA

Jiun-Ruey Hu
Section of Cardiovascular Medicine, Department of Internal Medicine, Yale School of Medicine, New Haven, CT 06510, USA

Minghao Liu and Gabrielle Page-Wilson
Endocrinology Division, Department of Medicine, Columbia University Medical Center, 650 West 168th St., Room 2012, New York, NY 10032, USA

Diane Hamele-Bena
Department of Pathology and Cell Biology, Columbia University Medical Center, Physicians and Surgeons Building, Room 404, 630 W 168th St., New York, NY 10032, USA

John Ausiello
Endocrinology Division, Department of Medicine, Columbia University Medical Center, Harkness Pavilion, 9th floor, 180 Fort Washington Ave., New York, NY 10032, USA

Moslem Sedaghattalab
Department of Internal Medicine, Yasuj University of Medical Sciences, Yasuj, Iran

Amir Hossein Doustimotlagh
Medicinal Plants Research Center, Yasuj University of Medical Sciences, Yasuj, Iran

Nern Hoong Kao and Adrian Jit Hin Koh
Department of General Surgery, Changi General Hospital, 2 Simei Street 3, Singapore

Chien Sheng Tan
Department of Histopathology, Changi General Hospital, 2 Simei Street 3, Singapore

Jolijn Van Cauwenberghe
Antwerp University Hospital, Department of Diabetology-Endocrinology, Wilrijkstraat 10, 2650 Edegem, Belgium

Sigri Beckers
Antwerp University Hospital, Department of Genetics, Wilrijkstraat 10, 2560 Edegem, Belgium

Peter Coremans
AZ Nikolaas, Department of Diabetology-Endocrinology, Moerlandstraat 1, 9100 Sint-Niklaas, Belgium

Yotsapon Thewjitcharoen, Ekgaluck Wanothayaroj, Chattip Thammawiwat, Sriurai Porramatikul, Soontaree Nakasatien, Sirinate Krittiyawong and Thep Himathongkam
Diabetes and Thyroid Center, Theptarin Hospital, Bangkok, Thailand

Chuleekorn Vorayingyong
Department of Dermatology, Theptarin Hospital, Bangkok, Thailand

Kumutnart Chanprapaph
Division of Dermatology, Department of Medicine, Ramathibodi Hospital, Bangkok, Thailand

Abigail M. Schmucker
Sidney Kimmel Medical College, thomas Jefferson University, 1025 Walnut Street, Philadelphia, PA 19107, USA

Dina E. Green and Philip M. Montemuro
Lankenau Medical Center, 100 East Lancaster Avenue, Wynnewood, PA 19096, USA

Mariangela Massaccesi and Francesco Miccichè
Fondazione Policlinico Universitario "A. Gemelli" IRCCS, Unità Operativa Complessa di Radioterapia, Dipartimento di Diagnostica per Immagini, Radioterapia Oncologica ed Ematologia, Roma, Italy

Maria Antonietta Gambacort and Vincenzo Valentini
Fondazione Policlinico Universitario "A. Gemelli" IRCCS, Unità Operativa Complessa di Radioterapia, Dipartimento di Diagnostica per Immagini, Radioterapia Oncologica ed Ematologia, Roma, Italy
Universitá Cattolica del Sacro Cuore Facoltà di Medicina e Chirurgia, Roma, Italy

Amna Khan
Avalon University of Medicine, Youngstown, OH, USA

Mario Rigante
Fondazione Policlinico Universitario "A. Gemelli" IRCCS, Unità Operativa Complessa di Otorinolaringoiatria, Dipartimento di scienze dell'invecchiamento, Neurologiche, Ortopediche e della testa-collo, Roma, Italy

Gianluigi Petrone
Fondazione Policlinico Universitario "A. Gemelli" IRCCS, Unità Operativa Complessa di Anatomia Patologica, Dipartimento di scienze della salute della donna, del bambino e di sanità pubblica, Roma, Italy

Elisabetta Lepre
Università Cattolica del Sacro Cuore Facoltà di Medicina e Chirurgia, Roma, Italy

J. L. Castedo
Department of Endocrinology, Diabetes and Metabolism of Centro Hospitalar Universitário de São João, Porto, Portugal

M. J. Ferreira, J. Pedro, D. Salazar and D. Carvalho
Department of Endocrinology, Diabetes and Metabolism of Centro Hospitalar Universitário de São João, Porto, Portugal
Faculty of Medicine of the Universidade do Porto, Porto, Portugal
Instituto de Investigação e Inovação em Sáude, Universidade do Porto, Porto, Portugal

A. Grangeia
Faculty of Medicine of the Universidade do Porto, Porto, Portugal
Department of Genetics of Centro Hospitalar Universitário de São João, Porto, Portugal

C. Costa
Portuguese Institute of Oncology, Porto, Portugal
Department of Pathology of Centro Hospitalar Universitário de São João, Porto, Portugal

J Aragão Rodrigues
Department of Pathology of Centro Hospitalar Universitário de São João, Porto, Portugal

M. M. Costa
Department of Endocrinology, Diabetes and Metabolism of Hospital Garcia de Orta, Porto, Portugal

Rahul Pansare and Sangeetha Nanthabalan
Department of Internal Medicine, St. Mary Mercy Hospital, Livonia, MI 48154, USA

Hala Mualla and Abid Yaqub
Division of Endocrinology, Diabetes and Metabolism, University of Cincinnati, 231 Albert Sabin Way, Cincinnati, OH 45267-0542, USA

Su Ah Bae
Cotton O'Neil Diabetes & Endocrinology Clinic, 3520 SW6th Ave, Topeka, KS 6660,USA

Fatima Zahra Zaher, Imane Boubagura, Sana Rafi, Ghizlane Elmghari and Nawal Elansari
Department of Endocrinology, Diabetes, Metabolic Diseases and Nutrition, Mohammed VI University Hospital, Marrakech, Morocco

Leena Shah, Emily V. Nosova and Khadeen Christi Cheesman
Division of Endocrinology, Diabetes, and Bone Disease, Department of Medicine, Icahn School of Medicine at Mount Sinai, New York, NY, USA

Joshua B. Bederson
Department of Neurosurgery, Icahn School of Medicine at Mount Sinai, New York, NY, USA

Sanket Shah
Department of Internal Medicine, Medical College of Wisconsin, Milwaukee, WI 53226, USA

Callie Torres
Department of Pathology & Immunology, Washington University in St Louis, St Louis, MO 63110, USA

Naser Gharaibeh
Department of Endocrinology, Mercy Hospital, 100 Mercy Way, Joplin, MO 64804, USA

Index

www.ingramcontent.com/pod-product-compliance
Lightning Source LLC
LaVergne TN
LVHW082201200926
848484LV00008B/2196
9798887405964